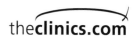

EMERGENCY MEDICINE CLINICS OF NORTH AMERICA

Ethical Issues in Emergency Medicine

GUEST EDITORS
Raquel M. Schears, MD, MPH and
Catherine A. Marco, MD

CONSULTING EDITOR
Amal Mattu, MD

August 2006 • Volume 24 • Number 3

SAUNDERS

An Imprint of Elsevier, Inc.
PHILADELPHIA   LONDON   TORONTO   MONTREAL   SYDNEY   TOKYO

W.B. SAUNDERS COMPANY
A Division of Elsevier Inc.

1600 John F. Kennedy Boulevard, Suite 1800 • Philadelphia, Pennsylvania 19103-2899

http://www.theclinics.com

EMERGENCY MEDICINE CLINICS   Volume 24, Number 3
OF NORTH AMERICA   ISSN 0733-8627
August 2006   ISBN 1-4160-3882-5
Editor: Karen Sorensen

Reprints. For copies of 100 or more, of articles in this publication, please contact the Commercial Reprints Department, Elsevier Inc., 360 Park Avenue South, New York, New York 10010-1710. Tel. (212) 633-3813; Fax: (212) 462-1935; e-mail: reprints@elsevier.com.

The ideas and opinions expressed in *Emergency Medicine Clinics of North America* do not necessarily reflect those of the Publisher. The Publisher does not assume any responsibility for any injury and/or damage to persons or property arising out of or related to any use of the material contained in this periodical. The reader is advised to check the appropriate medical literature and the product information currently provided by the manufacturer of each drug to be administered to verify the dosage, the method and duration of administration, or contraindications. It is the responsibility of the treating physician or other health care professional, relying on independent experience and knowledge of the patient, to determine drug dosages and the best treatment for the patient. Mention of any product in this issue should not be construed as endorsement by the contributors, editors, or the Publisher of the product or manufacturers' claims.

Emergency Medicine Clinics of North America (ISSN 0733-8627) is published quarterly by Elsevier Inc., 360 Park Avenue, South, New York, NY, 10010-1710. Months of issue are February, May, August, and November. Business and Editorial Offices: 1600 John F. Kennedy Boulevard, Suite 1800, Philadelphia, PA 19103-2899. Customer Service Office: 6277 Sea Harbor Drive, Orlando, FL 32887-4800. Periodicals postage paid at New York, NY, and additional mailing offices. Subscription prices are $175.00 per year (US individuals), $275.00 per year (US institutions), $235.00 per year (international individuals), $325.00 per year (international institutions), $215.00 per year (Canadian individuals), and $325.00 per year (Canadian institutions). International air speed delivery is included in all *Clinics'* subscription prices. All prices are subject to change without notice. POSTMASTER: Send address changes to *Emergency Medicine Clinics of North America*, Elsevier Periodicals Customer Service, 6277 Sea Harbor Drive, Orlando, FL 32887-4800. **Customer Service: 1-800-654-2452 (US). From outside of the US, call 1-407-345-4000.** **E-mail: hhspcs@harcourt.com.**

Emergency Medicine Clinics of North America is covered in *Index Medicus, Current Contents/Clinical Medicine, EMBASE/Excerpta Medica, BIOSIS, SciSearch, CINAHL, ISI/BIOMED,* and *Research Alert.*

Printed in the United States of America.

CONSULTING EDITOR

AMAL MATTU, MD, Program Director, Emergency Medicine Residency; Associate Professor, University of Maryland School of Medicine, Baltimore, Maryland

GUEST EDITORS

RAQUEL M. SCHEARS, MD, MPH, Assistant Professor, Department of Emergency Medicine, Mayo Clinic College of Medicine/St. Mary's Hospital, Rochester, Minnesota

CATHERINE A. MARCO, MD, Associate Professor, Medical College of Ohio, Toledo, Ohio

CONTRIBUTORS

LOUISE B. ANDREW, MD, JD, Co-Founder and First President, Coalition and Center for Ethical Medical Testimony, New York, New York

AMADO ALEJANDRO BÁEZ, MD, MSc, Instructor of Emergency Medicine, Department of Emergency Medicine and Division of Trauma, Burns and Surgical Critical Care, Brigham and Women's Hospital, Boston, Massachusetts; National Directorate of Emergencies and Disasters, Dominican Republic Ministry of Public Health

JILL M. BAREN, MD, MBE, FACEP, FAAP, Associate Professor, Departments of Emergency Medicine and Pediatrics, University of Pennsylvania School of Medicine; Attending Physician, Hospital of the University of Pennsylvania and The Children's Hospital of Philadelphia, Philadelphia, Pennsylvania

ROBERT A. BITTERMAN, MD, JD, President, Bitterman Health Law & Consulting Group, Inc., Charlotte, North Carolina; Vice-President, Emergency Physicians Insurance Company, Inc., Auburn, California

CAREY D. CHISHOLM, MD, Clinical Professor of Emergency Medicine, Indiana University School of Medicine, Department of Emergency Medicine, Indianapolis, Indiana

RITA K. CYDULKA, MD, MS, Vice Chair, Department of Emergency Medicine, MetroHealth Medical Center, Cleveland, Ohio; Associate Professor, Department of Emergency Medicine, Case Western Reserve University, School of Medicine, Cleveland, Ohio

ARTHUR R. DERSE, MD, JD, Clinical Professor of Bioethics and Emergency Medicine, Medical College of Wisconsin; Director for Medical and Legal Affairs and Associate

Director, Center for the Study of Bioethics, Medical College of Wisconsin, Milwaukee, Wisconsin

NICOLE M. FRANKS, MD, Assistant Professor, Department of Emergency Medicine, Emory University, School of Medicine, Atlanta, Georgia

MAUREEN GANG, MD, Assistant Professor, Coordinator for the Program in Ethics in Emergency Medicine, and Attending Physician, Department of Emergency Medicine, Bellevue Hospital/NYU Hospitals, New York University School of Medicine, New York, New York

JOEL MARTIN GEIDERMAN, MD, Clinical Professor, David Geffen School of Medicine at UCLA, Ruth and Harry Roman Emergency Department, Department of Emergency Medicine, Cedars-Sinai Center for Health Care Ethics, Burns and Allen Research Institute, Los Angeles, California

LEWIS R. GOLDFRANK, MD, Professor and Chair, Department of Emergency Medicine, New York University School of Medicine; Director, Emergency Medicine, Bellevue Hospital/NYU Hospitals, New York University School of Medicine; and Medical Director, New York City Poison Center, New York, New York

KENNETH V. ISERSON, MD, MBA, FACEP, FAAEM, Professor of Surgery, Department of Emergency Medicine, and Director, Arizona Bioethics Program, University of Arizona College of Medicine, Tucson, Arizona

GABOR D. KELEN, MD, Professor of Emergency Medicine and Chair, Department of Emergency Medicine, Johns Hopkins University, Baltimore, Maryland

ERICA KREISMANN, MD, Fellow in Ethics in Emergency Medicine and Instructor, Department of Emergency Medicine, Bellevue Hospital/NYU Hospitals, New York University School of Medicine, New York, New York

BO E. MADSEN, MD, Senior Resident, Department of Emergency Medicine, Mayo Clinic, Rochester, Minnesota; Former Head of Mission, European Community Humanitarian Office, Bosnia and Herzegovina

HAL MINNIGAN MD, PhD, Assistant Professor of Clinical Emergency Medicine, Indiana University School of Medicine, Department of Emergency Medicine, Indianapolis, Indiana

JOHN C. MOSKOP, PhD, Professor, Department of Medical Humanities, Brody School of Medicine at East Carolina University; Director, Bioethics Center, University Health Systems of Eastern Carolina, Greenville, North Carolina

PETER J. PRONOVOST, MD, PhD, Professor, Department of Anesthesiology & Critical Care Medicine, Johns Hopkins University School of Medicine, Baltimore, Maryland

TAMMIE E. QUEST, MD, Assistant Professor, Department of Emergency Medicine, Emory University, School of Medicine, Atlanta, Georgia

JUDY B. SHAHAN, RN, MBA, Research Associate, Department of Emergency Medicine, Johns Hopkins University, Baltimore, Maryland

TERRI A. SCHMIDT MD, MS, Professor, Department of Emergency Medicine, Center for Ethics in Health Care, Oregon Health & Sciences University, Portland, Oregon

JON W. SCHROCK, MD, Director, Observation Unit, Department of Emergency Medicine, MetroHealth Medical Center, Cleveland, Ohio; Senior Instructor, Department of Emergency Medicine, Case Western Reserve University, School of Medicine, Cleveland, Ohio

ROBERT C. SOLOMON, MD, Faculty, Emergency Medicine Residency, Ohio Valley Medical Center, Wheeling, West Virginia; Clinical Assistant Professor of Medicine, West Virginia School of Osteopathic Medicine, Lewisberg, West Virginia

SAMANTHA L. STOKES, MPH, Project Director, Removing Insult from Injury: Disclosing Adverse Events, Johns Hopkins Bloomberg School of Public Health, Baltimore, Maryland

ROBERT E. SUTER, DO, MHA, FACEP, Professor, Department of Emergency Medicine, Medical College of Georgia, Augusta, Georgia; Clinical Associate Professor of Surgery (Emergency Medicine), University of Texas-Southwestern, Dallas, Texas; Adjunct Professor, Emergency Medicine, Des Moines University, Des Moines, Iowa; Chair, Department of Emergency Medicine, Spring Branch Medical Center, Houston, Texas; Partner, Greater Houston Emergency Physicans, Houston, Texas; Past President, American College of Emergency Physicians, Dallas, Texas

MATTHEW D. SZTAJNKRYCER, MD, PhD, Associate Professor, Department of Emergency Medicine, Mayo Clinic, Rochester, Minnesota; Chief Medical Operating Officer, Disaster Medical Assistance Team MN-1

ALBERT W. WU, MD, MPH, Professor, Department of Health Policy and Management, Johns Hopkins Bloomberg School of Public Health, Baltimore, Maryland

CONTENTS

Neither law nor religion, bioethics absorbs and applies elements of both. Its theories, principles, and methods stem from various philosophical schools. Practitioners use case-based reasoning to apply bioethics to clinical situations, usually giving most weight to patients' autonomy and values, but also incorporating other relevant bioethical principles, including those encompassed in professional oaths and codes. Emergency clinicians must be able to recognize bioethical dilemmas, have action plans based on their readings and discussions, and have a method through which to apply ethical principles in clinical settings. This article provides an overview of ethical considerations and guidelines for emergency clinicians.

When ethical issues arise in emergency medical practice, many emergency physicians turn to the law for answers. Although knowing when and how the law applies to emergency medicine is important, the law is only one factor to consider among many factors. Additionally, the law may not be applicable or may not be clear, or the ethical considerations may seem to conflict with legal aspects of emergency medical treatment. Situations where ethics and the law may seem to be in conflict in emergency medicine are described and analyzed in this article, and recommendations are offered. In general, when facing ethical dilemmas in emergency medical practice, the emergency physician should take into account the ethical considerations before turning to the legal considerations.

EMTALA and the Ethical Delivery of Hospital Emergency Services 557
Robert A. Bitterman

Organizational Ethics 579
Robert E. Suter

Informed Consent and Refusal of Treatment: Challenges for Emergency Physicians 605
John C. Moskop

FORTHCOMING ISSUES

RECENT ISSUES

GOAL STATEMENT

The goal of *Emergency Medicine Clinics of North America* is to keep practicing physicians up to date with current clinical practice in emergency medicine by providing timely articles reviewing the state of the art in patient care.

ACCREDITATION

The *Emergency Medical Clinics of North America* is planned and implemented in accordance with the Essential Areas and Policies of the Accreditation Council for Continuing Medical Education (ACCME) through the joint sponsorship of the University of Virginia School of Medicine and Elsevier. The University of Virginia School of Medicine is accredited by the ACCME to provide continuing medical education for physicians.

The University of Virginia School of Medicine designates this educational activity for a maximum of 15 AMA PRA Category 1 Credits™. Physicians should only claim credit commensurate with the extent of their participation in the activity.

The Emergency Medicine Clinics of North America CME program is approved by the American College of Emergency Physicians for 60 hours of ACEP Category I credit per year.

The American Medical Association has determined that physicians not licensed in the US who participate in this CME activity are eligible for 15 AMA PRA Category 1 Credits™.

The American Medical Association has determined that physicians not licensed in the US who participate in this CME activity are eligible for AMA PRA category 1 credit.

Category 1 credit can be earned by reading the text material, taking the CME examination online at http://www.theclinics.com/home/cme, and completing the evaluation. After taking the test, you will be required to review any and all incorrect answers. Following completion of the test and evaluation, your credit will be awarded and you may print your certificate.

FACULTY DISCLOSURE/CONFLICT OF INTEREST

The University of Virginia School of Medicine, as an ACCME accredited provider, endorses and strives to comply with the Accreditation Council for Continuing Medical Education (ACCME) Standards of Commercial Support, Commonwealth of Virginia statutes, University of Virginia policies and procedures, and associated federal and private regulations and guidelines on the need for disclosure and monitoring of proprietary and financial interests that may affect the scientific integrity and balance of content delivered in continuing medical education activities under our auspices.

The University of Virginia School of Medicine requires that all CME activities accredited through this institution be developed independently and be scientifically rigorous, balanced and objective in the presentation/discussion of its content, theories and practices.

All authors/editors participating in an accredited CME activity are expected to disclose to the readers relevant financial relationships with commercial entities occurring within the past 12 months (such as grants or research support, employee, consultant, stock holder, member of speakers bureau, etc.). The University of Virginia School of Medicine will employ appropriate mechanisms to resolve potential conflicts of interest to maintain the standards of fair and balanced education to the reader. Questions about specific strategies can be directed to the Office of Continuing Medical Education, University of Virginia School of Medicine, Charlottesville, Virginia.

The authors/editors listed below have identified no professional or financial affiliations for themselves or their spouse/partner:
Louise B. Andrew, MD, JD; Amado A. Baez, MD, MSc; Jill M. Baren, MD; Robert A. Bitterman, MD, JD; Carey D. Chisholm, MD; Rita K. Cydulka, MD, MS; Arthur R. Derse, MD, JD; Nicole M. Franks, MD; Maureen Gang, MD; Joel M. Geiderman, MD; Lewis R. Goldfrank, MD; Kenneth V. Iserson, MD, MBA, FACEP; Gabor D. Kelen, MD; Erica Kreismann, MD; Bo E. Madsen, MD; Catherine A. Marco, MD; Amal Mattu, MD, FAAEM, FACEP; Hal Minnigan, MD, PhD; John C. Moskop, PhD; Peter J. Pronovost, MD, PhD; Tammie E. Quest, MD; Raquel M. Schears, MD; Terri A. Schmidt, MD, MS; Jon W. Schrock, MD; Robert C. Solomon, MD; Karen Sorensen, Acquisitions Editor; Samantha L. Stokes, MPH; Robert E. Suter, DO, MHA, FACEP; Matthew D. Sztajnkrycer, MD, PhD; and, Albert W. Wu, MD, MPH.

The author listed below has identified the following professional or financial affiliation for herself or spouse/partner:
Judy B. Shahan, RN, MBA is employed by Boston Scientific.

Disclosure of Discussion of non-FDA approved uses for pharmaceutical products and/or medical devices:
The University of Virginia School of Medicine, as an ACCME provider, requires that all faculty presenters identify and disclose any "off label" uses for pharmaceutical and medical device products. The University of Virginia School of Medicine recommends that each physician fully review all the available data on new products or procedures prior to instituting them with patients.

TO ENROLL

To enroll in the Emergency Medicine Clinics of North America Continuing Medical Education program, call customer service at 1-800-654-2452 or visit us online at www.theclinics.com/home/cme. The CME program is available to subscribers for an additional fee of $195.00

ELSEVIER
SAUNDERS

Emerg Med Clin N Am
24 (2006) xv–xvi

EMERGENCY
MEDICINE
CLINICS OF
NORTH AMERICA

Foreword

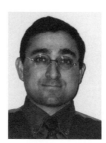

Amal Mattu, MD
Consulting Editor

Emergency medicine is changing rapidly. What first began as a specialty devoted to the concept of resuscitation and stabilization of the sickest of patients has evolved into a specialty that is often looked upon as the safety net for an imperfect health care system. At any hour of any day, every person has a doctor to turn to for whatever ails them, from the bumps and bruises of minor trauma to mild exacerbations of a chronic untreated condition to acute chest pain or stroke. That doctor is an emergency physician. As the specialty has evolved, however, emergency physicians have faced greater responsibilities and resulting challenges. Hospital overcrowding and limited resources have challenged the emergency physician's ability to deliver expedient and quality care. At the same time, increased pressure from the legal system has encouraged the frequent practice of "defensive medicine" rather than cost-effective medicine. Changes in academic centers and research funding have promoted frequent conflicts of interest among researchers and educators who work within the biomedical industry. With all of these changes, many ethical dilemmas have arisen for the individual practicing emergency physician as well as for the entire health care system.

In this issue of the *Emergency Medicine Clinics of North America*, Guest Editors Raquel Shears and Catherine Marco have assembled an outstanding team of authors to address many of these ethical issues in emergency medicine. Topics include clinical, research, medico-legal, and systems-based issues. The authors, almost all emergency physicians themselves, effectively guide the reader through these challenges and provide some practical

0733-8627/06/$ - see front matter © 2006 Elsevier Inc. All rights reserved.
doi:10.1016/j.emc.2006.06.001   *emed.theclinics.com*

solutions. The editors and authors are to be commended for providing this valuable addition to the *Emergency Medicine Clinics* series.

Amal Mattu, MD
Department of Emergency Medicine
University of Maryland School of Medicine
110 South Paca Street
6th Floor, Suite 200
Baltimore, MD 21201, USA

E-mail address: amattu@smail.umaryland.edu

ELSEVIER
SAUNDERS

Emerg Med Clin N Am
24 (2006) xvii–xviii

EMERGENCY
MEDICINE
CLINICS OF
NORTH AMERICA

Preface

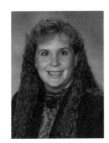 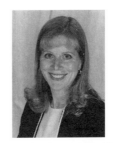

Raquel M. Schears, MD, MPH, FACEP   Catherine A. Marco, MD, FACEP
Guest Editors

Emergency physicians have basic instincts that can be relied on by the general public, as well as by health care professionals. Ask anyone in the United States. Where would they go for sudden health emergencies, the "perfect storm" of terrible circumstances? No time, no money, no ride? Come by ambulance, no problem. Society in its wisdom has voted to keep the house of medicine's lights on in the emergency department 24/7, shining brightly through all-cause calamity. Emergency physicians have carved out a noble niche, over the last few decades keeping a finger on the pulse of the people.

But helping the heart of humanity has evolved to encompass unique areas of ethical terrain, forced into sharper focus by three things. First, primary shifts in population demographics have emerged just as cultural sensitivity for personal values has deepened. Second, limitations to modern medicine persist but are increasingly buried beneath a high-tech exterior. And third, communicating about uncertainties in medical decision-making is made difficult by inflated patient expectations, more health care regulation, and provider perceptions of medico-legal risk. Thus the perennial ethics embedded in medical choice, limitation, and recourse actually give extra gravity to emergency department presentations and may potentiate volatile atmospheric conditions.

The intention of this issue of the *Emergency Medicine Clinics of North America* is to challenge us to expand our awareness of sensitive issues, to be more thorough in moral assessments, and, ultimately, to be better prepared to provide the best ethical care possible. In addition to some traditional moral concepts, this issue reflects on cutting-edge topics in ethics, including disaster triage and managing surge, conducting research that respects cultural diversity, treating age-related concerns, caring for impaired adults or colleagues, and much more. The contributing authors are nationally acclaimed experts chosen to mentor readers' contemplation and discussion of conceptual approaches in ethics. Their clinical experience with common ethical dilemmas, and their flexibility as researchers and educators, will complement new insights and improve ethical problem-solving skills among readers. Taken together, this issue addresses the confluence of knowledge gaps or other errors, moral perils of conflicting interests, and the relevance of medico-legal facts used to inform practice. Ultimately, endeavoring to model the good habits of ethical practice remains our goal, duty, and just reward.

Raquel M. Schears, MD, MPH, FACEP
Catherine A. Marco, MD, FACEP
Department of Emergency Medicine
Mayo Clinic/St. Mary's Hospital
200 First Street, SW
Rochester, MN 55905, USA

E-mail address: schears.rocky@mayo.edu

ELSEVIER
SAUNDERS

Emerg Med Clin N Am
24 (2006) 513–545

EMERGENCY
MEDICINE
CLINICS OF
NORTH AMERICA

Ethical Principles—Emergency Medicine

Kenneth V. Iserson, MD, MBA, FACEP, FAAEM*

*Department of Emergency Medicine and Arizona Bioethics Program, The University
of Arizona College of Medicine, 1501 North Campbell Avenue, Tucson, AZ 85724, USA*

Neither law nor religion, bioethics absorbs and applies elements of both. Its theories, principles, and methods stem from various philosophical schools. Practitioners use case-based reasoning to apply bioethics to clinical situations, usually giving most weight to patients' autonomy and values, but also incorporating other relevant bioethical principles, including those encompassed in professional oaths and codes [1]. Emergency clinicians must be able to recognize bioethical dilemmas, have action plans based on their readings and discussions, and have a method through which to apply ethical principles in clinical settings.

What is bioethics?

Ethics is the application of values and moral rules to human activities. Bioethics is a subset of ethics that provides reasoned and defensible solutions that incorporate ethical principles for actual or anticipated moral dilemmas facing clinicians in medicine and biology. Unlike professional etiquette, which relates to standards governing the relationships and interactions between practitioners, bioethics deals with relationships between practitioners and patients, practitioners and society, and society and patients [1].

Modern bioethics has developed during the last four decades largely because the law has often remained silent, inconsistent, or morally wrong on matters vital to the biomedical community. The rapid increase in biotechnology, the failure of both the legal system and the legislatures to deal with new and pressing issues, and, in the United States, the increasing liability crisis have driven the medical community to seek answers to some of the difficult questions practitioners have had to work through on a daily basis

---

* Arizona Bioethics Program, Box 245057, University of Arizona College of Medicine, 1501 N. Campbell Avenue, Tucson, AZ 85724.
E-mail address: kvi@u.arizona.edu

[1]. The clinical application of bioethics relies on case-based (casuistic) reasoning, in general favoring patients' autonomy and values, but also considering other relevant bioethical principles, including those values inscribed in communal ethics and professional oaths and codes. It is incumbent upon emergency physicians, whenever possible, to determine not only each patient's individual values, but also whether the patient subscribes to an individualistic or a communitarian ethic. Such determinations may help decide who the most appropriate decision makers will be if the patient lacks the capacity to make his or her own decisions.

Relationship between law and bioethics

Both the law and bioethics give us rules of conduct to follow. Yet, there are significant differences between the two. Laws stem from legislative statutes, administrative agency rules, or court decisions. They often vary in different locales and are enforceable only in the jurisdictions where they prevail. Ethics incorporates the broad values and beliefs of correct conduct. Although bioethical principles do not change because of geography (at least not within one culture), the interpretation of both ethical and legislative principles may evolve as societies change. But, while good ethics often makes good law, good law does not necessarily make good ethics. Most laws, while based loosely on societal principles, are actually derived from other laws. Ethical principles, however, are derived from the values of the society in which they are proposed.

Confusion often arises about the differences between law and bioethics for three reasons. The first is that Western, and especially US and Canadian, bioethics discussions often use legal cases to bolster their points because, unlike ethical discussions in most published medical cases, legal cases provide rich details for ethical discussion and deliberation. The second is that legal cases provide an insight into our social contract, demonstrating the level of societal acceptance of some knotty issues. Finally, in a democratic society, the law provides an avenue through which bioethical policy can be expressed and codified across a large region.

Law and ethics: similarities and differences

Significant overlap exists between legal and ethical decision-making (Table 1). Both ethical analysis (in bioethics committee deliberations) and the law (in the courts) use case-based reasoning in an attempt to achieve consistency. Legal and ethical dicta have existed since ancient times, have evolved over time, incorporate basic societal values, and form the basis for policy development within health care as well as in other parts of society.

The law and bioethics differ markedly, however, in some areas. For instance, the law operates under formal adversarial process rules, such as those in the courtroom, which allow little room for deviation, while

Table 1
Relationship between law and bioethics

Bioethics	Function	Law
✔	Case-based (casuistic)	✔
✔	Has existed from ancient times	✔
✔	Changes over time	✔
✔	Strives for consistency	✔
✔	Incorporates societal values	✔
✔	Basis for healthcare policies	✔
	Some unchangeable directives	✔
	Formal rules for process	✔
	Adversarial	✔
✔	Relies heavily on individual values	
✔	Interpretable by medical personnel	
✔	Ability to respond relatively rapidly to changing environment	

From Iserson KV. Principles of biomedical ethics. In: Marco CA, Schears RM, (editors.) Ethical issues in emergency medicine. The Emergency Clinics of North America 1999;17(2):285; with permission.

bioethics consultations are flexible enough to conform to the needs of each institution and circumstance and, rather than being adversarial, are designed to assist all parties involved in the process. The law also has some unalterable directives, sometimes called "black-letter laws," that require specific actions. Bioethics, while based on principles, is designed to weigh every specific situation on its own merits. Perhaps the key difference between bioethics and the law is that bioethics relies heavily on the individual's values—be they those of the patient or of the patient's surrogate. Also, even without the intervention of trained bioethicists, medical personnel can and should be able to make ethically sound decisions. The law does not consider individual values and generally requires lawyers for interpretation.

As previously noted, a reason for the development of bioethics, and a key difference between bioethics and the law, is the former's ability to respond to a rapidly changing health care environment.

Rights

Despite their differences, there is frequently concurrence between bioethics and the law on basic issues. On occasion, clarity within the law can lead to clearer thinking in bioethics (and vice versa). Both law and bioethics, for example, use the term *rights*, as in "patients' rights" and "the right to die." This term, often used to advance an ethical argument about medical care, is frequently misunderstood or applied erroneously. Having a *right* implies that a person, group, or the state has a corresponding moral and legal *duty*. Without a duty to act, there can be no rights. The rights can either be positive, dictating that a person or group act in a specific manner, or negative, requiring that they refrain from acting. Legal requirements, other authorities, or individual conscience can bestow rights, an act that requires a corresponding duty by those with the power to act, such as health care providers [2]. This obligation to act can be based upon an individual's personal values, professional position, or other commitment [3]. For the physician, this duty to act is a role responsibility, at least when holding oneself out as a physician—and possibly at all times. The role–duty link occurs "whenever a person occupies a distinctive place or office in a social organization, to which specific duties are attached to provide for the welfare of others or to advance in some specific way the aims or purposes of the organization" [4]. In this circumstance, performance is not predicated on a guarantee of compensation, but on a concern for another person's welfare [5]. The emergency physician has just such a duty.

Relationship between religion and bioethics

In homogenous societies, religions have long been the arbiters of ethical norms. Western societies, however, are multicultural, with no single religion holding sway over the entire populace. Therefore, a patient-value–based approach to ethical issues is necessary. Yet, religion still influences bioethics. Modern bioethics uses many decision-making methods, arguments, and ideals that draw from religious principles. In addition, clinicians' personal spirituality may influence their relationships with patients and families in crisis.

While various religions may appear dissimilar, most have a form of the Golden Rule, "Do unto others as you would have them do unto you," as a basic tenet. Other moral rules common to most religions are listed in Box 1. Problems surface when trying to apply religion-based rules to specific bioethical situations. For example, although "Do not kill" is generally accepted, the interpretation of the activities that constitute killing, active or passive euthanasia, or merely reasonable medical care varies among the world's religions, as it does among various philosophers [6].

Over time, the Western world, and especially the United States, has turned away from a uniform reliance on religious principles and toward secular principles for answers. The medical community has been no exception. Several such principles, such as autonomy, beneficence, nonmaleficence, and fairness, are now generally accepted. These have guided ethical thinking and have been instrumental in forming health care policies in the United States and other Western countries over the past three decades.

Ethical theories

Ethical traditions stretch back to earliest recorded history. Separate bodies of ethics, often encompassing a general system rather than a true theory, were developed in India and China, and within the Jewish, Christian, Islamic, and Buddhist religions. All these theories represent altruistic, rather than egoistic, attitudes toward mankind. Ethical theories represent the

---

Box 1. Commonly accepted moral rules

Moral rules govern actions that would be considered immoral
without an adequate moral reason. Such rules can justifiably
be enforced and their violation punished. Although none of
these rules is absolute, each requires that a person not cause
evil. Somewhat paradoxically, however, the rules may neither
require preventing evil nor doing good.

- Do not kill.
- Do not cause pain.
- Do not disable.
- Do not deprive of freedom.
- Do not deprive of pleasure.
- Do not deceive.
- Keep your promise.
- Do not cheat.
- Obey the law.
- Do your duty.

Adapted from Gert B. Morality: a new justification of the moral rules. New
York, Oxford University Press, 1988. p. 157; with permission.

---

grand ideas on which guiding principles are based, attempting to be coherent and systematic, while striving to answer fundamental, practical questions: What ought I do? How ought I live? Ethicists normally appeal to
these principles, rather than the underlying theory, when defending a particular action. Western bioethics continues to encompass a number of theories,
some quite contradictory. Some of the most commonly cited include:

Natural law. This system, often attributed to Aristotle, posits that man
should live life according to an inherent human nature. It can be contrasted with man-made, or judicial, law. Yet, they are similar in that
both may change over time, despite the frequent claim that natural
law is immutable [7].

Deontology. This theory holds that the most important aspects of our
lives are governed by certain unbreakable moral rules. Deontologists
hold that these rules may not be broken, even if breaking them may improve an outcome. In other words, they may do the "right" thing, even
though the consequences of that action may not be "good." The famous
philosopher, Immanuel Kant, is often identified with this theory. One
example of a list of "unbreakable" rules is the Ten Commandments [8].

Utilitarianism. One of the more functional and commonly used theories,
utilitarianism, sometimes called consequentialism or teleology, promotes good or valued ends, rather than using the right means. This

theory instructs adherents to work for those outcomes that will most advantage the majority of those affected in the most impartial way possible. Utilitarianism is often simplistically described as advocating methods to achieve the greatest good for the greatest number of people. It is often advocated as the basis for broad social policies [9].

Virtue theory. This theory asks what a "good person" would do in specific real-life situations. This recently revived theory stems from the character traits discussed by Aristotle, Plato, and Thomas Aquinas. They discuss such timeless and cross-cultural virtues as courage, temperance, wisdom, justice, faith, and charity. Recently, the Society for Academic Emergency Medicine took the unusual step of adopting a virtue-based code of conduct (Box 2) [10].

Other theories. Other ethical theories are rarely applied within the scope of bioethics, and each has serious, if not fatal, flaws. Rights theory is based on respecting others' rights. The social contract tradition is based on the implicit agreement we make with others to exist in a cooperative society. Prima facie duties, although less rigid than deontology, lays down certain duties each person has toward others. Egoism advocates that each person live so as to further his or her own interests, a theory in direct opposition to altruism.

Values and principles

Where are values and principles learned?

Values are the standards by which we judge human behavior. They are, in other words, moral rules, promoting those things we think of as good and minimizing or avoiding those things we think of as bad. We learn these values, usually at an early age, from observing behavior and through secular (including professional) and religious education. While many of these learned values overlap, each source often claims moral superiority over the others, whether the values stem from generic, cultural, or legal norms; religious and philosophical traditions; or professional codes [11]. Societal institutions incorporate and promulgate values, often attempting to rigidify old values even in a changing society. In a pluralistic society, clinicians often treat individuals having multiple and differing value systems and they must be sensitive to others' beliefs and traditions.

Ethical values stem from ethical principles. These principles are "action guides" derived from ethical theories, each consisting of various "moral rules," which are our learned values [12]. For example, the values of dealing honestly with patients; fully informing patients before procedures, therapy, or research participation; and respecting the patient's personal values are all subsumed under the principle of autonomy (respect for persons).

A question that naturally arises is whether ethical principles are universal. This is an important question in bioethics, since clinicians must treat

Box 2. Society for Academic Emergency Medicine Ethical Code: a code of conduct for academic emergency medicine

As a member of the Society for Academic Emergency Medicine (SAEM), I am committed to serve humanity. I will practice my art with conscience and virtue, keeping patient welfare my first consideration. I will be considerate, forthright, and just in all of my dealings with patients and colleagues, regardless of their power, position, or station in life. I will maintain the utmost respect for human dignity. I will strive to safeguard the public health and protect the vulnerable. I will advance the ideals of the profession, and I will not abuse the privilege of my knowledge or position. In addition to these general professional obligations,

As a **researcher** of emergency medicine, I vow

- *Competence*, conducting scientifically valid research that, before all else, benefits patients and society.
- *Compassion*, attending humanely to the comfort and dignity of all subjects, animal or human.
- *Respect*, securing the safety, privacy and personal welfare of human subjects, and offering informed choice whenever possible.
- *Impartiality*, treating fairly all those associated with the research process, including subjects and nonsubjects, coinvestigators, and potential authors, and being neither too eager to promote nor too quick to condemn new scientific concepts.
- *Integrity*, reporting promptly any scientific fraud or misconduct, publishing only accurate, uninflated results, and resisting conflicts of interest and the lure of personal gain.
- *Responsibility*, advancing the boundaries of emergency medical science and taking care to use prudently the resources entrusted to me for this purpose.

As a **teacher** of emergency medicine, I vow

- *Altruism*, generously sharing the art and science of emergency medicine for the betterment of others and the honor of the calling.
- A *commitment to excellence*, maintaining my technical expertise and moral sensitivity through continued study and practice.
- *Respect*, giving all who seek to learn emergency medicine the dignity due a colleague.
- *Fairness*, treating all students and fellow teachers equitably, in a manner free of prejudice, abuse, or coercion.

- *Honesty*, imparting truth and uncertainty openly, and identifying clearly for my patients all trainees and students involved in their care.
- *Mentorship*, nurturing and encouraging the requisite technical, intellectual, and moral virtues of the profession in students of every kind through my words and deeds.

By keeping these promises, may I bring honor to myself and my profession, enriching the lives of patients, students, and colleagues.
From Larkin GL, SAEM Ethics Committee. A code of conduct for academic emergency medicine. Acad Emerg Med 1999;6:45; with permission.

patients from a variety of cultural backgrounds. Philosophers once scorned the idea that there were contradictory ethical principles in different cultures. Yet, today, there is a growing acceptance that such differences exist [13]. This discussion, however, will concentrate on those ethical principles generally accepted in Western cultures.

Although each individual is entitled and perhaps even required to have a personal system of values, there are certain values that have become generally accepted by the medical community, courts, legislatures, and society at large. Although some groups disagree about each of these, this dissension has not affected their application to medical care. A respect for patients (often described as patient autonomy) has been considered so fundamental that it is often given overriding importance. Other frequently cited values are beneficence and nonmaleficence.

Why are patient values important?

A key to making bedside ethical decisions is to know the patient's values. As members of democracies with significant populations practicing a number of religions and subgroups of those religions, Western emergency medical practitioners must behave in a manner consistent with the values of each patient. While many people cannot answer the question, "What are your values?," physicians can get an operational answer by asking what patients see as the goal of their medical therapy and why they want specific interventions. The underlying question must be: "What is the patient's desired outcome for medical care?" Responses from patients represent concrete expressions of patient values. In patients too young or incompetent to express their values, it may be necessary for physicians to make general assumptions about what the normal person would want in a specific situation or to rely on surrogate decision-making. However, with patients who are able to communicate, care must be taken to discover what they hold as their own, uncoerced values. A typical, ethically dangerous scenario involves a patient who refuses lifesaving medical intervention "on religious grounds." Commonly, the spouse is at the bedside, does most of the talking, and may be influencing the patient's decisions. In those cases, it is incumbent on the clinician to re-question the patient to assess his or her real values in that situation.

Not only religion, but family, cultural, and other values contribute to patients' decisions about their medical care. Without asking, there is no way to know what decision a patient will make. It is important to note that religion influences modern secular bioethics, which uses many religion-originated decision-making methods, arguments, and ideals. In addition, clinicians' personal spirituality may allow them to relate better to patients and families in crisis.

Clinicians' and institutional values

Institutions, including health care facilities and professional organizations, also have their own value systems. Health care facilities, although relatively well standardized under the requirements of regulatory bodies and government agencies, often have specific value-related missions. Religiously oriented or affiliated institutions may be the most obvious of these, but charitable, for-profit, and academic institutions also have specific role-related values. The values that professional organizations aspire to are often set forth in their ethical codes, described later in this article.

On a wider, but individual basis, some medical centers deny treatment (or at least admission through the emergency department) on internal medicine, family practice, and pediatric teaching services based on arbitrary resident work limits. "Capping" is commonly used to describe prescribed resident work limits, a relatively new practice that, in its current form, is damaging the physician educational system and possibly the professionalism of medicine. It involves two elements: (1) restricting residents' work hours, and (2) limiting the number of patients that can be admitted or the number of inpatients for whom residents can be responsible [14].

Clinicians have their own ethical values, as do professional organizations and health care institutions. Conscience clauses permit clinicians to "opt out" when they feel that they have a moral conflict with professionally, institutionally, or legally required actions. These conflicts, which may have a religious, philosophical, or practical basis, prevent them from following the normal ethical decision-making algorithm. When such conflicts exist, it is morally and legally acceptable, within certain constraints, for the individual to follow a course of action based upon his or her own value system. The constraints generally require that there be the provision of timely and adequate medical care for the patient, which may be particularly difficult to achieve in emergency medicine. The most common conflict has been about whether to provide emergency contraception. Consensus generally discourages delaying necessary medical treatments, including emergency contraception, since patients often have no choice about the emergency department to which they go and cannot know the practitioners' attitudes about such treatment in advance [15,16]. When conflicts over values exist, however, it is essential for the practitioner to recognize the patient's identity, dignity, and autonomy to avoid the error of blindly imposing one's own values on others.

While it is tempting to use the latest instruments or medications, physicians have a duty to maintain competency in new technologies and be informed of new medications to decrease any potential risks before subjecting their patients to them. Since there is relatively little oversight of individual practitioners in this area, it remains substantially a matter of personal ethics [17].

Over the millennia, personal values have dictated whether a physician would remain with his or her patients during extreme or catastrophic circumstances. Physicians, even such legends of medicine as Galen, often fled to save their own lives. In the era of modern epidemics of unknown virulence and etiology, the question of whether physicians will stay and treat patients remains a personal moral decision. This issue is of special concern for emergency physicians in the front line of these medical assaults.

Autonomy

Definition and basis

Individual freedom is the basis for the modern concept of bioethics. This freedom, usually spoken of as "autonomy," is the principle that a person should be free to make his or her own decisions. It is the counterweight to the medical profession's long-practiced paternalism (or parentalism), wherein the practitioner acted on what he thought was "good" for the patient, whether or not the patient agreed. The principle of autonomy does not stand alone, but is derived from an ancient foundation for all interpersonal relationships—a respect for persons as individuals.

Physicians have only grudgingly begun to accept patient autonomy in recent years. From three perspectives, this is understandable. First, accepting patient autonomy means that physicians' roles must change. They must be partners in their patients' care rather than the absolute arbiters of the timing, intensity, and types of treatment. Second, they must become educators, teaching their lay patients enough about their diseases and treatments to make rational decisions. Finally, and most distressing to clinicians, is accepting that some patients will make what clinicians consider to be foolish choices. For physicians dedicated to preserving their patients' well being, allowing people to select what the physician considers poor treatment options (such as refusing treatment or opting for ineffective regimens) may be both frustrating and disheartening. Yet, allowing these "foolish" choices is part of accepting the principle of patient autonomy. If clinicians fully understand patient autonomy, much of the rest of clinical bioethics naturally follows.

Communitarianism—an alternate view of life

Both a philosophical and a political value, communitarianism is the belief that the standards of justice must be based on the life and traditions of a particular society and how that society views the world. Key to this concept is the understanding that cultural factors can affect how people prioritize and justify rights. This different prioritization becomes vitally important during ethical dilemmas, when values often conflict. The application of one set of values instead of another may lead to radically different outcomes. In contrast to the Western emphasis on autonomy, communitarians cleave to the Aristotelian view that "Man is a social animal, indeed a political animal, because he is not self-sufficient alone, and in an important sense is not self-sufficient outside a polis."

Typical communities may be related to one another by geographical location, a morally significant history, or may work together for common goals in a trusting and altruistic manner. In practice, communitarian values are found in many patients presenting to emergency departments who have close family interrelationships and whose sense of self is bound to their communities. This example of communitarianism most frequently occurs with patients from outside the United States. Given the Western emphasis on autonomy, the best way to function with those patients displaying a communitarian ethic is to recognize this as their autonomous wish and to follow it. This means accepting the communitarian ethic of involving family in consultations and relying on senior or other family members for making decisions affecting the patient.

Decision-making capacity, consent, and surrogates

When patients cannot make their own health care decisions, others must make such decisions for them. Two questions arise: When do patients lack such capability? Who then makes the decision?

Patients may exercise their autonomy only if they have the mental capacity to do so. Justice Benjamin Cardozo stated this principle of both bioethics and the law early in the last century: "Every human being of adult years and sound mind has a right to determine what shall be done with his own body ..." [18]. Only if we understand how to determine decision-making capacity can we use the principle of patient autonomy in clinical practice. In emergency medicine, questions of decision-making capacity frequently arise for issues of informed consent, patient refusals (often in the emergency medical services system), and patient discharge from the emergency department.

We often mistakenly use the word *competency* when we mean *capacity*. "Competency," like the word "insanity," is a legal term and can only be determined by the court. Decision-making capacity, though, refers to a patient's ability to make *specific* decisions about his health care, as determined by his clinician. Decision-making capacity is always decision relative (for a specific decision or related type of decision) rather than global (all decisions). Having decision-making capacity relates to the patient's level of understanding of that decision, which in turn is related to both the seriousness of the potential outcomes and the complexity of the information presented. Unless a patient is unconscious, he is unlikely to lack decision-making capacity for at least the simplest decisions.

To have adequate decision-making capacity in any one circumstance, individuals must understand the options, the consequences of acting on the various options, and the costs and benefits to them of these consequences in terms of their personal values and priorities (Box 3) [19,20]. Disagreement with the physician's recommendation is not by itself grounds for determining that the patient is incapable of making a decision. In fact, even refusing lifesaving medical care may not prove the person incapable of making valid decisions if the refusal is based on firmly held beliefs, as is sometimes the case with patients who are Jehovah's Witnesses. Using medications, such as antipsychotics, to restore decision-making capacity carries the danger of simultaneously diminishing a patient's discriminatory thought processes. Standards for determining adequate decision-making capacity in these instances is a difficult and unresolved area of emergency medicine and psychiatric practice [21].

If patients lack capacity to participate in some decisions about their care, surrogate decision-makers must become involved. These surrogates may be designated by the patient's advance directives or detailed in institutional policy or law. (Some countries do not recognize surrogate decision-making [22].) Surrogate decision-makers may include spouses, adult children, parents (of adults), and others, including the attending physician. On occasion, bioethics committees or the courts will need to intervene to help determine the decision maker.

Children represent a special situation. Individuals less than the age of majority (or unemancipated) are usually deemed incapable of making independent medical decisions, although they are often asked to give their assent to the decision, allowing them to "buy in" to their medical treatment plan. In those cases, the physician–parent–child relationship is triadic, with parents

---

Box 3. Components of decision-making capacity

- Knowledge of the options
- Awareness of consequences of each option
- Appreciation of personal costs and benefits of these consequences in relation to relatively stable values and preferences (When ascertaining this, ask the patient why they made a specific choice.)

Adapted from Iserson KV, Sanders AB, Mathieu D, et al, editors. Ethics in emergency medicine, 2nd edition. Tucson (AZ): Galen Press; 1995. p. 52.

in the unusual position of being able to make choices based on quality of life [23]. In many cases, when deciding which children have decision-making capacity, the same rules that apply to adult capacity apply to children. The more serious the consequences, the more children are required to understand the options, consequences, and values involved.

Emergency physicians often operate within variable degrees of uncertainty, with less-than-ideal information, and under severe time constraints. Therefore, they must often quickly decide whether patients lack "decision-making capacity," the ability to make their own health care decisions. While this is obvious in the unconscious or delirious patient, it is often less so when the patient remains verbal and at least somewhat coherent. Decisions in emergency situations must often be made rapidly and, unlike other medical venues, bioethics consultation may not be readily available.

Limitations on autonomy

Personal autonomy has limitations. Within emergency medicine, this often arises in the context of patients who are actively suicidal or homicidal. These patients, even though they may desire to leave the emergency department or to refuse treatment, cannot do so. In these cases, beneficence, for the patient and society, trumps autonomy. The same holds true with patients involved in physician-assisted suicide who present to the emergency department after an unsuccessful suicide attempt. Patients can be allowed to die (passive euthanasia) if there is sufficient time to "consider the morally relevant features of the situations, including the patient's decision-making capacity and desires, current condition and medical history, and the nature of the suicide attempt." The luxury of time usually does not exist in these cases, so lifesaving interventions must be provided, at least until more information can be ascertained. Treatment can then be withdrawn. In no cases should emergency physicians administer lethal drugs or otherwise assist such patients to complete the suicide [24,25].

Other bioethical principles

In addition to autonomy, other bioethical principles guide the actions of emergency clinicians. The following are short descriptions of some of these.

Beneficence

Beneficence, doing good, has long been a universal tenet of the medical profession at the patient's bedside. Most health care professionals entered their career to apply this principle. Outside typical emergency medicine practice, beneficence is the guiding principle behind Good Samaritan actions when emergency department physicians render aid after motor vehicle crashes, on airplanes, after disasters, and in other situations without expectation of recompense [26]. In emergency departments, this principle guides physician behavior in the face of epidemics carrying potential personal risk, such as was initially true with hantavirus, severe acute respiratory syndrome, and AIDS.

Nonmaleficence

Nonmaleficence is the philosophical principle that encompasses the medical student's principal rule, "First, do no harm." This credo, often stated in the Latin form, *primum non nocere,* derives from knowing that patient encounters with physicians can prove harmful as well as helpful. This principle includes not doing harm, preventing harm, and removing harmful conditions. Within emergency medicine, nonmaleficence also includes the concept of security. That means protecting the emergency clinician and the clinician's team, as well as the patient, from harm [27].

Confidentiality versus privacy

Stemming at least from the time of Hippocrates, confidentiality is the presumption that what the patient tells the physician will not be revealed to any other person or institution without the patient's permission. Health care workers have an obligation to maintain patient confidentiality. Occasionally, the law, especially public health statutes that require reporting specific diseases, injuries, mechanisms, and deaths, may conflict with this principle. The Health Insurance Portability and Accountability Act of 1996, a US federal law designed to further protect patient information, has, paradoxically, made obtaining the information needed for patient care in emergency departments more difficult.

Long used in emergency departments, drug-seeker lists can be seen as violations of patient confidentiality. These lists can directly harm patients, especially when patient entry and clinician access to these lists are not properly controlled [28]. Rarely discussed, however, are similar computer lists of prior emergency department visits that can be easily generated from most emergency department computer systems.

In another recent development, part of the "reality TV" fad, emergency department activities are being filmed for public viewing. Filming emergency department patients, whether for medical records, education, peer review, or for "reality television," strains the nature of confidentiality, since these records can easily be distributed or misused. Although good reasons exist to allow such filming with patient acquiescence [29], the standard is now to abstain from such filming for commercial purposes and to require patient or surrogate consent for educational purposes [30].

Privacy, often confused with confidentiality, is a patient's right to be afforded sufficient physical and auditory isolation so that others cannot view or hear them when interacting with medical personnel. Emergency department overcrowding, patient and staff safety, and emergency department design limit patient privacy in many cases.

The increasing use of telemedicine to render advice and eventually to guide procedures at remote sites also places a strain on both patient privacy and confidentiality. Suggested ethical guidelines for such practice can facilitate the use of these new technologies without sacrificing either patient rights or physician duties [31].

Personal integrity

Personal integrity involves adhering to one's own reasoned and defensible set of values and moral standards, and is basic to thinking and acting ethically. Integrity includes a controversial value within the medical community—truth telling. Many who feel that the patient has the right to know the truth no matter what the circumstances have championed absolute honesty. Yet, honesty does not have to be the same as brutality, and must be tempered with compassion. Perhaps truth telling is not universally accepted within the medical profession because of poor role models, lack of training in interpersonal interactions, and bad experiences, rather than a discounting of the value itself [32]. The issues surrounding truth telling become somewhat murky in cases involving a third party, such as a sex partner who is being exposed to an infectious disease [32].

Distributive justice (fairness)

Distributive justice relates to fairness in the allocation of resources and to the physician's obligations to patients. This value is the basis of and is incorporated into society-wide health care policies. The concept of comparative or distributive justice suggests that a society's comparable individuals and groups should share similarly in the society's benefits and burdens. Yet, for individual clinicians to arbitrarily limit or terminate care on a case-by-case basis at patients' bedsides is an erroneous extrapolation of the idea that there may be a need to limit health care resource expenditures [33]. Distributive justice is a policy, rather than a clinical, concept.

In emergency medical practice, the most direct application of distributive justice is in triage. Triage situations exist on a continuum, ranging from the daily triage performed in emergency departments to the absence of triage after the use of weapons of mass destruction. While utilitarian ethics are normally invoked to justify triage, it actually involves a combination of utility and strict equality, depending on patients' apparent disease or injury severity [34]. A unique aspect of triage in area-wide disasters is the priority given to health care workers, public safety personnel, and community leaders, who can be returned to duty to either help decrease morbidity and mortality or to help stabilize social order [35,36].

Medical and moral imperatives in emergency medicine

Emergency clinicians, both in the prehospital care and emergency department environments, operate with four imperatives: (1) to save lives when possible, (2) to relieve pain and suffering, (3) to comfort patients and families, and (4) to protect staff and patients from injury. All but the last of these are also imperatives for most other clinicians, although saving lives may occur more often and more dramatically in emergency medical settings than in most other settings.

The imperative to save lives causes the most conflict between emergency and ICU clinicians. Emergency physicians know that some of the intubations and resuscitations they perform are unwanted by patients or surrogates. Nearly all emergency physicians have gotten calls from irate intensive care clinicians or private practitioners berating them for resuscitating patients "who should not have been resuscitated." Many families have heard these physicians berate the emergency department and ambulance staffs for their over-aggressive resuscitative efforts. Yet, the lifesaving imperative begins when the ambulance is called.

Emergency medical service personnel are required to attempt resuscitations except when there is no chance that life exists (eg, decapitation, rigor mortis, charred beyond recognition, or decomposition). They usually have little leeway in whom to resuscitate. The real answer is for primary physicians to educate the families of homebound hospice-type patients to not call the ambulance (or police) when the person dies, but rather to call the clinician to pronounce the person dead.

Recently, the emergency medicine community has developed a method to avoid medical interventions, even when the ambulance is inadvertently called. Prehospital advance directives, which are made by patients or surrogates, and prehospital do-not-attempt-resuscitation orders, which are issued by physicians, have proved very successful where they have been implemented [37,38]. The orders usually specify that intubation, artificial ventilations, cardioversion, and cardiopulmonary resuscitation should not be performed on an individual. Some focus on providing comfort care, even if life-support measures are declined [39]. Arizona is the only state that allows the use of prehospital advance directives and prehospital do-not-attempt-resuscitation orders for children [40].

The last imperative, safety, is nearly unique to emergency medical clinicians. Both in the prehospital and emergency department settings, clinicians often encounter dangerous situations, be they from the environment (eg, fires, extreme cold, floods), patients, or families. While most clinicians try to accommodate "patient rights," their priorities must be their own safety and the safety of their coworkers when safety questions arise. That does not imply that clinicians should ignore patient safety, but only that they should first ensure their own safety if they and their colleagues are at risk (often from the patient).

Ethical oaths and codes

Through the years, the medical profession has codified its ethics more rigorously than any other professional group, incorporating many standard bioethics principles into the profession's ethical codes and oaths. For generations, the existing part of the Hippocratic Oath set the ethical standard for the medical profession (Box 4). Yet, its precepts clash with modern bioethical thinking, and many subsequent professional codes have included what may best be termed economic guidelines and professional etiquette along with ethical precepts [41].

Many current medical ethical codes have been criticized for being more professional management guidelines than ethical codes. Bioethics and professional etiquette are two distinct bodies of values and standards. Bioethics deals with relationships between practitioners and patients, practitioners and society, and society and patients. Professional etiquette relates to standards governing the relationships and interactions among practitioners. Although the two areas occasionally overlap, they rely upon different standards, different values, and different methods of solving problems.

Most modern ethical codes prescribe only the same basic moral behavior for members to follow that is expected by the society at large, and do not require any higher level of duty or commitment. In fact, many of the ethical issues that would seem important to medical specialties are usually not addressed in their codes. Even when topics of interprofessional interactions are excluded, existing medical professional codes differ markedly (Table 2). All, however, try to give a "bottom line" course of action below which the medical practitioner may not pass.

In the spirit of returning to basic bioethical principles, the American College of Emergency Physicians (Box 5), the Emergency Medicine Residency Association (Box 6), and the Society for Academic Emergency Medicine (see Box 2) have adopted patient-focused bioethical codes. In 2001, the American Medical Association also revised its *Ethical Principles*.

Applying bioethics

Moral reasoning, used in bioethics, is one of the three basic reasoning strategies (ie, moral, deductive, and inductive) [42]. Yet, to apply bioethical principles to a clinical situation, one first must recognize that a bioethical problem exists. To do this, practitioners must read and discuss the issues and specific situations both to be able to recognize bioethical issues within clinical cases and to formulate plans for dealing with them.

Although physicians like to reduce all clinical situations to "medical problems," today's complex medical environment often produces problems that are inexorably intertwined with fundamental bioethical dilemmas. Some are obvious, but many are more difficult to recognize. The key to

Box 4. Hippocratic Oath

I swear by Apollo Physician and Asclepius and by Health [the god
   Hygiea] and Panacea and all the gods as well as goddesses,
   making them judges [witnesses], to bring the following oath
   and written covenant to fulfillment, in accordance with my
   power and my judgment;
to regard him who has taught me this *techné* [art and science] as
   equal to my parents, and to share when he is in need of
   necessities, and to judge the offspring [coming] from him equal
   to [my] male siblings, and to teach them this *techné*, would
   they desire to learn [it], without fee and written covenant,
and to give a share both of rules and of lectures, and of all the
   rest of learning, to my sons and to the [sons] of him who has
   taught me and to the pupils who have both made a written
   contract and sworn by a medical convention but by no other.
And I will use regimens for the benefit of the ill in accordance
   with my ability and my judgment, but from [what is] to their
   harm or injustice I will keep [them].
And I will not give a drug that is deadly to anyone if asked [for it],
   nor will I suggest the way to such a counsel.
And likewise I will not give a woman a destructive pessary.
And in a pure and holy way I will guard my life and my *techné*.
I will not cut, and certainly not those suffering from stone, but I
   will cede [this] to men [who are] practitioners of this activity.
Into as many houses as I may enter, I will go for the benefit of the
   ill, while being far from all voluntary and destructive injustice,
   especially from sexual acts both upon women's bodies and
   upon men's, both of the free and of the slaves.
And about whatever I may see or hear in the treatment, or even
   without treatment in the life of human beings—things that
   should not ever be blurted out outside—I will remain silent,
   holding such things to be unutterable [sacred, not to be
   divulged].
If I render this oath fulfilled, and if I do not blur and confound it
   [making it to no effect] may it be [granted] to me to enjoy the
   benefits both of life and of *techné*, being held in good repute
   among all human beings for time eternal. If, however, I
   transgress and perjure myself, the opposite of these.

From von Staden H. "In a pure and holy way": personal and professional conduct in the Hippocratic Oath. J Hist Med Allied Sci 1996;51:406–8; with permission.

Table 2
Comparison of six ethical codes

	SAEM	ACEP	EMRA	AMA[a]	AOA[b]	Hippocratic Oath
Protect patient confidentiality	c	X	X	X	X	X
Maintain professional expertise	X	X	X	X	X	X
Committed to serve humanity	X	X	X	X	X	
Patient welfare primary concern	X	X	X	X		X
Considerate to patients, colleagues	X	X	X	X		X
Respect human dignity	X	X	X	X		X
Safeguard public health	X	X	X	X		
Protect vulnerable	X	X		X	X	X
Advance professional ideals	X	X	X	X		X
Honesty	d	X		X	X	
Report incompetent, dishonest, impaired physicians	d	X	X	X		
Moral sensitivity	X	X		X		
Obtain necessary consultation				X	X	X
Altruism in teaching	X			X		X
Fairness to students, colleagues	X	X				X
Obey, respect the law			X	X	X	
Prudent resource use	X	X				
Work to change laws for patient benefit				X	X	
Not abuse privileges	X					X
Respect for students	X					X
Choose whom to serve except in emergencies				X	X	
Ensure beneficial research with competence, impartiality, compassion	X					
No abortion						X
No euthanasia						X
Do not compromise clinical judgment for money			X			
Universal access to healthcare				X		
Preserve human life						X

The American Association of Emergency Medicine's ethical code deals primarily with questions of professional etiquette, including conflicts of interest. The American College of Osteopathic Emergency Physicians and the Canadian Association of Emergency Physicians do not have an ethical oath or code.

Abbreviations: ACEP, American College of Emergency Physicians; AOA, American Osteopathic Association; AMA, American Medical Association; EMRA, Emergency Medicine Residents's Association; SAEM, Society for Academic Emergency Medicine.

[a] The American Medical Association has both a relatively brief *Principles of Medical Ethics* (nine points) and an extensive *Code of Medical Ethics.*

[b] The American Osteopathic Association has both a *Code of Ethics* and an interpretation of some of its sections.

[c] The SAEM code addresses research subject privacy, but not confidentiality—an unusual oversight.

[d] The SAEM code deals primarily with research when addressing these issues.

Box 5. American College of Emergency Physicians principles of ethics for emergency physicians

The principles section of the *Code of Ethics for Emergency Physicians*, the first of three sections in the code, lists 10 ethics guidelines for emergency physicians to follow in their emergency medicine practice. The following is the principles section only: The basic professional obligation of beneficent service to humanity is expressed in various physician oaths. In addition to this general obligation, emergency physicians assume more specific ethical obligations that arise out of the special features of emergency medical practice. The principles listed below express fundamental moral responsibilities of emergency physicians. Emergency physicians shall:

1. Embrace patient welfare as their primary professional responsibility.
2. Respond promptly and expertly, without prejudice or partiality, to the need for emergency medical care.
3. Respect the rights and strive to protect the best interests of their patients, particularly the most vulnerable and those unable to make treatment choices due to diminished decision-making capacity.
4. Communicate truthfully with patients and secure their informed consent for treatment, unless the urgency of the patient's condition demands an immediate response.
5. Respect patient privacy and disclose confidential information only with consent of the patient or when required by an overriding duty such as the duty to protect others or to obey the law.
6. Deal fairly and honestly with colleagues and take appropriate action to protect patients from health care providers who are impaired, incompetent, or who engage in fraud or deception.
7. Work cooperatively with others who care for, and about, emergency patients.
8. Engage in continuing study to maintain the knowledge and skills necessary to provide high quality care for emergency patients.
9. Act as responsible stewards of the health care resources entrusted to them.
10. Support societal efforts to improve public health and safety, reduce the effects of injury and illness, and secure access to emergency and other basic health care for all.

From American College of Emergency Physicians. Code of ethics for emergency physicians. Dallas (TX): American College of Emergency Physicians; 1997; with permission.

Box 6. Emergency Medicine Residents' Association code of ethics

Emergency Medicine Residents' Association Principles of Medical Ethics preamble

These principles are intended to aid physicians individually and collectively in maintaining a high level of ethical conduct. They are not laws, but standards by which a resident physician may determine the propriety of his conduct in his relationship with patients, with colleagues, with members of allied professions, and with the public.

1. The principal objective of the medical profession is to render service to humanity with full respect to the dignity of man. Physicians should merit the confidence of patients entrusted to their care, rendering the full measure of service and devotion.
2. Physicians should strive continually to improve medical knowledge and skill, and should make available to their patients and colleagues the benefits of their professional attainments.
3. The medical profession should safeguard the public and itself against physicians deficient in moral character or professional competence. Physicians should observe all laws, uphold the dignity and honor of the profession, and accept its self-imposed disciplines. They should expose, without hesitation, illegal or unethical conduct of fellow members of the profession.
4. A physician should not dispose of his services under terms and conditions that tend to interfere with or impair the free and complete exercise of his/her judgment and skill, or tend to cause a deterioration of the quality of medical care.
5. A physician may not reveal the confidences entrusted to him in the course of medical attendance, or the deficiencies he may observe in the character of patients, unless he is required to do so by law or unless it becomes necessary to protect the welfare of the individual or of the community.
6. The honored ideals of the medical profession imply that the responsibilities of the physician extend not only to the individual but also to the society where these responsibilities deserve his interest and participation in activities that have the purpose of improving both the health and well-being of the individual and the community.

From Article VIII, Emergency Medicine Residents' Association Bylaws, Dallas, TX: EMRA, 2003; with permission.

recognizing bioethical issues and applying ethical principles and virtuous behavior is preparation for both their obvious and their subtler presentations. In the same way that physicians must prepare for other critical events encountered in medicine, physicians must read, discuss, and think about how to face these issues when they present. This strategy leads not only to personal preparation, but also to more general policies that help guide everyone faced with difficult bioethical issues.

Prioritizing principles: the bioethical dilemma

In the abstract, bioethical principles often appear simple. However, clinicians usually adhere not only to basic bioethical principles, but also, at least tacitly, to ethical oaths, codes, and statements of a number of professional, religious, and social organizations. This can make for a confusing array of potentially conflicting bioethical imperatives. Since bioethical principles seem to be neither universal nor universally applied, those principles that are most patient-centered normally hold sway.

Even then, applying bioethical principles in practice can be confusing. When two or more seemingly equivalent principles or values seem to compel different actions, a bioethical dilemma exists. This situation is often described as "being damned if you do and damned if you don't," where taking any course of action or taking no action at all could potentially result in harm of one kind or another. In the following actual case, the attending physician can be said to be on the horns (two prickly but seemingly equal choices) of a dilemma. The physician seems to have only two options for action and they both involve a number of conflicting bioethical principles.

Case

The emergency medical service transported a 43-year-old woman to the emergency department after a bus struck her. Although tachycardic and in obvious pain from pelvic and leg injuries, she was awake, alert, and fully responsive to all questions. Her abdomen was rapidly distending with a large amount of intraperitoneal fluid on a focused-assessment-with-sonography-in-trauma (FAST) exam. As the operating room was being readied, a surgery resident asked the patient to consent for the blood transfusions she would need to survive. She refused, saying, "I am a Jehovah's Witness and will not take blood or blood products." The resident instructed that the blood be sent back to the blood bank.

The emergency physician then approached the patient and asked her what she had been told. She lucidly explained that she was simply told that she "needs blood before surgery." She agreed to surgery, but declined the blood. When asked whether she had been told that she would die within the half hour, she asked if all other options had been tried. When told that they had—saline had been administered and a cell saver outside the operating room was not an option—she simply said, "Well, I don't want to die; give me the blood." As it turned out, the 30-minute estimate was too generous; with her injuries, she would have died sooner. If, with the demonstrated decision-making capacity for this decision, she had still opted not to receive blood, it would have been withheld.

The patient immediately began receiving blood and went to the operating room. She eventually received dozens of units of blood and fresh frozen plasma, but survived her injuries in a fully functional condition.

Case discussion

This patient demonstrated decision-making capacity, including knowledge of the options presented, understanding of the risks and benefits to her of the options, and the ability to state how her choices—first one, then the other—meshed with her stable values. The problem, of course, is that "informed consent" must include the information necessary to make a reasoned decision. As in all parts of medicine, a little knowledge can be a dangerous thing. In this case, the resident had learned a little about patient autonomy, but had inadequate knowledge about giving informed consent, which almost cost this patient her life. Nevertheless, these actions fell within a morally acceptable range: They passed the Impartiality Test, Universalizability Test, and Interpersonal Justifiability Test, described below.

Clinical practice

Emergency clinicians often must make ethical decisions with little time for reflection or consultation. While bioethics committees now have an increasing ability to give at least limited "stat" consultations, even these often do not meet the need for a rapid response. For that reason, the author developed a rapid decision-making model for emergency clinicians, based on accepted biomedical theories and techniques (Fig. 1). On occasion, this model may also be applicable to those working in critical care.

The following rules of thumb give the emergency medicine practitioner a process to use for emergency ethical decision-making even in cases where there is not time to go through a detailed, systematic process of ethical deliberation. While somewhat oversimplified, this approach offers guidance to those who are under severe time pressures and who wish to make ethically appropriate decisions.

When using this approach, one must first ask: Is this an instance of a type of ethical problem for which I have already worked out a rule? Or, is it similar enough to such cases that the rule could be reasonably extended to cover it? In other words, if there had been time in the past to think coolly about the issues, discuss them with colleagues, and develop some rough guidelines, can the rules worked out at that time be used in this case? If the current case fits under one of those guidelines that you have arrived at through critical reflection, and you do not have time to analyze the situation any further,

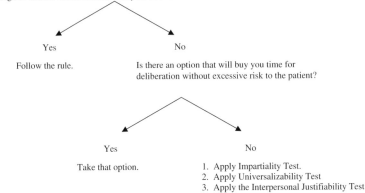

Is this a type of ethical problem for which you have already worked out a rule or is it at least similar enough so that the rule could reasonably be extended to cover it?

Yes   No

Follow the rule.   Is there an option that will buy you time for
                                                 deliberation without excessive risk to the patient?

Yes   No

Take that option.   1. Apply Impartiality Test.
                                                   2. Apply Universalizability Test
                                                   3. Apply the Interpersonal Justifiability Test

Fig. 1. Rapid decision-making model. (*From* Iserson KV. An approach to ethical problems in emergency medicine. In Iserson KV, Sanders AB, Mathieu D, editors. Ethics in Emergency Medicine, 2nd Edition. Tuscon, AZ: Galen Press, Ltd. p. 45; with permission.)

then the most reasonable step would be to follow that rule. In ethics, this step follows from casuistry, or case-based learning.

Such predetermined rules, of course, must be periodically evaluated. Practitioners must question whether the results obtained when they follow this rule remain appropriate. Are they compatible with the intention of the rule and with the values that underlie it? This reevaluation only emphasizes that it is unrealistic and ethically irresponsible to believe that one can work out ethical rules to be mechanically applied during an entire professional career. Similarly, it would be unrealistic and irresponsible to continue to perform a medical procedure just as one learned it in medical school, regardless of its efficacy or whether better techniques had been subsequently developed.

But, suppose that the practitioner faces an emergency case that does not fit under any previously generated ethical rule. At this point, the practitioner should ask herself if there is an option that will buy her time for deliberation. If there is such a strategy, and it does not involve unacceptable risks to the patient, then it would be the reasonable course to take. Using a delaying tactic may provide time to consult with other professionals, including the bioethics committee and the family, before developing an ethically appropriate course of action.

If there is no delaying tactic that can be used without unreasonable risk to the patient, then a set of three tests can be applied to possible courses of action to help make a decision. These are often what people use instinctively when confronted with ethical issues, whether medical or otherwise. The three tests, the Impartiality Test, the Universalizability Test, and the Interpersonal Justifiability Test, are drawn from three different philosophical theories.

Impartiality Test. Would you be willing to have this action performed if you were in the patient's place? This is, in essence, a version of the

Golden Rule and is intended to correct one obvious source of moral error—partiality, or self-interested bias.

Universalizability Test. Would you be comfortable if all clinicians with the same background and in the same circumstances act as you are proposing to do? This generalizes the action and asks whether developing a universal rule for the contemplated behavior is reasonable—an application of Kant's categorical imperative. The usefulness of this test is that it can help eliminate not only bias and partiality, but also short-sightedness. Justifying one particular instance that falls under a rule is not sufficient for justifying the practice of acting on that rule.

Interpersonal Justifiability Test. Using a theory of consensus values as a final screen for the proposed action, this test asks you to provide good reasons to justify your actions to others [43]. Will peers, superiors, or the public be satisfied with the answers? Also, can you give reasons that you would be willing to state publicly?

When ethical situations arise that allow no time for further deliberation, it is probably best to act on the rule or perform the action that allows all three tests to be answered in the affirmative with some degree of confidence. Once the crisis has subsided, however, the practitioner should review the decision with the aid of colleagues and bioethicists to refine his emergency ethical decision-making abilities. In particular, it is crucial to ask whether the decision-making process has served the most basic ethical values. Were the actions taken in the emergency situation consonant with showing the kind of respect for patient autonomy that you believe appropriate? Were the ethical decisions really in the patient's best interest, or were you unduly influenced by the interests of others or considerations of your convenience or psychological comfort? Were people treated fairly, justly, and equitably?

Ethical problems, like emergency clinical problems, require action for resolution. Ideally, one would have extensive discussions and reflect in advance of each ethical decision. Discussions and reflection, of course, are not possible for many emergency care decisions. Nevertheless, by making a sincere effort to anticipate recurring types of problems, subjecting them to ethical analysis in advance, and conscientiously reviewing decisions after they have been made, the emergency care professional can better fulfill his or her ethical responsibilities. That a decision is an emergency decision, therefore, does not remove it from the realm of ethical evaluation.

What is the difference between withholding and withdrawing treatment?

As the ambulance screams to a halt and the medics bring in a patient in critical condition, only rarely will emergency physicians have enough information to make a judgment that intervention would be futile (see next section). They usually lack vital information about their patients' identities, medical conditions, and wishes. Therefore, they must intervene quickly to try to save a life [44,45]. Only later, when relatives arrive or medical records become available, may they discover that the patient has a terminal disease or near death, did not want resuscitative efforts, or even has excruciating pain and was wishing for death. Yet, due to the limited information available when the patient arrives in the emergency department, the emergency physician's mandate to attempt resuscitation is morally justifiable.

Ethicists usually do not distinguish between withholding treatment and withdrawing treatment (through an act of omission) [46]. Yet, in emergency medicine, the difference between withholding and withdrawing life-sustaining medical treatment is significant. The justification for this difference stems, in part, from the nature of emergency medical practice and the unique manner in which clinicians apply many ethical principles. While a clear moral distinction between withholding and withdrawing treatment may be absent from other medical areas, emergency medical care's unique circumstances continue to make this distinction relevant and morally significant.

In the usual medical setting, withholding further medical treatment is done quietly, often without input from the patient or surrogate decision-maker, while withdrawing ongoing medical treatment can be more obvious and difficult. This situation is reversed in the emergency medical setting. Withholding emergency medical treatment is much more problematic than withdrawing unwanted or useless interventions later. Society has specific expectations of emergency medical practitioners. Due to the nature of emergency medicine, both in the prehospital and the emergency department settings, the distinction between withdrawing and withholding medical treatment has never disappeared and is not likely to disappear in the future [45].

While lifesaving medical interventions may not be appropriate in all cases, emergency clinicians, whenever possible, should provide patients with palliative care. The purpose of palliative interventions is not to prolong the dying process, but rather, when death is inevitable, to make it as comfortable for the patient as possible. As the Steinberg Report notes, terminal patients have the right to receive state-of-the-art palliative care [47]. Palliation often includes analgesics, and may include diuretics, sedation, oxygen, paracentesis or thoracentesis, or other medications or procedures to alleviate suffering. While medical personnel may withdraw or withhold treatment, they should never withdraw or withhold care. While medical practitioners, surrogate decision-makers, and sometimes patients find it emotionally easier to forego new interventions than to withdraw ongoing treatment, no orders, policies, or directives should ever prevent emergency physicians from caring for their patient (ie, alleviating discomfort). As patient advocates, emergency physicians may need to "push" to have the patient admitted to a hospital, hospice, or nursing home, or to get ancillary personnel (eg, social workers, home health nurses) to intervene for the patient.

Is futility an issue in emergency care?

Emergency physicians, nurses, and emergency medical system personnel may, in some circumstances, feel that further medical interventions are futile. This commonly used but still controversial concept has been described as a judgment about "odds and ends." That is, efforts with very low odds of achieving desired ends [48]. Some have suggested replacing the nebulous term "futility" with seemingly more specific adjectives for medical interventions, such as "nonbeneficial," "ineffective," "medically inappropriate," or "with a low probability of success" [49]. Yet, for now, "futility" remains a common part of the medical vernacular, and so should be discussed in that way.

Only three circumstances meet the most commonly accepted definition of futility [50]. The first, which clinicians can only identify in a very limited set of circumstances, is when the intervention is effective in <1% of identical cases, based on the medical literature. Emergency department thoracotomies for blunt trauma are just such a circumstance. However, individual clinician's experiences cannot be relied upon, since they are often skewed due to selective memory, limited numbers of similar cases, and other biases. A common scenario with survival rates approaching 0% is the out-of-hospital cardiac arrest that is not witnessed or arrives from a long-term care facility [51].

The second futile circumstance is physiological futility, when known anatomical or biochemical abnormalities will not permit successful medical interventions. Examples generally accepted by emergency medical systems as reasons not to intervene or provide transport to hospitals include rigor mortis, algor mortis, patients burned beyond recognition, or injuries incompatible with life (eg, decapitation). These, along with prolonged normothermic resuscitative attempts without success, prolonged "down time" with an isoelectric ECG, or pulseless electrical activity are the criteria often used to help determine whether emergency medical personnel can pronounce death on the scene. Emergency medical services, in these instances, need not expend valuable resources in a futile resuscitative effort.

The third category, based on the patient's values, when known, is that intervention will not achieve the patient's goals for medical therapy. Since this course is based on knowing the patient's values related to medical treatment, it is necessary to have talked with the patient in advance, which is rare in the emergency department setting; to have received surrogate-supplied information or decisions; or to have access to the medical record. The danger is that differences in values between caregivers and patients may lead to over- or under-treatment. Communication, if necessary using a third party, may help resolve these issues.

A fourth futility category, qualitative futility, has been discussed, but is only applicable when based on the patient's values. A case of qualitative futility is that where medical interventions will not lead to an acceptable quality of life [52]. Recognizing that, the American College of Emergency Physicians assert, "Physicians are under no ethical obligation to render treatments that they judge have no realistic likelihood of medical benefit to the patient" [53].

The futility concept, however, should not be used to deny care to dying patients. Even terminal patients have medical emergencies that require intervention. The goal is to ease pain and suffering. How that is accomplished depends upon the patient, the medical condition causing discomfort, and the patient's value system.

Bioethics committees and consultants

In most large hospitals, multidisciplinary bioethics committees have been established to help resolve bioethical dilemmas. Meanwhile, many smaller hospitals now have bioethics consultants. Not only do committees and consultants review bioethical dilemmas, they also act to reconfirm prognoses and to mediate between dissenting parties. The four roles that bioethics committees should perform are (1) concurrent case reviews (consultations), (2) retrospective case reviews, (3) policy development, and (4) education [54]. Not all committees are capable of performing all of these tasks. Some, however, are able to provide "stat" consultations for emergency medicine practitioners.

Education

Trainees constitute a group vulnerable to abuses. The educational milieu creates the opportunity for tension and conflict, since trainees will not possess the knowledge, skills, or experience to function smoothly in the clinical arena. Due to the imbalance in power and authority between them and their instructors, trainees may be subject to exploitation, harassment (sexual and otherwise), and pressures to act unprofessionally [55–57]. The basic principle of respect for persons applies to trainees as well as to patients and research subjects.

One area in which ethical rules are too often overlooked is that involving advice to medical students on choosing a specialty and the subsequent residency application and interviewing processes. In emergency medicine, as in all other specialties, egos often overwhelm clinicians' duty to sensitively and honestly counsel medical students about their future careers. Residency programs in relatively undersubscribed specialties also bend rules to attract residents [58].

Trainees also have a basic ethical duty: to avoid dishonesty in their nonclinical education and when working with patients. The Society for Academic Emergency Medicine cites six ethical principles for educators to follow (see Box 2) and the American College of Emergency Physicians promotes ethical guidelines for education in its *Code of Ethics* [59]. The Council of Emergency Medicine Residency Directors specifically identifies the need for education to avoid potential "conflicts of interest that may arise from the promotion and marketing efforts of industry, primarily the pharmaceutical industry" [60].

Research

Basic bioethical research principles stem from the same sources as do clinical bioethics. The primary principle is respect for persons as individuals. While seemingly obvious, the principles have been reiterated numerous times over the past 50 years, beginning with the *Nuremberg Code* and finding clearer expression in the *Declaration of Helsinki* and its subsequent revisions [61,62]. In the research arena, good ethical conduct also means good science, since it is morally repugnant to subject patients to discomfort, not to mention risk, if the results of a study will be meaningless.

Many countries have established special review boards to oversee research protocols. However, some have called into question the performance of these review boards [62a]. Ethical constraints also surround the publication of research, with ethical guidelines now in place covering such topics as data falsification, redundant publications, requirements for patient informed consent, plagiarism, requirements for authorship, and unethical research [63]. The Society for Academic Emergency Medicine cites six ethical principles for researchers to follow (see Box 2) and the American College of Emergency Physicians promotes ethical guidelines in its *Code of Ethics* [59].

A well-recognized ethical problem for research related to emergency medicine and critical care has been the inability to get informed consent for many studies involving emergent interventions in patients with medical crises and diminished consciousness. A revised *Declaration of Helsinki* permits such research using surrogate decision-makers and increased institutional review board review [64]. In the United States, federal rules now permit waivers for informed consent in these situations if the institutional review board first does an intensive assessment, including community consultation meetings. This last requirement has proven troublesome, since it has not been well defined or previously used. Researchers have now developed models for successfully identifying, organizing, and using these groups [65–67].

Proactive bioethics

What are proactive ethics? How can emergency physicians change the rules?

In every medical system, practitioners find that they repeatedly face identical ethical dilemmas. The normal reaction is to gripe about it and often to get an incomplete and sometimes unsatisfactory solution from administrators, lawyers, bioethics committees, or others. There is a better solution. Proactive ethics involves changing the rules under which emergency personnel operate. Easier done in some settings than in others, the process requires that all stakeholders, those with a vested interest in an equitable solution, first to come to the table and reach a compromise. Such groups will often include physicians, nurses, emergency medical personnel, lawyers, religious authorities, and representatives of affected groups (eg, an organization of elder individuals in the case of issues about the aged).

Proactive ethics falls in the realm of public policy, an area in which emergency physicians are particularly well suited to play roles. One example of a process stemming from proactive ethics led to a landmark prehospital advance directive law, which markedly reduced the number of unwanted resuscitation attempts in the emergency medical service [38]. It also led to an extensive statutory surrogate list and a simplified set of advance directives.

Summary

Ethics is the application of values and moral rules to human activities. Bioethics, a subset of ethics, provides reasoned and defensible guidelines that incorporate ethical principles for actual or anticipated moral dilemmas facing clinicians in medicine and biology. Bioethics differs from both law and religion, although it incorporates some elements of both disciplines.

Multiple ethical theories guide philosophers and bioethicists, although altruism overlies all philosophies. With altruism as a guide, emergency clinicians must assess each patient's values and, whenever possible, make decisions based on them. Clinicians must also take their personal, professional, and institutional values into consideration in the decision-making process. Professional oaths and codes may help clinicians clarify their own values.

Patients with the capacity to do so may make their own health care decisions. Assessing decision-making capacity and knowing how to use surrogate decision-makers are key skills for emergency clinicians. As with other scenarios in emergency medicine, common ethical dilemmas should be studied and discussed in advance so morally appropriate actions can be taken when they occur in the clinical setting. The Rapid Decision-Making Model helps guide clinicians to take actions within the scope of moral acceptability, even if they have not worked out decision rules in advance. Bioethics committees, rarely used by emergency clinicians, can often help, concurrently or retrospectively, in improving the decision-making process.

The most important and effective action to take in resolving recurrent bioethical dilemmas is to address them proactively, working to change the emergency medical system, the medical system, or the law. It is always a tragedy when clinicians know what should be done, but are prevented from doing the right thing due to systematic constraints.

References

[1] Iserson KV. Bioethics. In: Marx JA, Hockberger RS, Walls RM, et al, editors. Rosen's Emergency Medicine: Concepts and Clinical Practice. 5th edition. St. Louis (MO): C.V. Mosby; 2002. p. 2725–33.

[2] Feinberg J. Social philosophy. Englewood Cliffs (NJ): Prentice-Hall; 1973.

[3] Black HC. Black's law dictionary. 5th edition. St. Paul (MN): West Publishing; 1979.

[4] Hart HLA. Punishment and responsibility. Oxford (United Kingdom): Oxford University Press; 1976.

[5] Ladd J. Legalism and medical ethics. J Med Ethics 1979;4(1):70.

[6] McCormick RA. Theology and bioethics. Hastings Cent Rep 1989;19(2):5.

[7] Buckle S. Natural law. In: Singer P, editor. A companion to ethics. Oxford (United Kingdom): Basil Blackwell; 1991. p. 161–74.

[8] Davis NA. Contemporary deontology. In: Singer P, editor. A companion to ethics. Oxford (United Kingdom): Basil Blackwell; 1991. p. 205–18.

[9] Goodin RE. Utility and the good. In: Singer P, editor. A companion to ethics. Oxford (United Kingdom): Basil Blackwell; 1991. p. 241–8.

[10] The Society for Academic Emergency Medicine. Code of honor—an oath for academic emergency medicine. Lansing (MI): Society for Academic Emergency Medicine; 1998.

[11] Graber GC. Basic theories in medical ethics. In: Monagle JF, Thomasma DC, editors. Medical ethics. Rockville (MD), Aspen Publishing; 1997.

[12] Beauchamp TL, Childress JF. Principles of Biomedical Ethics. 3rd edition. New York: Oxford University Press; 1989. 6–9.

[13] Foot P. Moral relativism. In: Krausz M, Meiland JW, editors. Relativism—cognitive and moral. Notre Dame (IN): University of Notre Dame Press; 1982. p. 152–66.

[14] Iserson KV. Resident "capping": rationale, ethics and effects. Submitted for publication.

[15] Faúndes A, Brache V, Alvarez E. Emergency contraception—clinical and ethical aspects. Int J Gynecology and Obstetrics 2003;82:297–305.

[16] Cook RJ, Dickens BM. Access to emergency contraception. J Obstet Gynaecol Can 2003; 25(11):914–6.

[17] Iserson KV, Chiasson PM. The ethics of applying new medical technologies. Seminars in Laparoscopy 2002;9(4):222–9.

[18] Schloendorff v Society of New York Hospital, 105 NE 92 93 (1914).

[19] Drane JF. Competency to give an informed consent. JAMA 1984;252(7):925.

[20] Buchanan AE. The question of competence. In: Iserson KV, Sanders AB, Mathieu D, editors. Ethics in Emergency Medicine. 2nd edition. Tucson (AZ): Galen Press; 1995. p. 61–5.

[21] Geiderman JM. Ethics seminars: consent and refusal in an urban American emergency departments: two case studies. Acad Emerg Med 2001;8:278–81.

[22] Naess A-C, Foerde R, Steen PA. Patient autonomy in emergency medicine. Med Health Care Philos 2001;4:71–7.

[23] Bridges J, Hanson R, Little M, et al. Ethical relationships in paediatric emergency medicine: moving beyond the dyad. Paediatric Emergency Medicine 2001;13:344–50.

[24] Moskop J, Iserson KV. Emergency physicians and physician-assisted suicide, part I: a review of the physician-assisted suicide debate. Ann Emerg Med 2001;38(5):570–5.

[25] Moskop J, Iserson KV. Emergency physicians and physician-assisted suicide, part II: emergency care for patients who have attempted physician-assisted suicide. Ann Emerg Med 2001;38(5):576–82.

[26] Dachs R. Curbside consultation. Responding to an in-flight emergency. Am Fam Physician 2003;68(5):975–6.

[27] Iserson KV. Ethics of wilderness medicine. In: Auerbach P, editor. Wilderness medicine: management of wilderness and environmental emergencies. 3rd edition. St. Louis (MO): C.V. Mosby; 1995. p. 1436–46.

[28] Drug-seeker lists are dangerous at best, require tight administrative controls. ED Manag 2004;16(3):25–8.

[29] Iserson KV. Film: exposing the ER. Ann Emerg Med 2001;37(2):220–1.

[30] Marco CA, Larkin GL. Filming of patients in academic emergency departments. Society for Academic Emergency Medicine position statement. Available at: http://www.saem.org/newsltr/2001/may.june/filmingp.htm. Accessed June 17, 2004.

[31] Iserson KV. Telemedicine: a proposal for an ethical code. Camb Q Health Ethics 2000;9(3): 404–6.

[32] Novack DH, Detering BJ, Arnold R, et al. Physicians' attitudes toward using deception to resolve difficult ethical problems. JAMA 1989;261:2980.

[33] Landesman BM. Physician attitudes toward patients. In: Iserson KV, Sanders AB, Mathieu D, editors. Ethics in Emergency Medicine. 2nd edition. Tucson (AZ): Galen Press; 1995. p. 350–7.

[34] Iserson KV, Moskop J. The ethics of triage: distributive justice in clinical medicine. In process.

[35] Pesik N, Keim ME, Iserson KV. Terrorism and the ethics of emergency medical care. Ann Emerg Med 2001;37(6):642–6.

[36] Iserson KV, Pesik N. Ethical resource distribution after biological, chemical or radiological terrorism. Camb Q Health Ethics 2003;12:455–65.

[37] Marco CA, Schears RM. Prehospital resuscitation practices: a survey of prehospital providers. J Emerg Med 2003;24(1):87–9.

[38] Iserson KV. A simplified prehospital advance directive law: Arizona's approach. Ann Emerg Med 1993;22(11):1703–10.

[39] Schears RM, Marco CA, Iserson KV. "Do not attempt resuscitation" (DNAR) in the out-of-hospital setting. Ann Emerg Med 2004;44(1):68–70.

[40] Arizona Revised Statutes. Title 36, Chapter 32: living wills and health care directives.

[41] Ethical statements—overview. In: Iserson KV, Sanders AB, Mathieu D, editors. Ethics in Emergency Medicine. 2nd edition. Tucson (AZ): Galen Press; 1995. p. 429–32.

[42] Croskerry P. The cognitive imperative: thinking about how we think. Acad Emerg Med 2000;7(11):1223–31.

[43] Gauthier DP. Morals by agreement. Oxford (United Kingdom): Clarendon Press; 1986.

[44] Sanders AB. Unique aspects of ethics in emergency medicine. In: Iserson KV, Sanders AB, Mathieu D, editors. Ethics in emergency medicine. 2nd edition. Tucson (AZ): Galen Press; 1995.

[45] Iserson KV. Withholding and withdrawing medical treatment: an emergency medicine perspective. Ann Emerg Med 1996;28(1):51.

[46] Barilan YM. Revisiting the problem of Jewish bioethics: the case of terminal care. Kennedy Inst Ethics J 2003;13(2):141.

[47] Israeli Ministry of Health. Available at: http://www.health.gov.il/pages/steinberg.htm [in Hebrew]. Accessed. June 15, 2006.

[48] Caplan AI. Odds and ends: trust and the debate over medical futility. Ann Intern Med 1996; 125:688–9.

[49] Marco CA, Larkin GL, Moskop JC, et al. Determination of "futility" in emergency medicine. Annals of Emergency Medicine 2000;35(6):604–12.

[50] Jecker NS, Schneiderman LJ. Futility and rationing. Am J Med 1992;92(2):189.

[51] Awoke S, Mouton CP, Parrott M. Outcomes of skilled cardiopulmonary resuscitation in long-term facility: futile therapy? J Am Geriatr Soc 1992;40:593.

[52] Brody BA, Halevy A. Is futility a futile concept? J Med Philos 1995;163:287.

[53] American College of Emergency Physicians. Nonbeneficial ("futile") emergency medical interventions [policy statement]. Dallas (TX): American College of Emergency Physicians; approved 1998, reaffirmed 2002.

[54] Iserson KV, Goffin F, Markham JJ. The future functions of ethics committees. Hospital Ethics Committee Forum 1989;1(2):63–76.

[55] Schmidt TA. Faculty-student relationships. In: Iserson KV, Sanders AB, Mathieu D, editors. Ethics in Emergency Medicine. 2nd edition. Tucson (AZ): Galen Press; 1995. p. 114–9.

[56] Baldwin DC Jr, Daugherty SR. Do residents also feel "abused"? Perceived mistreatment during internship. Acad Med 1997;72(10 Suppl. 1):S51–3.

[57] Baldwin DC Jr, Daugherty SR, Rowley BD. Residents' and medical students' reports of sexual harassment and discrimination. Acad Med 1996;71(10 Suppl):S25–7.

[58] Iserson KV. Bioethics and graduate medical education: the great match. Camb Q Health Ethics 2003;12(1):61–5.

[59] American College of Emergency Physicians. Code of ethics for emergency physicians. Dallas (TX): American College of Emergency Physicians; 1997.

[60] Keim S, Perina DG. Council of emergency medicine residency directors' position on interactions between emergency medicine residencies and the pharmaceutical industry. Acad Emerg Med 2004;11(1):78.

[61] Iserson KV, Sanders AB, Mathieu D, editors. Ethics in Emergency Medicine. 2nd edition. Tucson (AZ): Galen Press; 1995. p. 463.

[62] Recommendations guiding medical doctors in biomedical research involving human subjects adopted by the 18th World Medical Assembly, Helsinki, Finland, 1964, and revised periodically. Handbook of WMA Declarations. (Switzerland): World Medical Association. Available at: http://www.wma.net/e/policy/b3.htm. Accessed June 15, 2006.

[62a] Emanuel EJ, Wood A, Fleischman A, et al. Oversight of human participants research: identifying problems to evaluate reform proposals. Ann Intern Med 2004;141(4):282–91.

[63] Bailar JC III, Angell M, Boots S, et al. Ethics and Policy in Scientific Publication. Bethesda (MD): Council of Biology; 1990.

[64] World Medical Association. Ethical principles for medical research involving human subjects. Eur J Emerg Med 2001;8:221–4.

[65] Dix ES, Esposito D, Spinosa F, et al. Implementation of community consultation for waiver of informed consent in emergency research: one institutional review board's experience. J Investigative Medicine 2004;52(2):113–6.

[66] Raju TNK. Waiver of informed consent for emergency research and community disclosures and consultations. J Investigative Medicine 2004;52(2):109–12.

[67] Biros MH. Research without consent: current status, 2003. Ann Emerg Med 2003;42:550–64.

EMERGENCY
MEDICINE
CLINICS OF
NORTH AMERICA

Emerg Med Clin N Am
24 (2006) 547–555

Ethics and the Law in Emergency Medicine

Arthur R. Derse, MD, JD[a,b]

[a]Center for the Study of Bioethics, Medical College of Wisconsin,
8701 Watertown Plank Road, Milwaukee, WI 53226-0509, USA
[b]Department of Emergency Medicine, Medical College of Wisconsin,
8701 Watertown Plank Road, Milwaukee, WI 53226-0509, USA

Case example

A man presents to the emergency department with chest pain, and an electrocardiogram shows evidence of cardiac ischemia. After medical treatment in the emergency department, the patient's pain is relieved, and his electrocardiogram no longer shows ischemic changes. His cardiac enzymes are elevated, however. The physician explains to the patient that he needs to be admitted to the hospital for more treatment and diagnostic evaluation. The patient refuses. The emergency department physician explains the risks of leaving without treatment, and the patient states that he understands the risks, but that he needs to be somewhere and it is important that he be there. He refuses to explain further. After a short evaluation of the patient's mental status and a review of the laboratory values, the emergency department physician decides that the patient is not incapacitated by drugs or alcohol. She knows that the patient has a legal right to refuse treatment. She has the patient sign a form stating that he is leaving against the emergency department physician's medical advice and tells the patient that he is always welcome to return. The next day the emergency department physician discusses the case with the emergency department chairperson. The emergency department chairperson tells her that she has covered her legal bases. The emergency department physician wonders, however, even if she has followed the law, whether she has done the right thing in allowing the patient to leave with known myocardial damage and an unknown cardiac status.

E-mail address: aderse@mcw.edu

doi:10.1016/j.emc.2006.05.004
emed.theclinics.com

Ethics and its relation to the law

Ethics is the branch of practical philosophy that answers the question, "What ought to be done, all things considered?" The relationship between law and ethics is a dynamic one in a pluralistic society. Ethical guidance for individuals may come from many sources, including personal character, religious belief, social expectations, and philosophical reflection. The law has been recognized as a blunt instrument for social regulation, and important goals of society may be reinforced with laws that are tailored to reach those goals. Ultimately, society must differentiate the actions it wishes to enforce with legal sanctions in the form of civil or criminal penalties from the actions that society, on the whole, thinks are matters that are personal choices that do not significantly harm others, or that society cannot or will not enforce. It is important that physicians be caring and compassionate toward their patients, and that they engender trust from patients. Patients should be interested in their own well-being and should act in partnership with physicians in making decisions about their health care. It is practically impossible to legislate such behavior on the part of physician or patient. Additionally, the law may not be the best means to help resolve difficult ethical dilemmas in patient care. The problem for ethical issues in medical practice is that the language of the law, with its emphasis on rights and individual autonomy, has been an inapt tool to describe and resolve some complex interactions and dilemmas in patient care [1]. In the case example described, the patient may have exercised his legal right, and the physician may have been legally protected by her actions, but the physician was left wondering whether she did the right thing (ie, whether the best ethical outcome was achieved).

When emergency physicians are confronted with difficult ethical dilemmas, they often turn to the law to answer the questions. Although knowing when and how the law applies to emergency medicine is important, the law is only one factor to consider among many factors [2]. The emergency department is not always an ideal place to reflect on difficult ethical issues [3]. Recognizing that ethical issues are likely to arise in emergency medical practice that may involve legal factors, the emergency physician should have a framework for ethical decision making that can be applied to the situation at hand. The emergency physician should consider the ethical issues first and then turn to the law for its contribution to guidance for action. Generally, the law is supportive of the same action that an analysis of ethical concerns would recommend. This is not always the case, however. In some cases in emergency medical practice, the ethics and the law may be at variance. The following sections describe the US legal system and give examples of ethical issues when the law and ethics may seem to conflict in emergency medical practice, along with analyses and recommendations.

United States Law

US law can be divided into three types: statutory, common, and administrative. Statutory law is the law that legislatures codify into statutes, or written law. One can open a state's statute books and find the law often spelled out in black and white (although often in complex legislative language). An example of statutory law is a state's law that requires the reporting of child abuse to authorities. Common law is the law that has developed over centuries that is not spelled out in statute books, but is interpreted by judges and applied to actual, litigated cases. An example is the law of medical malpractice. Typically, legislatures do not specify what constitutes medical malpractice. That is determined by juries applying the common law that requires finding in a specific set of facts a duty by a physician to a patient, a breach of that duty by the physician, causation of harm by the physician, and damages. The elements have been developed by judges through case law over many years and often vary to some degree by state. The third type of law is administrative law. Administrative law is law that has been enabled by legislation and issued by executive agencies in the form of regulations. An example of administrative law is the Drug Enforcement Administration regulations that control the prescription of narcotics and other scheduled drugs.

US law also can be divided into federal and state laws. The Drug Enforcement Administration regulations are examples of a federal law, and medical malpractice law and child abuse statutes are examples of state laws. Generally, federal law takes precedence over state laws. The bulk of laws applicable to emergency physicians are state laws. A patient's legal right to refuse medical treatment, as outlined in the case presentation, is regulated by state law. A significantly increasing number of federal laws also apply to emergency physicians in such areas as federal insurance payment programs (eg, Medicare and Medicaid). The federal privacy law, the Health Insurance Portability and Accountability Act (HIPAA), was passed in part because privacy advocates argued that state laws were inadequate in protecting patient privacy. The Emergency Medical Treatment and Active Labor Act (EMTALA), a federal law, requires that the patient in the case example be evaluated for an emergent condition by the emergency department and emergency physician [4].

**Emergency department physician–patient relationship
and Good Samaritan statutes**

Ethically one could argue that physicians should not be legally liable for their charitable care. The legal duty by an emergency department physician to a patient is easily formed, however, and, contrary to what many emergency department physicians hope, liability is not absolved by the fact that the physician is offering charitable care. Emergency physicians have

come to understand that charitable care comes with the same liability exposure as compensated care.

Although the emergency department physician–patient relationship is
easily formed, there are other situations where the emergency physician
can choose to form the relationship. If an off-duty emergency physician
comes to the scene of an accident or emergency, in all but two states in
the United States, he or she is not legally obligated to give medical assistance. Emergency physicians are ethically obligated to help, but that ethical
obligation in almost all states is not legally enforceable. Additionally, physicians who did help could be held liable for any negligence by acts or omissions in their provision of charitable care. This glaring conflict between the
lack of a legal duty to help and liability exposure if an emergency physician
did help led to the passage of laws known as Good Samaritan laws, which
gave physicians immunity for acts or omissions while rendering emergency
care in good faith at an accident or emergency when responding to the accident or emergency was not part of the physician's regular duties. Some
states also specify that the care must be rendered without compensation
to qualify for the immunity.

Federal law has delineated the emergency department physician–patient
relationship further. Numerous egregious examples of patients being refused
emergency treatment by emergency physicians in an emergency department
or being transferred inappropriately were one of the motivating factors for
the passage of EMTALA.

Refusal by patients of emergency medical treatment

In the case example at the beginning of this article, the patient refused
emergency medical evaluation and treatment of cardiac ischemia. Although
the patient might have a legal right to refuse treatment, it could be argued
that ethically the physician should be more than persuasive in convincing
the patient to stay for evaluation and treatment, perhaps even be insistent
and unwilling to accept the patient's refusal. Why should a patient be able
to refuse lifesaving medical treatment? That question would have made sense
to an American physician in the first half of the twentieth century and still
makes sense to many US physicians and physicians from many other cultures. In the United States, paternalism, the principle that the physician
knows what is best for the patient and can override the patient's wishes,
has been surpassed by the bioethical principle of autonomy, which respects
patient choices to refuse treatment. In the above-described case, strong moral
persuasion on the part of the physician is warranted, but in the final analysis,
the patient who has the capacity to make medical decisions is ethically and
legally able to refuse even life-sustaining medical treatment [5].

The patient's strong right to be free from unwanted treatment is balanced
by another reality: The physician does have the obligation to ensure the

patient has the ability to make medical decisions because patients who are incapacitated cannot make a decision to refuse medical treatment. Patients may be incapacitated by external factors, such as drugs or alcohol, or by psychiatric illness or dementia. Medical decision-making capacity consists of the ability of the patient to take in information about the medical decision, compare it against his or her internal values, make a choice consistent with those values, and communicate the choice to the physician [6]. If the patient has decision-making capacity, the patient has the right to refuse treatment.

A simple refusal by a patient needs to be followed by a conversation and examination to the extent possible ascertaining that the patient has the decision-making capacity to refuse medical treatment. Often it is pointed out ironically by ethicists that physicians typically are concerned with patient decision-making capacity when the patient refuses treatment [7], but physicians are rarely concerned about decision-making capacity when the patient agrees with the proposed therapy. This is true, but it is based on another reality: Physicians recommend treatments that are beneficial to the patient, so even if the patient is not able to make a decision, the patient presumably would benefit from the treatment. When patients refuse treatment, it may be to their detriment, so the need to confirm a patient's decision-making capacity is paramount.

Patients who refuse treatment have the ethical and legal right to be informed of the consequences of their refusal [8]. Patients also may waive this right, however. Legally, a signature on an "against medical advice" form may be helpful as a signification that the patient has understood the consequences of refusal and is assuming the risks associated with refusal. Informed refusal is similar to informed consent in that it is a process of communication. Having a witness to the discussion may be helpful as another marker that the discussion occurred and that the patient refused. Some patients may wish to leave without being informed of the risks of refusal. This is a difficult situation in which the law and ethics may conflict. Emergency physicians should ensure that the patient does have decision-making capacity to refuse before allowing the patient to leave. It may be argued that the danger of allowing patients with impaired decision-making capacity to leave and possibly harm themselves or others outweighs the added burden to the patient with decision-making capacity to allow the emergency physician to determine that the patient in fact does have decision-making capacity, before the patient leaves. Nonetheless, this situation is one where the emergency department physician may have to choose between the risks of being sued by those who have been harmed by a patient who left the emergency department while incapacitated (or by the patient or his or her survivors) versus the risks of being sued by a patient who was detained by the emergency physician until the patient's decision-making capacity could be assured. It is best to choose the course of action one can best defend ethically because either course may result in liability.

Limitation of treatment at the end of life

The legal right of a patient to refuse emergency medical treatment is one that is embodied in the US Constitution in the liberty interest of the 14th Amendment [9]. As noted, patients can refuse even life-sustaining medical treatment. This includes resuscitation, ventilation, and blood products [10]. Emergency physicians have tended to treat all emergent conditions, including those that are expected at the end of life, using the maxim, "always err on the side of life." Any discussion about discontinuing these treatments, they would argue, can occur in the ICU after the treatment is begun. The principle of autonomy also applies to patients facing life-threatening medical problems, however. The principle of autonomy has been recognized by courts to allow Jehovah's Witnesses without terminal conditions to refuse lifesaving transfusions [11]. This autonomy to refuse life-sustaining medical treatment should be respected especially for patients who have terminal illnesses. For patients who express that they do not want certain life-sustaining medical treatment (eg, through prehospital do-not-resuscitate orders or for patients without decision-making capacity, through other documentation including advance directives such as a living will or power of attorney for health care), these wishes should be respected. This should be done not only because of ethical respect for the patient's autonomy, but also because there are legal ramifications for not respecting the patient's wishes, including actions for battery, lack of consent, and medical malpractice [12].

Foregoing life-sustaining treatment does not mean emergency physicians should do nothing. Patients at the end of life may be treated with comfort measures and be admitted to the hospital for comfort care or to the hospice service if the hospital has one. Erring on the side of life is still a good maxim, but like all good maxims, it has some important exceptions.

Managing pain at the end of life

Emergency physicians have long been reluctant to treat patients with chronic pain, concerned that patients may become addicted to narcotics, and that emergency department physicians may be feeding an already established addiction. There is much truth to this, as some studies show a high number of so-called drug-seeking patients in the emergency department [13]. Opioid treatment for chronic pain patients aside, emergency physicians also have been reluctant to treat patients with cancer or other end-of-life conditions with narcotics with the rationale that the emergency department physician may cause addiction to narcotics in the patient, and that the emergency department physician may hasten the patient's death through the narcotic side effect of depressed respirations.

Patients who are facing the end of life should be thought of in a different category than other chronic pain patients. First, the addiction issue is moot in end-of-life care. Patients may need to be on long-term pain medication to ease the pain from the disease that is causing their eventual death, and the risks of addiction are far outweighed by the benefit of pain relief. Second, the intent of the physician in providing end-of-life patients opiates is to relieve pain. If the patient should die as a result of a known, rare but unintended risk of respiratory depression, the physician is not culpable under the philosophical principle of double effect. To be protected under the principle of double effect, the unintended but foreseen side effect (respiratory depression, which rarely causes death) must be proportional to the intended good effect (pain relief) [14].

Although these principles of pain treatment at the end of life have been long recognized in ethics at the end of life, regulatory agencies have taken some time to catch up. There has been a significant change in the understanding of medical examining boards, which recognize that patients in end-of-life care who have pain may need large doses of opioids for their appropriate treatment [15].

Futile treatment

Legally and ethically, emergency physicians are not required to provide treatment that would be ineffective. There is a controversy in the bioethical literature, however, as to whether and under what circumstances emergency department physicians should be required by patients or families to provide treatment that the patient or family demand, but the emergency department physician considers "futile." Futility has been notoriously difficult to define. It is important that quality-of-life decisions not be conflated with the determination of futility, which should be physiologically based. The determination of what kind of life is worth living is left to the patient with decision-making capacity, or to the surrogate (eg, guardian or agent of the power of attorney for health care), rather than to the physician.

Nonetheless, at some point in the dying process, further life-sustaining measures become ineffective. Although the determination of futility is a problem more often for physicians who treat hospitalized patients, patients may arrive in the emergency department for whom the emergency physician will determine that nothing more can be done—including resuscitation—other than comfort measures. So-called slow codes (providing less than timely therapy) and show codes (providing less than effective therapy for the benefit of the family) should not be done. Rather, the family should be informed that the patient would not benefit from life-sustaining measures, and comfort measures should be provided to the patient, recognizing that the process of dying includes the final common pathway of cardiopulmonary arrest.

Physician-assisted suicide and the emergency physician

The issue of physician-assisted suicide has split public and physician opinion [16]. It also has split the nation into 49 states that prohibit the measure through statutory or common law and one state, Oregon, that has legalized it. In all other states, patients may not be assisted in suicide under any circumstances. In most jurisdictions, patients who attempt suicide cannot refuse life-sustaining measures in the immediate interval when their life is in jeopardy and they are under emergency detention for the suicide attempt. Ethically, this can be justified under the best interest standard to treat patients when they are not capable of decision making because of suicidal ideation.

In Oregon, competent patients who are residents of the state and are determined to have 6 months or less to live are able to be prescribed a lethal dose of medication, which may be taken only voluntarily by the patient. Should such a previously competent patient arrive in an emergency department in Oregon with respiratory depression or cardiopulmonary arrest, physicians would not be required to resuscitate such a patient, but instead would provide comfort care [17]. As other states consider whether to follow Oregon's lead, emergency physicians need to be prepared to weigh the law and their consciences in deciding how to respond to failed, but legal assisted suicide attempts [18].

Summary

When confronted with difficult ethical dilemmas, emergency physicians often turn to the law to provide definitive answers to their questions. The law is only one factor to consider among others. The law may not be applicable or may be unclear. The emergency physician should consider the ethical issues first and then turn to the law for its contribution to guidance. In most situations, ethics and the law, if it applies, are concordant. In the examples in this article, the ethical considerations may seem to conflict with legal aspects of emergency medical treatment. In general, when facing ethical dilemmas in emergency medical practice, the emergency physician should take into account the ethical considerations before turning to the legal considerations. Ultimately, if the ethical choice and the law do conflict, the emergency physician must make the best decision under the circumstances and be prepared to defend the decision.

References

[1] Schneider CE. Bioethics in the language of the law. Hastings Cent Rep 1994;24:16–22.
[2] De Ville K. "What does the law say?" Law, ethics and medical decision making. West J Med 1994;160:478–80.
[3] Sanders AB. Unique aspects of ethics in emergency medicine. In: Iserson KV, Sanders AB, Mathieu D, editors. Ethics in emergency medicine. 2nd edition. Tucson: Galen Press; 1995. p. 7–10.
[4] Emergency Medical Treatment and Labor Act of 1986, 42 USC 1395 dd. Publication 99-272.
[5] Derse AR. Consent: explicit and presumed—patient refusal of emergency care: autonomy and informed consent: case commentary. In: Iserson KV, Sanders AB, Mathieu D, editors. Ethics in emergency medicine. 2nd edition. Tucson: Galen Press; 1995. p. 95–105.

[6] Junkerman C, Schiedermayer D. Competence and decision making capacity. In: Practical ethics for students, interns, and residents: a short reference manual. 2nd edition. Frederick (MD): University Publishing Group; 1998. p. 16–9.

[7] President's Commission for the Study of Ethical Problems in Medicine and Biomedical and Behavioral Research. Making health care decisions, vol. 1. Washington (DC): Government Printing Office; 1982. p. 62.

[8] Truman v. Thomas, 27 Cal. 3d 285, 611 P.2d 902, 165 Cal. Rptr 308 (1980).

[9] Cruzan v. Missouri Department of Health, 497 US 261, 111 L.Ed.2d 224, 110 S.Ct 2841 (1990).

[10] Meisel A. The legal consensus about forgoing life-sustaining treatment: its status and prospects. Kennedy Inst Ethics J 1993;2:309–45.

[11] Wons v. Public Health Trust of Dade County, 500 So.2d 679 (Fla.App. 3 Dist, 1987).

[12] Anderson v. St. Francis-St. George Hospital WL 582645 (Ohio, 1996).

[13] Geiderman JM. Keeping lists and naming names: habitual patient files for suspected non-therapeutic drug–seeking patients. Ann Emerg Med 2003;41:873–81.

[14] Sulmasy DP, Pellegrino ED. The rule of double effect: clearing up the double talk. Arch Intern Med 1999;159:545–50.

[15] Hoffman DE, Tarzian AJ. Achieving the right balance in oversight of physician prescribing for pain: the role of state medical boards. J Law Med Ethics 2003;31:21–40.

[16] Ore. Rev. Stat. §127.800–127.995 (1995).

[17] Schmidt TA, Zechnich AD, Tilden VP, et al. Oregon emergency physicians' experiences with, attitudes toward, and concerns about physician-assisted suicide. Acad Emerg Med 1996;3: 938–45.

[18] Moskop JC, Iserson KV. Emergency physicians and physician-assisted suicide: Part I and II. a review of the physician-assisted suicide debate. Ann Emerg Med 2001;38:570–82.

ELSEVIER
SAUNDERS

Emerg Med Clin N Am
24 (2006) 557–577

EMERGENCY
MEDICINE
CLINICS OF
NORTH AMERICA

EMTALA and the Ethical Delivery of Hospital Emergency Services

Robert A. Bitterman, MD, JD[a,b]

[a]Bitterman Health Law & Consulting Group, Inc., 4500 Swing Lane,
Charlotte, NC 26226-3422, USA
[b]Emergency Physicians Insurance Company, Inc., 11760 Atwood Road,
Suite 5, Auburn, CA 95603, USA

"Medicine is, at its center, a moral enterprise grounded in a covenant of trust [1]."

The Emergency Medical Treatment and Active Labor Act (EMTALA) is the federal law that governs virtually all facets of hospital-based emergency medical care in the United States [2]. This article considers the ethical issues related to the government's application of EMTALA and the practice behavior of physicians and hospitals in response to the mandates of the law through three of EMTALA's primary elements: medical screening and stabilization of patients presenting to the emergency department, accepting patient transfers from other hospitals, and providing on-call physician services to the emergency department.

It is commonly perceived that EMTALA exists because of egregious "unethical" behavior of health care providers [3–5]. Hospitals and physicians were denying indigent patients access to examination or treatment at hospital emergency departments or transferring patients, "dumping" them, from private hospitals to public institutions for purely economic reasons, even though the transferring physicians and hospitals were capable of providing the necessary care these individuals needed. Whether one judges such conduct to be unethical depends, however, on exactly how one defines acceptable *ethical* behavior by hospitals and physicians. Raising the specter that someone's conduct is unethical conjures up such pejorative connotations about one's character that it is essential to establish an unambiguous meaning to the portrayal.

E-mail address: robertbitterman@earthlink.net

0733-8627/06/$ - see front matter © 2006 Elsevier Inc. All rights reserved.
doi:10.1016/j.emc.2006.05.003   *emed.theclinics.com*

Classic ethics

The classic dictionary definition of *ethical,* which is virtually the same in *Webster's, Stedman's Medical,* or *Black's Law* dictionaries, is "conforming to accepted professional standards of conduct." This definition begs the two questions: (1) What are the existing professional standards? (2) Are those standards truly acceptable to patients, society, or even the medical profession itself?

During the heyday of managed care in the late 1990s, it was common practice for insurance companies to require "prior authorization" for payment before a hospital could examine or treat one of its enrollees in the emergency department. Prior authorization procedures were unarguably illegal under EMTALA and clearly jeopardized the health and safety of patients, but, at least temporarily, hospitals and physicians were complicit in allowing the managed care entities to implement such predatory practices. It became an "accepted professional standard," but one that was hardly prudent for patients [6].

The medical profession eventually rejected prior authorization procedures, using the law (EMTALA) to dismantle it, but principally because it was believed to be unethical [7,8]. It was believed that all individuals presenting to the emergency department should be examined to determine if they had an emergency medical condition and, if so, provided emergency medical treatment, regardless of their insurance status.

Physicians in the United States, from the beginning of colonial American society, have always felt obligated—morally, ethically, or otherwise—to provide care to those in "distress," or in "time of necessity," regardless of a patient's ability to pay [9]. The American Medical Association (AMA) Code of Medical Ethics states: "A physician shall, in the provision of appropriate patient care, except in emergencies, be free to choose whom to serve, with whom to associate, in the environment in which to provide medical services" [10]. The American College of Emergency Medicine (ACEP) and all medical specialties in the United States agree with the AMA that physicians have an ethical duty to treat any patient in an emergency, but that they are free to choose whom to serve in nonemergency situations [11].

This definition of ethical behavior can be labeled "classic ethics." It should not be called *medical* or *professional* ethics because, as is discussed subsequently, although it may conform to the standards of most in the medical profession, it may not be a high enough standard for physicians or a standard acceptable to Americans.

The failure of physicians and hospitals to live up to their classic ethical duties prompted Congress to impose EMTALA in the mid-1980s [12,13]. Americans would not tolerate individuals in the throes of an emergency denied access to emergency departments because they could not pay, or mothers delivering babies at the roadside because private hospitals refused to act responsibly and instead elected to transfer them to public hospitals for financial reasons. It took an act of Congress to determine that refusal to provide examination and treatment of individuals presenting to emergency departments was simply unconscionable. Hospitals and physicians had succumbed to the economic strain on their medical practice and forgotten that their primary role, particularly as physicians, is to be patient advocates [14].

Congress understood why indigent patients were turned away: the substantial growth in the provision of uncompensated care by hospitals and physicians. House Rep. Pete Stark of California, one of the leading proponents of EMTALA, said: "Patient dumping is but a symptom of a much larger problem. Thirty-seven million Americans are without health insurance. Low income sick people are finding it increasingly difficult to get needed health care, and the burden of caring for them is falling on fewer and fewer hospitals" [15]. Presently, the number uninsured is about 47 million [16].

Nevertheless, Congress used its financing power through the Medicare program to force hospitals and physicians to examine all patients presenting to a Medicare-participating hospital and to stabilize patients with emergency medical conditions. EMTALA represented the first time Congress used the Medicare statute to define a standard of care for hospital emergency services and to regulate directly the delivery of health care to non-Medicare patients [17]. Substantively, EMTALA created a federal right to emergency care.

However, health care is not a fundamental *right* in the United States, and it never can be, for one quintessential reason: No person has the right to take the services or resources of another without their consent—a physician's services are his or hers alone to provide voluntarily. It should be self-evident that all people are endowed with certain unalienable rights, including liberty and the freedom from indentured servitude (paraphrasing the Declaration of Independence of the Second Continental Congress, July 4, 1776, and the prohibition of slavery by the Thirteenth Amendment to the Constitution of the United States.)

Health care *is* a fundamental *need*. Health is essential for a productive workforce, stable family structure, and basic human happiness. Society should endeavor in all ways possible to provide health care services to all denizens* in need regardless of economic status.

The countervailing arguments regarding health care as a right are epitomized in the following two passages:

---

* The word *denizens*, as opposed to citizens, is used intentionally. All hospitals and physicians, but particularly emergency physicians, routinely provide substantial amounts of care to illegal aliens or other noncitizens in the United States. Whether one adheres to traditional "classic ethics" or "fiduciary ethics," as described later, emergency health care should be provided to citizen and noncitizen alike in US emergency departments (analogous to physicians in time of war—witness presently Afghanistan and Iraq—treating all injured individuals based solely on their need for immediate medical attention, regardless of their status as US soldier, enemy combatant, or civilian casualty.)

The concept of medical care as the patient's right is immoral because it denies the most fundamental of all rights; that of a man to his own life and the freedom of action to support it. Medical care is neither a right nor a privilege: it is a service that is provided by doctors and others to people who wish to purchase it. If the right to health care belongs to the patient, he starts owning the services of a doctor without the necessity of either earning them or receiving them as a gift from the only man who has the right to give them: the doctor himself.—Robert M. Sade, MD [18].

Physicians who limit their practice to insured and paying patients declare themselves openly to be merchants rather than professionals. This demeans the individual physician and cheapens the profession. ... It also fosters the myth that physicians as a group are greedy and self serving rather than dedicated and altruistic. Most important, it deprives a large segment of our fellow humans of care. Physicians who value their professionalism should treat patients on the basis of need, not remuneration. Physicians who do not, deserve the contempt and censure of their colleagues.—Peter H. Elias MD [19,20].

The advent of EMTALA did not lead to universal access to emergency care or universal classic ethical behavior. Sensational publicity and horror stories about denial of emergency care continued to capture attention in the United States. President Clinton went on national television to decry the morals and behavior of Ravenswood Hospital in Chicago after its staff refused to leave the hospital's emergency department to help a young boy who had been shot and fatally wounded in the alley next door. NBC's "Dateline" ran an exposé condemning the failure of a half-dozen tertiary hospitals in Oklahoma City to accept a critically injured patient in transfer from a community facility. *USA Today, Time* magazine, and the *Los Angeles Times* ran articles describing the unresponsiveness of on-call physician specialists and the problems hospitals are experiencing in delivering emergency services. Previously, US society condemned such behavior as immoral, shameful, and unacceptable, but largely without consequence. Now it is a violation of a federal right, EMTALA, and the consequences are severe [6].

Regulatory ethics

The economics of uncompensated care coupled with the EMTALA mandate (and exacerbated by malpractice liability) has led to a new definition of ethical behavior related to emergency care, a minimalist or "legalistic" ethos. Under this ethical standard, hospitals and physicians accept or treat emergency patients only if and only to the extent that the law requires them to do so. Clinical examples best elucidate what are escalating trends:

- A hospital screens all patients who present to its emergency department, but whenever it determines the patient does not have an emergency medical condition, the hospital refuses to provide further care to the patient until the patient pays for the services. "No Emergency? Go Elsewhere" was the headline of an article describing this practice. Some of these hospitals arrange for the patient to receive care "elsewhere"; others tell the patient to leave [21].

- A group of orthopedic surgeons is required to take emergency department call by hospital rules or medical staff by-laws; however, the orthopedists refuse to come into the emergency department or accept any patient in follow-up who does not need immediate stabilizing care, as defined by law, EMTALA. These physicians refuse to accept patients with complex trimalleolar ankle fractures, as long as there is no acute neurovascular compromise or compartment syndrome present. The patient needs surgery to fix the fracture, but it is legally "stable" in a splint, so the orthopedic surgeons refuse to care for the patient unless payment is assured [22].
- Tertiary medical centers accept in transfer only the patients it must accept by law. All other transfers of indigent patients are refused. Some referral hospitals contend that they do not have to accept inpatients with emergency conditions that the transferring hospital lacks the capability to manage because EMTALA now ends when the patient is admitted [23]. The higher level medical centers have the capability and the capacity to treat the patient's emergency condition, but they refuse to do so when the patient is uninsured.

This mercantile or business approach to providing emergency care, in line with the previous comments of Elias [19], threatens to erode the moral-based behavior of classic ethics and replace it with one of "rule following, and behaviors determined only by the law" [24].

Sir William Osler cautioned against such an approach, stating: "The Practice of Medicine is an Art, not a Trade; a Calling, not a Business; a Calling in which your Heart will be Exorcised equally with your Head" [25].

There have always been, and will always be, economic, political, and personal obstacles that collide with the medical profession's ethical duties to patients in need. Physicians should expose, condemn, eliminate, or at least minimize any influences in conflict with their ethical duties. The practice of medicine is a special kind of human endeavor, one dedicated to the care of others rather than self-interest. The physician's role in society always must be one of patient advocate, always acting in a patient's best interest regardless of the external forces at play.

To draw from the language of law, the substance of patient advocacy is to act as a *fiduciary*. A fiduciary has a "duty to act for someone else's benefit, while subordinating one's personal interests to that of the other person" [26]. The term is derived from Roman law and means a person holding the character of a trustee or guardian.

A fiduciary relationship between the patient and physician is based on the expectations that physicians at all times will put the needs of the patient first, over and above the interests of the physician or any third party (eg, the hospital, on-call physicians, inpatient nursing unit, insurance company). It is a relationship founded on a covenant of trust, the highest standard of duty implied by law, and should be the standard of ethics adopted by a profession whose patients entrust their lives. It dates back to Hippocrates and Asklepios (1500 B.C. to 500 B.C.), and only by continually advocating for patients can physicians sustain the integrity of the profession despite modern-day pressures [27].

As noted by a past president of the AMA, "The covenant [of trust] constitutes the last line of defense between our patients and shoddy care delivered by a profession subverted by economic incentives to deliver such care" [28].

The physician needs to decide which definition of ethical standards he or she wishes to espouse—classic ethics, legal ethics, or fiduciary ethics—and apply that standard to the scenarios discussed subsequently or to difficult encounters in daily practice. Only then can it be determined if the actions of the government, hospital boards or administrators, and physicians are ethically acceptable.

1. Medical screening and stabilization of patients presenting to the emergency department

The medical screening examination and stabilization mandates of EMTALA require all Medicare-participating hospitals with an emergency department to evaluate all individuals who come to the emergency department to determine if an emergency medical condition is present. If the hospital determines that an emergency medical condition exists, it must stabilize the patient or transfer the patient to a hospital that can stabilize the patient.

This section of the law is essentially a nondiscrimination statute. EMTALA was Congress' solution to the problem of the discriminatory denial of access to emergency health care for the indigent, the uninsured, and illegal aliens. When it enacted EMTALA, Congress realized the enormous financial burden it was imposing on hospitals. Sen. David Durenberger of Minnesota, speaking on EMTALA, said: "Access should be the government's responsibility at the federal, state, and local levels. We cannot and should not expect hospitals to be this nation's National Health Service" [29]. But by enacting EMTALA, that is precisely what Congress did. Rather than address the real issue of uncompensated care, Congress simply decreed universal access for all and forced health care providers to assume fiscal responsibility for taking care of the poor under threat of $50,000 fines, new civil liability, or loss of provider participation in the Medicare and Medicaid programs [30].

There is no right to health care under the Constitution of the United States, and Congress understood that the 13th Amendment prohibited it from forcing hospitals and physicians to provide medical services to the poor [31]. Instead, it economically coerced hospitals to comply with its edict through the Medicare program [2]. Hospitals actually "voluntarily" agree to comply with EMTALA, by accepting participation in Medicare. The government said, in essence, "Hospitals, if you want our money, you play by our rules." EMTALA is one of its rules.

But what has EMTALA wrought? Since EMTALA was enacted, emergency department use has surged from 85 million visits per year to almost 115 million visits per year, whereas more than 560 hospitals and 1200 emergency departments closed, as did many trauma centers, maternity wards, and tertiary referral centers [16,32–36]. Of the remaining trauma centers, 90% are currently overwhelmed. Ninety percent of larger hospitals have saturated their capacity for treating patients, primarily because of the lack of money to support inpatient critical care beds and the nurses to staff them. Emergency medical services diversion is rampant, most emergency departments are overcrowded, waiting times have increased 33%, and the number of individuals seeking emergency care who leave the emergency department before being seen has tripled in some areas of the United States [32–36]. The total uninsured population has increased from 13% to almost 18% (37 million to 47 million individuals) and is expected to reach 20% to 22% of all individuals in the United States by the end 2010 [16,33,37]. Liability costs are soaring, and malpractice insurance may not even be available in some states, such as Pennsylvania, North Carolina, or Florida.

EMTALA is nothing but a giant unfunded government mandate,*and its uncompensated care burden decimates hospitals in domino fashion, toppling hospitals in poor payer-mix areas first, inner cities and rural areas, then spreading to the surrounding communities. Besides closing down entirely, closing units within the hospital, diverting ambulances, or making patients wait excessively long for emergency care, hospitals and physicians have taken other steps to avoid EMTALA's economic burden.

---

* In fairness to the US government, this statement is not entirely true. The Balanced Budget Act of 1997 provided about $25 million/year for emergency care mandated by EMTALA, and the Medicare Modernization Act of 2003 provides $1 billion over 4 years to help offset the EMTALA costs of treating undocumented aliens [38,39]. Additionally, the practice expense portion of Medicare payments to emergency physicians includes a small allotment for uncompensated care. There are also a few other ways the government provides funding for indigent care, but the overall dollars committed are grossly inadequate to cover the estimated $26 billion per year in EMTALA-related uncompensated care provided by hospitals and physicians [40,41]. Emergency physicians provide an estimated $138,000 per year per *each* physician in uncompensated EMTALA-mandated services—about $3 billion for our the specialty of emergency medicine alone [42].

Providing walk-in care through urgent care centers is one way to avoid EMTALA. If physicians own and operate the urgent care center, EM-TALA does not apply, because the urgent care center does not meet EM-TALA's definition of a hospital department [2]. Hospitals also legally can structure these entities to avoid EMTALA's reach and limit their EM-TALA exposure to the uninsured only at their main facility's overcrowded emergency department (where the less urgent, and more frequently unin-sured, patients must overcome long waits to be seen) [2,23]. Many large health care systems across the United States already have taken this step to protect the financial health of their outpatient centers and overall mission.

Another way hospitals circumvent EMTALA's unfunded mandate is to, in essence, adopt "legalistic ethics" and provide only the least amount of care required by the law to patients presenting to its emergency department. "Screen and street" or "No Emergency? Go Elsewhere!" becomes their op-erating credo [21,43,44].

In these emergency departments, all patients are triaged, and the lower acuity patients are screened by physicians or physician assistants to deter-mine if an emergency medical condition is present. If not, the patient is asked to pay for the care before it is provided or to leave the hospital. Some of these hospitals arrange to provide the care the patients need at their clinics, public health facilities, or through other predetermined avenues. Some hospitals just instruct the patients to find services elsewhere on their own or provide a "resource book" and let the patients search themselves for an alternative source of care. Sometimes the hospital is reticent even to assist the patient in finding care elsewhere for fear of liability; they want the decision to stay or leave to be the patient's and do not be viewed as having coerced the patient to leave and subsequently sued if adverse con-sequences result [21,43,44].

Some examples where an emergency department refused to provide med-ical care unless the patient paid money in advance include the following:

- A 3-year-old girl with a 2-hour-old 1 cm facial laceration
- A 24-year-old with a tender wrist after falling down on the sidewalk
- A 4-year-old boy with a bug in the ear
- A 35-year-old with a small abscess to the thigh from an insect bite
- A 42-year-old with a toothache
- A 19-year-old man with a sticky yellow urethral discharge

Is it an ethical practice for emergency physicians to turn away these types of patients for financial reasons, when one has not made alternative arrange-ments for the patient's care, and one (usually) knows that they would not be able to obtain the services elsewhere on a timely basis?

Simply referring patients away from the emergency department, without making alternative arrangements for the patients to receive care, may be a vi-olation of the ACEP Code of Ethics for Emergency Physicians, which states:

"Emergency physicians have an ethical duty to act as advocates for the health needs of indigent patients and to assist them in finding appropriate care," and "[e]mergency physicians shall embrace patient welfare as their primary professional responsibility" [45].

If emergency departments arrange alternative avenues for these patients to receive the medical attention they need on a reasonably timely basis, that is an acceptable ethical practice. There are many other just as appropriate and perhaps more appropriate locations and service models to provide episodic urgent or semiemergent care. It does not matter *where* the care is provided, just that it *is* provided.

The "screen and street" hospital's real goal is discourage future use of its emergency department by the uninsured in its community. If other hospitals in their community are screening away patients, they feel compelled to do the same, lest they be the remaining magnet for the uninsured. In Houston, Texas, most of the hospitals now screen away emergency department patients in some fashion [46].

Hospitals particularly want to avoid the financially devastating admissions of extremely ill indigents or illegal aliens, which literally can determine if the hospital ends the year in the black or the red [47]. Patients are less likely to come to a hospital's emergency department if they know there is a financial price tag attached to each visit. Such programs can save a hospital $1 million/y by decreasing its uncompensated-care costs 20% [21,43,44]. Some hospitals pressure its contract emergency physician group to participate, subtly suggesting loss of the group's contract if the physicians do not begin screening patients away, sometimes putting the physicians' ethical beliefs in conflict with their economic interests.

The denial of health care services and limitation of resources is a societal decision that should be determined in the political arena, not at the bedside. The specialty of emergency medicine and its reputation were built on the premise that emergency physicians are always there, 24/7/365, to care for anyone and everyone needing medical attention [48]. Emergency physicians and hospital partners are truly society's health care safety net; shouldn't these physicians, as the last line of protection for the disadvantaged and the disenfranchised, manifest a higher degree of ethics? When patients are sick and vulnerable, they expect their physicians to be their advocate, their trusted guardian, their fiduciary: Physicians should figure out ways to provide care to these individuals, not be the ones turning them away.

2. Accepting patient transfers from other hospitals

EMTALA requires hospitals with specialized capabilities or facilities to accept appropriate transfers from other hospitals, if they have the capacity to treat the individual. Consider two representative scenarios:

- A 62-year-old man presents to the emergency department with an ischemic stroke and is admitted and started on warfarin by the hospital's on-call neurologist. The patient subsequently falls, hits his head, and develops an expanding subdural hematoma. The hospital lacks a neurosurgeon on staff, so the neurologist calls the nearby university hospital and asks it accept the patient in transfer to see a neurosurgeon. The university hospital contends, under the Centers for Medicare and Medicaid (CMS) new regulations, that EMTALA ends when a patient is admitted, and it does not have a legal duty to accept the patient. It refuses the transfer if the patient is medically indigent, but accepts if he covered by insurance.
- Emergency medical services and the police bring a 25-year-old woman to a small community hospital emergency department after she tried to kill herself with an acetaminophen and benzodiazepine overdose. The emergency physician appropriately manages her overdose and "stabilizes" her emergency psychiatric condition, her suicidality, by arranging for a sitter or restraining her as necessary to prevent her from harming herself again. The hospital has no inpatient psychiatric services and no psychiatrist on-call, so the emergency physician seeks to transfer the patient to a private hospital that has the capability and capacity to manage the patient's suicidal ideation. The private hospital claims it does not have to accept the patient under EMTALA because the patient is "stable"; it refuses the transfer after learning the patient is uninsured.

In each scenario, the hospital is adopting a legalistic approach to avoid caring for indigent patients, regardless of the potential serious adverse medical consequences to the patients. It is analogous to former Vice-President Al Gore's statement when the propriety of his campaign fundraising was questioned: "There is no controlling legal authority," which seemed to be the guiding principle by which he judged his behavior rather than an ethical covenant of trust between himself and the people he was supposed to represent [49].

In each instance, the hospital and physicians could treat a patient in need of real emergency care yet refused. Were they acting in the best interest of the patient, as the patient's guardian, or were they putting their own interest ahead of that of the patients? Classic ethics, fiduciary ethics, or just basic compassion for a fellow human being obliges providers to act otherwise.

This behavior, called *reverse dumping,* is what prompted Congress to add the transfer acceptance mandate to EMTALA (also called its nondiscrimination clause) [6,12,13]. It was not part of the original law, but when Congress learned that larger referral hospitals were refusing to take transfers of patients with emergency conditions from other hospital emergency departments, it amended the law [6,12,13]. It is inconceivable that CMS regulators or legislators would allow hospitals to revert to reverse dumping based on the distinction between a patient admitted and a patient still considered an "emergency department patient."

The legalistic ethical approach adopted by these hospitals is most likely legally mistaken. A recipient hospital's duty to accept patients in transfer under EMTALA is not legally derivative of another hospital's duties under the law. In other words, just because EMTALA ends for one hospital when it admits the patient does not mean the law does not apply to a different hospital when asked to accept an appropriate transfer of a patient who needs emergency care. It is an independent duty.

The language of EMTALA's transfer acceptance mandate does not differentiate inpatients from emergency department patients, and it does not differentiate stable versus unstable patients (the psychiatric example). It should be interpreted to mean that if the patient has an emergency medical condition (as that term is defined by law) that the current hospital cannot manage, a receiving hospital with the capability and capacity to care for the emergency medical condition must accept the patient in transfer, regardless of the location of the patient in the sending hospital and regardless of whether the patient is currently stable or unstable.

To interpret the law otherwise would lead to the absurd behavior of physicians and hospitals refusing to admit patients from the emergency department if a transfer seemed potentially indicated, or accepting hospitals refusing to accept critically ill or injured inpatients because of their insurance status. Imagine if internists or neurologist refused to admit stroke patients from the emergency department if the hospital lacked neurosurgeons because of the possibility that the patient may bleed from anticoagulation or tissue plasminogen activator therapy and require neurosurgical intervention. Emergency departments in smaller hospitals would come to a standstill, and larger hospitals would be inundated with transfer requests.

To date, CMS has declined to opine on the legality of the psychiatric scenario presented earlier. It did not contemplate the ramifications to the law's transfer acceptance mandate when it declared in its new regulations that EMTALA ends for a hospital when it admits an emergency department patient. Until CMS addresses these issues directly or until an appellate court decides which interpretation is correct, hospitals have to rely on their conscience and ethical constitution in deciding whether to accept patients with emergency conditions in transfer.

3. Providing physician on-call services to the emergency department

Current state of the on-call crisis

The on-call issue is complex highly politically and economically charged, and EMTALA is only one reason driving the diminishing availability of on-call services by US physician specialists. The uncompensated care burden, malpractice liability issues, decreased reimbursement from Medicare and Medicaid, difficulties obtaining payment from managed care entities, and lifestyle issues are more or equally compelling reasons physicians avoid emergency department on-call services. EMTALA creates contentious relationships, however, between hospitals and their medical staffs: Ostensibly the law requires hospitals to provide on-call physicians, but it does not require physicians to take call [3].

Additionally, hospitals are directly responsible for the all the actions of its on-call physicians, imposing tremendous new liability for hospitals, which forces the hospital to take an active roll in managing the provision of on-call services. Under EMTALA, the hospital must control the behavior of its medical staff, who may not be willing to provide on-call services or accept patients in transfer on the hospitals' behalf.

Physicians now recognize the onerous burdens and penalties of EMTALA and bewail the fact that they have lost control over their own practices. They no longer can define their practice to a local community or, regional referral area or limit the volume of cases they must accept. They have no choice over which patients they must accept and treat when on-call. As the neurosurgeons have learned, when on-call for one hospital they are literally on-call for the entire United States. If any hospital anywhere lacking a neurosurgeon asks them to accept a patient with a neurosurgical emergency, they have a legal duty under EMTALA to accept that patient in transfer.

In response, physicians have devised ways to avoid emergency department services. Many physicians have cut down the number of call days they provide hospitals. Physicians also have curtailed their hospital privileges specifically to minimize their exposure to emergency department patients and on-call duties. General surgeons drop trauma privileges, orthopedic surgeons drop privileges to care for hand injuries or open long-bone fractures, and neurosurgeons drop intracranial privileges to avoid patients with head trauma or intracranial hemorrhages (the most common neurosurgical presentations to the emergency department). If these physicians do not have the privileges to treat certain maladies at their own hospital, they do not have to accept patients with those maladies in transfer from other hospitals under EMTALA's nondiscrimination clause [50–53].

Additionally, many primary care physicians have relinquished all hospital privileges and practice only office-based care primarily so that they do not have to take emergency department call. Certain subspecialists, such as ophthalmologists and plastic surgeons, have done the same to avoid emergency department patients because they no longer need hospital-based resources to practice [50–53]. Physicians also have responded to EMTALA burdens by resigning privileges from certain hospitals altogether, most notably smaller or rural hospitals, leaving entire communities without specialty coverage and forcing them to transfer many emergency department and inpatients out to larger medical centers [50–53].

Alternatively, physicians built specialty hospitals (or urgent care centers) without an emergency department so that they specifically could circumvent EMTALA. That way they could avoid the uninsured and high liability of emergency department patients and avoid EMTALA's requirement to accept uninsured patients in transfer from other hospitals that lack their specialty expertise. (The law applies only to Medicare-participating hospitals that offer emergency services) [3–5]. However, CMS and its technical advisory group have proposed advising the EMTALA regulations to require specialty hospitals to accept appropriate patient transfers, even if they do not operate an ED or offer emergency services.

In the Medicare Reform bill of November 2003, Congress imposed an 18-month moratorium on the creation of new specialty hospitals or expansion of existing ones, ostensibly because of concern over self-referral and anti-kickback issues [38,39]. The real reason federal and state legislators are worried about specialty hospitals is the potential impact on community general hospitals. If specialty hospitals siphon off all the paying patients, the general hospitals fear insolvency owing to the crush of uninsured care (assuming they cannot compete adequately with the specialty hospitals). It should not shock the conscience of anyone that no one is competing to provide services to the medically indigent in a country with a market-driven health care economy. Politicians want to restrain specialty hospitals or require them to operate full-service emergency departments and provide care to uninsured patients, rather than address the real issue of uncompensated care. EMTALA should not be the solution to Congress's failure to establish a national health care policy or refusal to pay for its mandated services [54,55].

Should the government force hospitals to provide on-call coverage?
(EMTALA's on-call provision)

CMS is aware of the difficulties hospitals face in maintaining available on-call expertise. In its most recent EMTALA regulations, CMS attempted to improve access to physician services by allowing hospitals the flexibility ("maximum flexibility") to provide on-call coverage … "in accordance with the resources available to the hospital, including the availability of on-call physicians" [23]. Many hospitals and particularly specialty physicians took this to mean that the hospital only had to provide on-call coverage to the extent the physicians were willing to provide availability. Hospitals also used the "with the resources available" clause to eliminate or decrease on-call coverage, rather than pay physicians to take call in certain specialties. Consequently, the new regulations only accelerated the loss of specialty call coverage across the United States [56].

The real issue is whether EMTALA actually requires hospitals to force members of its medical staff to provide on-call services. The relevant statutory language requires hospitals "to maintain a list of physicians who are on-call for duty after the initial examination to provide treatment necessary to stabilize an individual with an emergency medical condition" [57], which is an EMTALA-related requirement, not an actual part of the EMTALA statute itself. The CMS regulations state "each hospital must maintain an on-call list of physicians on its medical staff in a manner that best meets the needs of the hospital's patients ... in accordance with the resources available to the hospital, including the availability of on-call physicians" [23].

This language should be interpreted to mean that hospitals are required only to maintain a list of the physicians who have voluntarily or contractually agreed to take call so that the emergency department is prospectively aware of what on-call physician resources are available for any given day. The language of the statute states "to maintain a list of physicians who are on-call"; it does not say that the hospital must provide on-call physicians.

EMTALA was intended to require hospitals to provide the same services to all patients seeking emergency care, regardless of their insurance status; it was not intended to require hospitals to provide a certain defined level of services, for instance 24/7 physician services of particular specialties, such as neurosurgery and orthopedics, or 24/7 diagnostics such as CT and ultrasonography. Each hospital is unique, with varying capitalization, ancillary resources, and physician staffing; each hospital should be allowed to determine and define the scope of services it offers through its emergency department (unless mandated otherwise by state law). EMTALA requires only that whatever level of services is available through the emergency department is equally available to all, regardless of insurance status or other potential discriminatory factors.

Nevertheless, it seems CMS is set on actually forcing hospitals to compel its physicians to take call under threat of termination from the medical staff. In the preamble to its new regulations, CMS states the following [23]:

> We will continue to investigate such situations in response to complaints and will take appropriate action if the level of on-call coverage is unacceptably low.
> We further note that physicians who practice in hospitals do so under privileges extended to them by those hospitals, and that hospitals facing a refusal by physicians to assume on-call responsibilities or to carry out the responsibilities they have assumed could suspend, curtail, or revoke the offending physician's practice privileges.

CMS has not clearly articulated whether hospitals must force physicians to take call. The "maximum flexibility" allowed under the new rules may mean that "maximum uncertainty" will continue to exist regarding what is required of hospitals and physicians concerning their on-call duties and will continue to make it difficult for emergency physicians to arrange timely access to specialty care for patients.

CMS does require that "each hospital must maintain an on-call list of physicians on its medical staff in a manner that *best meets the needs* of the hospital's patients ..." [23]. This "best meets the needs" language is vague and creates a slippery slope of near-impossible compliance and unlimited, inconsistent retrospective enforcement and civil litigation. No hospital possibly can know in advance what it must do to ensure compliance with the law. No hospital possibly can provide on-call coverage that "best meets the needs" of all of the hospital's emergency department patients, regardless of the qualifying language in the regulations regarding "resources available to the hospital, including the availability of on-call physicians."

If the statutory language requires hospitals to provide on-call coverage, how much coverage is adequate? What if one hospital requires its three orthopedists to take call every third night to achieve 24/7 coverage, but another hospital's board of trustees believes that no physician should be required to provide unfunded mandated medical services (indentured servitude from the physician's perspective) or be exposed to potential devastating liability more than once per week? Which of these hospitals "best meets the needs" of its patients? Does one violate EMTALA and the other not? The second hospital would transfer patients more frequently, almost certainly provoking the receiving hospital to complain it is being "dumped on," inciting a CMS investigation.

Every decision the hospital makes with respect to how much on-call coverage is enough—how many days per month must each physician take call, whether to allow simultaneous call at multiple hospitals, whether to allow a general surgeon to do short elective operations while on-call, even whether to grant "senior physicians" exemption from call duties—subjects the hospital to termination from Medicare, civil monetary penalties, and civil liability for failure to stabilize individuals owing to failure to produce the appropriate on-call specialist. (Such lawsuits already exist, and the plaintiff attorneys typically use CMS's regulatory language to frame their claims.) CMS's "best meets the needs" language is nothing but an invitation to litigation for civil damages against hospitals for adverse outcomes related to lack of on-call coverage.

If CMS holds that EMTALA mandates that hospitals force their medical staff to take call, it will only accelerate the already increasing practice of hospitals being forced to pay for on-call coverage. Hospitals will justifiably expect the government to fund the expense resulting from the mandated on-call coverage.

Alternatively, physicians will resign from as many hospital staffs as possible and concentrate their services at only the larger hospitals where the complement of physicians is sufficient to lessen the burden of providing on-call services. Many communities will be left without medical specialties, and many more patients will have to be transferred to larger hospitals to receive specialty care. Eventually, the larger hospitals will be at capacity (most are already at or over capacity now) and will not be able to accept patients in transfer, forcing patients to seek care from further and further hospitals, jeopardizing their health and safety. Hospitals will continue to abandon acute care specialty services, such as trauma care, or will close altogether under the burden of the combined cost of providing uncompensated physician and hospital emergency care and increased liability exposure. Perhaps in the future some hospitals will refuse to participate in the Medicare program, just to avoid the obligations of EMTALA.

Should physicians voluntarily take call for hospital emergency departments?

The original Code of Ethics adopted by the AMA in 1847 at its inaugural meeting states that the preeminent duty of a physician is to "come when called" to care for patients during an emergency [58]. Today's physicians also should honor the call to help care for patients with emergencies. It should be an individual decision, however, motivated by each physician's conscience, ethical integrity, and commitment to serve the community. Which physicians take call, how often they take call, the scope of a physician's on-call responsibilities, and whether they will honor that commitment in a classic, legalistic, or fiduciary ethical manner should be determined in advance so that the emergency department is always prospectively aware of what services it does and does not have available on any given night.

Peer pressure, professional and societal expectations, financial inducements, and hospital relationships all play a role in determining the ultimate amount of on-call services provided by physicians. Strong physician leadership or strong hospital board leadership may be effective in increasing on-call coverage of a community's emergency department. Whether emergency department call coverage is required in exchange for medical staff privileges and whether the hospital provides consideration for on-call services (eg, stipends or malpractice liability insurance) should be between the physicians and the hospital, however, without government intervention. CMS should allow social, political, and economic forces to determine a hospital's on-call contingent.

Forcing physicians to provide emergency care, whether as emergency physicians or on-call physicians, not only pilfers their services and time, but it also diminishes the spiritual satisfaction of giving their professional expertise to the less fortunate, freely through their own benevolence. It is hoped that most emergency physicians would continue to provide a substantial amount of voluntary care to the poor regardless of government mandates, just as they always did before enactment of EMTALA in 1985.

If CMS forces hospital and physicians to provide on-call services, hospitals are in a much better position to fund the on-call coverage than physicians. Hospitals are rightfully viewed as valued community resources, and as such, they have endowments and fund-raising campaigns and may receive some subsidy for indigent care through Medicare, Medicaid, or state and county governments. Physicians have no access to such capital accounts.

Role of society in the ethical delivery of emergency care: should society expect or force physicians and hospitals to provide emergency services and on-call services?

> What, in the history of the American medical profession, aside from the profession's own rhetoric, should lead a thoughtful person to expect from physicians a conduct significantly distinct from the conduct of other purveyors of goods and services? Society should not expect private physicians or private hospitals (for-profit or not) to absorb the cost of whatever social pathos washes onto their shores. We as a society have a moral duty to compensate the providers of health care for treating the poor. If providers do give some charity care, our thanks to them.—W.E. Reinhardt [59].

When Congress passed EMTALA, it was ethically correct to insist on access to emergency care for everyone, regardless of their economic status. Congress took only half the step necessary to ensure access, however; it ignored the essential element of financing its mandated care. Instead, it nationalized US hospital emergency departments and simply "took" the resources and services of hospitals and the services of emergency physicians and on-call physicians without providing reasonable compensation. Is it ethical for society through its elected officials to refuse to pay for the services it requires to be provided by law?

The government and society can only "take" so much from hospitals and physicians before hospitals shut down and physicians withdraw from emergency department call lists or limit services at particular hospitals to avoid an excessive burden of uncompensated care and liability. It is reasonable to expect physicians to grant a degree of altruism, but beyond a certain point the pendulum swings too far, and it becomes untenable to provide particular services simply because it becomes economically nonviable to maintain that service. EMTALA is essentially ensured mutual destruction because hospitals cannot limit their exposure to uninsured EMTALA-mandated services, and any hospital left standing is required to accept patients in transfer other hospitals cannot handle, owing to the fact that they have closed specialty units or all the physician specialists have left or refuse to take emergency department call because of the uncompensated care burden and liability issues.

EMTALA and its unfunded mandate have effectively forced hospitals and physicians into unethical behavior, or the lowest common denominator—legalistic ethics—just to survive. Overburdened uncompensated emergency department costs? Institute "screen and street" tactics. Overwhelmed with uncompensated transfers to tertiary or academic medical centers? Refuse to accept transfers unless absolutely forced to do so by law (or simply refuse out of spite and dare the authorities to catch you, calculating that the potential penalties are far outweighed by the uncompensated admissions avoided). Too many uncompensated emergency department cases when on-call? Take less call, accept only the true emergencies required by EMTALA, and refuse all others in need of specialty care.

> If you allow the business world to treat us [physicians] as journeymen, then journeymen we will become.—Former US Surgeon General C. Everett Koop, MD.

Hospitals and physicians should not be the ones deciding who receives and who does not receive health care in the United States. It is a societal decision, and hospitals and physicians should not be the rationing tool for a society unwilling to address its health care needs forthrightly. In some sense, the fact that physicians have been so willing to give so much uncompensated care [33,37,40,41,42,47] has allowed the United States to put off addressing the issue of access to care for the uninsured.

Physicians should be held to a high ethical standard in the care of individual patients, and their ethical duties should run to their individual patients, not society as a whole. It is the responsibility of society to address the global ethical issues of access and financing of health care.

Physicians can be faulted and blamed for submitting to external pressures and forgetting their fiduciary duties and the trust granted to them by patients. If physicians do not continue to act in the best interests of patients, society will again, as it did with EMTALA, legislate morality and in some way force physicians to provide socially acceptable medical care. Most of the external forces threatening the medical profession are direct results, however, of the attempts to control health care costs and the government abdicating its responsibility to pay for mandated services.

Why isn't emergency care a fundamental essential community service, exactly like police and fire protection? Society does not expect its firemen to leave their families at night or disrupt their private enterprises during off days to put out fires without appropriate compensation. Why does it expect physicians to do exactly that and require them to pay for their own liability protection should an adverse outcome occur? If society wants to mandate and force hospitals and physicians to provide health care to the indigent, including the emergency care required by EMTALA, an ethical society should pay for it.

Summary

Health care, especially emergency health care, is a fundamental need of society, but can never be a fundamental right because no individual has the right to take the services of others without their consent. Physicians must assume an ethical role as protectors and guardians of patients' health care needs and as fiduciaries always place their patient's interests ahead of their own. The specialty of emergency medicine, as the portal of last resort in the US health care safety net, has a unique and venerable role to play in the delivery of emergency services, and emergency physicians should hold fast their commitment to be there at all times for all individuals in need. Emergency physicians should fight to preserve access to emergency care and avoid denying services to patients or rationing care without express societal sanction. If physicians fail, inevitably patients suffer, but so too does the integrity of the medical profession [60,61].

EMTALA would not have occurred if physicians had remembered their obligation to put patients first and had the courage and strength to act on this principle. Society also has a responsibility, however, to fund adequately the health care it needs. EMTALA represents an anomalous "right" to emergency health care, but its escalating uncompensated care burden will destroy hospitals and ultimately access to the health care delivery system if society fails to address this issue. If society values access to emergency care, there should be a *quid pro quo*—adequate funding, qualified liability immunity, or some other form of consideration.

Many politicians and community leaders deplore physicians who refuse to provide uncompensated emergency services, and it is true that some have forgotten the essence of what it means to be a physician. It is equally appalling, however, for Congress and society as a whole, as Senator Durenberger stated on the senate floor in 1985, to knowingly appropriate hospital and physician services as the nation's national health care policy. In the long run, it is undeniably destined to fail, and all citizens, insured and uninsured alike, will find it increasingly difficult to obtain timely, competent emergency care.

References

[1] Crawshaw R, Rogers DE, Pellegrino ED, et al. Patient-physician covenant. JAMA 1995;273: 1553.
[2] 42 USC §1395dd.
[3] Himmelstein DU, Woolhandler S, Harnley M, et al. Patient transfers: medical practice as social triage. Am J Public Health. 1984;74:494–7.
[4] Schiff RL, Ansell DA, Schlosser JE, et al. Transfers to a public hospital: a prospective study of 467 patients. N Engl J Med 1986;314:552–7.
[5] See generally Rothenberg KH: Who cares? The evolution of a legal duty to provide emergency care. Houston Law Review 1989;26:21.
[6] Bitterman RA. Providing emergency care under federal law: EMTALA. American College of Emergency Physicians; Dallas, TX: 2001. A supplement addressing the impact of the new 2003 EMTALA regulations was published in May 2004.
[7] Derlet RW, Hamilton B. The impact of HMO care authorization policy on an emergency department before California's new managed care law. Acad Emerg Med 1996;3:338–44.
[8] Wood JP. Emergency physicians' obligations to managed care patients under COBRA. Acad Emerg Med 1996;3:794.
[9] New Jersey Medical Society. Instruments of Association of the New Jersey Medical Society. New Brunswick (NJ): New Jersey Medical Society; 1766.
[10] American Medical Association Code of Ethics [emphasis added]. In: Baker R, editor. The codification of medical morality: historical and philosophical studies of the formalization of medical morality in the eighteenth and nineteenth centuries. Dordrecht (the Netherlands): Kluwer Academic Publishers; 1995:75, 86.
[11] American College of Emergency Medicine (ACEP). Code of ethics for emergency physicians. Ann Emerg Med 1997;30:365–72.
[12] Bitterman RA. A critical analysis of the federal COBRA hospital "antidumping law": ramifications for hospitals, physicians, and effects on access to healthcare. University of Detroit Mercy Law Review 1992;70:125–90.

[13] Hyman DA. Patient dumping and EMTALA: past imperfect/future shock. Health Matrix J Law-Medicine 1998;8:29–56.

[14] Council on Ethical and Judicial Affairs, American Medical Association. Ethical issues in managed care. JAMA 1995;273:330–5. The council maintained that physicians, no matter what their payment (or managed care) structure, must remain primarily dedicated to the care of individual patients.

[15] 131 Congressional Record 13903 (October 23, 1985) (statement of Rep. Pete Stark).

[16] McCaig LF, Burt CW. National Hospital Ambulatory Medical Care Survey: 2003 Emergency Department Summary. Centers for Disease Control, Division of Health Care Statistics, 2005. Available at: www.cdc.gov/nchs. Accessed May 28, 2005.

[17] Hudson T. New patient transfer amendments pose problems for hospitals. Hospitals 1990;3: 46–9.

[18] Sade RM. Medical care as a right: a refutation. N Engl J Med 1971;285:1281.

[19] Elias PH. Physicians who limit their office practice to insured and paying patients. N Engl J Med 1986;314:391.

[20] Baker RB. American independence and the right to emergency care. JAMA 1999;281: 859–60.

[21] Scheck A. No emergency? Go elsewhere. Emergency Medicine News 2005;28:1, 20, 21.

[22] Phipps v Bristol Regional Medical Center, 1997 US App LEXIS 17919 (6th Cir 1997).

[23] 42 CFR 489.24;42 CFR 489.20 (EMTALA regulations) Emphasis added. See 68 Fed Reg 2003;68:53,221–64. The new regulations were effective November 10, 2003.

[24] Pellegrino ED. Character, virtue, and self interest in the ethics of the professions. J Contemp Health Law Policy 1989;5:53–73.

[25] Osler W. Equanimities with other addresses. 3rd edition. Philadelphia: Blakeston Company; 1932.

[26] Black's Law Dictionary. 8th edition. Eagan, MN: West-Thompson; 2004.

[27] Bailey JE. Asklepios: ancient hero of medical caring. Ann Intern Med 1996;124:257–63.

[28] Ring JJ. Past President, American Medical Association. Letters to the editor. JAMA 1995; 274:1265.

[29] Statement of Sen. Durenberger. 131 Congressional Record 13903 (October 23, 1985).

[30] 42 USC §1395dd(d).

[31] Without the voluntary participation by hospitals, EMTALA would be a violation of the 13th Amendment, the prohibition against slavery or indentured servitude, and the "taking without just compensation" clause of the 5th Amendment.

[32] McCaig LF, Nghi L. National Hospital Ambulatory Medical Care Survey: 2000 emergency department summary. Hyattsville (MD): US Department of Health and Human Services, National Center for Health Statistics; 2002. 326:1–32.

[33] Bureau of the Census. Health insurance coverage, 1997. Washington (DC): Government Printing Office; 1998:60–202.

[34] Fields W, editor. Defending America's Safety Net. Dallas (TX): American College of Emergency Physicians; 1999.

[35] Lambe S, Washington DL, Fink A, et al. Trends in the use and capacity of California's emergency departments, 1990–1999. Ann Emerg Med 2002;39:389–96.

[36] Derlet RW. Overcrowding in emergency departments: increased demand and decreased capacity. Ann Emerg Med 2002;39:430–2.

[37] See generally Kuttner A. The American health care system: health insurance coverage. N Engl J Med 1999;340:163–8.

[38] Balanced Budget Act of 1997 (Public Law 105–33).

[39] Medicare Prescription Drug Improvement and Modernization Act. (Public Law 108–173, December 8, 2003).

[40] Burt CW, Arispe IE. Characteristics of emergency departments serving high volumes of safety-net patients: United States, 2000. National Center for Health Statistics. Vital Health Stat 2004;13:155.

[41] Weissman JS. The trouble with uncompensated hospital care. N Engl J Med 2005;352:12.
[42] Kane CK. Impact of EMTALA on physician practices. AMA Center for Health Policy Research; Washington, D.C.: 2004.
[43] Connolly C. Some finding no room at the ER: screening out non-urgent cases stirs controversy. Washington Post, April 26, 2004, p. A01.
[44] Rapaport L. MedCenter to steer patients away. The Sacromento Bee, February 4, 2005.
[45] American College of Emergency Physicians. Code of ethics for emergency physicians. Ann Emerg Med 1997;30:365–72.
[46] ED screening changes put pressure on competitors. ED Management, April 2005, p. 40–2.
[47] Truhe JV. Uncompensated care for nonresidents—an emerging fiscal and policy minefield. In-House Counselor (American Health Lawyers Association) 2000;6:6.
[48] Marx JA. The rightness of emergency medicine. J Emerg Med 2004;27:307–12.
[49] Pellegrino ED. Character, virtue, and self interest in the ethics of the professions. J Contemp Health Law Policy 1989;5:53–73.
[50] General Accounting Office. Impact of EMTALA on hospital emergency departments, the delivery of emergency care, and CMS/OIG enforcement. GAO-01-747; June 22, 2001.
[51] Wanerman R. The EMTALA paradox. Ann Emerg Medicine 2002;40:464–9.
[52] Bitterman RA. Explaining the EMTALA Paradox [editorial]. Ann Emerg Med 2002;40: 470–5.
[53] General Accounting Office. Medical malpractice: implications of rising premiums on access to health care. GAO-03-0836; August 2003.
[54] Iglehart JK. The uncertain future of specialty hospitals. N Engl J Med 2005;352:1405–7.
[55] Iglehart JK. The emergent: a physician-owned specialty hospital. N Engl J Med 2005;352: 78–84.
[56] Robert Wood Johnson/ACEP Survey of ED Directors: On-call specialist coverage of US emergency departments. September 2004. The RWJ/ACEP Survey confirms empiric evidence that CMS's recent on-call regulations only accelerated physician and hospital abandonment of on-call services, increased the risk of harm to patients needing specialty care, caused more delay in patient access to specialty care, and increased the number of patient transfers.
[57] 42 USC 1395cc (a) (1) (I) (iii).
[58] American Medical Association. Code of ethics. In: Baker R, editor. The codification of medical morality: historical and philosophical studies of the formalization of medical morality in the eighteenth and nineteenth centuries. Dordrecht (the Netherlands): Kluwer Academic Publishers; 1995. p. 75, 86.
[59] Reinhardt WE. For-profit enterprise in healthcare. Institute of Medicine 1986;210:213.
[60] Kassier JP. Our endangered integrity—it can only get worse. N Engl J Med 1997;337:1666–7.
[61] Kassier JP. Managing care—should we adopt a new ethic? [editorial]. N Engl J Med 1998; 339:397–8.

ELSEVIER
SAUNDERS

Emerg Med Clin N Am
24 (2006) 579–603

EMERGENCY
MEDICINE
CLINICS OF
NORTH AMERICA

Organizational Ethics

Robert E. Suter, DO, MHA, FACEP*

*Department of Emergency Medicine, Medical College of Georgia, 1120 15th Street, Augusta,
GA 30912, USA*
*Emergency Medicine, University of Texas-Southwestern, 5323 Harry Hines Boulevard,
Dallas, TX 75391-8579, USA*
*Emergency Medicine, Des Moines University, 3200 Grand Avenue,
Des Moines, IA 50312, USA*
*Department of Emergency Medicine, Spring Branch Medical Center, 8850 Long Point,
Houston, TX 77005, USA*
*Greater Houston Emergency Physicians, 211 Highland Cross, Suite 275,
Houston, TX 77073, USA*
*American College of Emergency Physicians, P.O. Box 619911,
Dallas, TX 75261-9911, USA*

Over the centuries the development of the concept of ethics within medicine focused on the role of the individual practitioner of medicine. The tradition of the solo medical practice and the simple relationship of the individual doctor and patient clearly defined our thinking about ethical issues on both a practical and theoretical basis well into the last century.

The increasing size and complexity of the health care system has led to a delivery system that is dominated by organizations, rather than individual practitioners. In emergency medicine, this starts with the groups of providers that staff an individual emergency department (ED); hospital or multiple group structures that may oversee these single EDs; and associations that represent the interests of emergency physicians and patients on a regional, national, or even international level.

By its very nature, the management of these organizations cannot help but have an influence on both the relationship between practitioners and the relationship between physicians and their patients. Policies and procedures, the design of compensation and incentives, and formal values or

Special thanks to Davis Mellick, Department of Emergency Medicine, Medical College of Georgia, for his extraordinary assistance in researching references for this chapter.

* PO Box 619911 Dallas, TX 75261-9911.

E-mail address: rsuter@acep.org

lack thereof, all impact these relationships and the ethical quality of any decisions that are made within an organization.

Recognition of this simple fact has led to the study and promotion of organizational ethics over the past several decades. This movement, which actually began in the health care sector, has grown to transcend it. In spite of the increasing discussion of business ethics, nowhere more important is the integration of ethics into an organization than it is in health care organizations.

Because emergency patients have sometimes been described as patients without choices, this integration of ethics into practice is even more critical. Unlike the classic doctor-patient relationship, where a thoughtful discussion of risks and benefits occurs in a setting that allows for reflection, family input, and second opinions, the emergency patient is often in a more dependent relationship with the emergency physician or other providers for the clinical care they need [1]. Given this relative decrease in traditional protections to patient autonomy, organizations providing emergency care have an organizational obligation to ensure that providers do not abuse this more dependent relationship, and that patients are protected by other mechanisms. This effectively means that emergency medicine organizations, like hospitalists and others who care for patients in similar "captive" situations, must take the lead in providing ethical guidelines and monitoring of practitioners, striving to do so at a higher level than may be necessary in other clinical settings [2–4].

In this chapter, we will discuss the application to the concept of organizational ethics and its application to emergency medicine organizations. These entities include hospital-managed emergency departments, small ED groups, larger emergency medicine corporations, emergency medicine support companies, prehospital emergency medical services (EMS), and specialty organizations.

Definition and principles

Organizational ethics includes both corporate and business ethics, or, put another way, both the corporate values and the financial practices of the organization. They relate to all aspects of the organization including mission, vision, governance, and leadership [5]. Within health care, organizational ethics encompasses the professional and moral codes of the organization's conduct. In the case of a patient care facility or clinical organization, it constitutes the behavior it should follow as it interacts with patients, families, visitors, providers, and staff. In the case of other organizations, it may reflect the conduct toward employees, contractors, or members [6]. Does it treat employees fairly? Are the contracts it signs, including those for patient care reimbursement, morally acceptable? These and similar questions are a step removed from clinical ethics, yet obviously have an impact on patient care [7].

The influence of all of these factors on the patient has lead to a logical and rational argument by scholars that in our current health care environment, health care organizations now practice medicine [8]. In recognition of the significance of this area, in 1996 the Joint Commission on the Accreditation of Health Care Organizations (JCAHO) promulgated an accreditation standard requiring each health care organization to develop and operate under a code of organizational ethics [9].

Much of the recent attention given to organizational ethics in health care has been focused on financial compliance programs. While compliance programs are important, an organizational ethics strategy must be broader than compliance programs that typically focus on legal and regulatory requirements [5].

Because clinical and organizational ethics can overlap, it is sometimes difficult to address one without addressing the other. Clinical topics might include end of life, pain management, organ donation, maternal fetal health, treatment refusal, mental health, and care of vulnerable populations. Organizational issues such as informed consent, research, marketing, access, conflict of interest, financial management, and public policy are embedded into these topics, and provide a means for them to be addressed by individuals within the organization.

Similar to clinical ethics, there are guiding principles that should be used to guide ethical organizational behavior (Box 1). These principles should be considered, implicitly or explicitly, in every decision made by the organization and its representatives.

Although a relatively new concept, organizational ethics actually fits easily into the framework of the traditional ethical principles of respect for persons, beneficence, and justice. Respect is earned by organizational leaders who model ethical behavior, and by staff who replicated these behaviors. Beneficence is achieved by organizations hiring and maintaining ethical staff, developing an ethical culture, and implementing programs in an ethical

---

Box 1. Principles of organizational ethics [10]

- Duty to individual patients
- Financial incentives
- Quality of care
- Duty to practitioners within the organization
- Due process
- Fairness
- Duty to the community
- Shepherd scarce resources

manner. Justice is demonstrated when action is taken to recognize ethical behaviors, and misconduct is dealt with swiftly and forcefully [10].

Current problems in organizational ethics

Business scandals have been at the top of the headlines over the past decade, and health care organizations have not been exempt. These scandals have caused an ethical crisis in many organizations with a concomitant moral collapse of trust among regulators. Dealing with these concerns is not merely about law, but also about ethics. Just as a focus on business law characterized the emergence of corporations after the industrial revolution 100 years ago, today's challenges call for addressing the more fundamental cause of basic business ethics.

The forfeiture of trust in health care organizations is not merely a result of the flurry of corporate scandals. Rather, it is the result of slow erosion over decades. Several combined causes are to blame, including the increasing role of market forces, such as managed care, and the constant tension that is inherent to access, cost, and quality within the structure of the health care system.

Unfortunately, our nation's organization of the delivery of care often seems to facilitate a fragmentation rather than integration of these important issues. For example, achieving fiscal responsibility entails competing dilemmas; cost reductions may be achieved by constraining services or decreasing access; expanding access typically increases costs whereas lowering costs often entails a reduction of services [5]. Interestingly, it has been shown that large corporations demonstrating a practical commitment to ethical conduct have improved long-term financial performance [11].

The challenge: regaining trust

A crucial role for organizational ethics in health care is to regain lost trust and to recover the confidence of providers, staff, and communities. An organizational commitment to developing and maintaining a foundation of stewardship and integrity should inspire the decision-making processes and standards of conduct for personnel throughout the organization. Of course, while there are examples of health care organizations, including those in emergency medicine, that have lost the trust of some, there are also those whose daily behaviors are already influenced by these principles [5].

Values

Arguably, the only way to create an organization that consistently exhibits ethical behavior is to create a values-driven organization. The management theory behind values-driven organizations is full of hyperbole. The text *Built to Last* written by two researchers from the Stanford

University Graduate School of Business, identified 18 "visionary companies." The primary tenet of these companies was identified as the use of core values, "essential and enduring tenets, not to be compromised for financial gain or short term expediency." Examples are "innovation and absolute integrity" (3M), and "service to the customer above all else" (Nordstrom). The thesis is that these companies with core values and purpose are built to last, and will survive with or without great leaders [12].

Core values should reflect and honor organizational traditions, serve as a bridge between the mission and management decisions, create a unique moral identity, and create organizational pride. Dedication to core values gives organizations strategic focus and provides stability in a crisis. They can and should be the major component of the organizational "soul," and help to both recruit a workforce looking for more than a paycheck, and a client base looking for something beyond basic service provision.

Creating a values-driven health care organization is not necessarily a straightforward task. In clinical organizations, some providers may identify more with the values ascribed to their specific profession, while in professional organizations, other providers may feel more affinity to supporting the values of the clinical organization. Although it is unlikely that the values of these different types of organizations would be in direct conflict, they could be sufficiently disparate to create challenges to achieving uniform buy-in [13].

This is an important issue for emergency medicine organizations and providers that work within the confines of a broader health care entity. Most emergency physicians are not hospital employees, but rather, have a relationship with their hospital though an employment or contractor relationship with a group that contracts with the hospital. While they may have a contractual obligation to abide by that health care organization's ethical policies, they are not members of the organization per se. This creates both opportunities and challenges to the development of organizational ethics for the contracting physician group or emergency medicine support organization. This is especially true if the physician group or organization has relationships with multiple hospitals that have differing ethical values or policies.

Ethical organizations use values to guide all activities of the organization. Core values should promote a culture that promotes the open discussion of ethical dilemmas and the use of a fair process to resolving ethical conflicts. In this regard, organizations must prevent and address ethical mistakes in the same way that they are charged with preventing medical mistakes [13].

Organizations that are not values driven can be fragmented, lacking a unified strategic focus, cohesiveness of purpose, and strong internal social ties, attributes that are lauded by management theorists. Solidarity is a goal and end result of these attributes. Interestingly, solidarity is not necessarily valued by all of the personality types commonly found in health care organizations. Physicians in particular may value autonomy above solidarity to the extent that presents special challenges to health care organizations attempting to implement a values-driven approach to management [13].

Creating an organizational ethics program

Mission, value, and vision statements

The relative strengths of an organization should be expressed as formal mission, vision, and values statements. The mission statement should express the organization's purpose or reason for existence and describes what they do and for whom. The vision is a broader statement that provides an overall direction or portrait of where the organization sees itself or its interests in the future. The values are the organization's basic philosophy, principles, and ideals. Each of these sets the ethical tone for the organization, and therefore it is critical that ethical principles be incorporated into all three in a substantial and thoughtful way, not just by adding the word "ethics" to the statements. Then, having written these documents, and with continued input and buy-in from stakeholders, everyone must strive to "live them," ensuring that they are the cornerstone of the organization [13].

Most organizations already have mission statements, and many have formal organizational values. Those organizations that have developed a values-driven approach to functioning have a good start to the implementation of an organizational ethics plan. Similarly, organizations that have developed mission statements, values, or philosophy statements have a base from which to start. These documents should be reviewed very early in the process of developing or reviewing the comprehensive organizational plan (COP) to ascertain how well they cover ethical issues, and to determine what sorts of modifications might be necessary to accomplish this goal [13].

The goal should be to create the three basic elements of an organizational ethics program: education, consultation, and policy development/review [14]. Competence in ethics requires moral responsiveness, moral reasoning, and moral leadership. The organizational ethics program provides the structure and processes to develop and maintain this competence. The organizational mission is supported by providing consistency; addressing the multiple loyalties of staff, customers, and governing authorities; and by recognizing priorities and the need for financial stability [14].

Stewardship and integrity are the foundation for organizational ethics in health care. Stewardship first requires that the trust of those served be treasured by the organization as the necessary context for pursuing a prudent use of limited resources. It invites the organization to recall mission as the context that will inspire ethical financing, delivery, and care. In this sense, it fosters commitment, trust, and integrity by abiding to stated organizational values. While most ethics strategies focus on actual behavior, organizations need to plan and integrate ethical principles corresponding to the mission, fostering a virtuous community with appropriate ethical principles, decision-making processes, and conduct [5].

Infusing ethics into organizational behavior

In the case of established organizations beginning a new organizational ethics program, the effort might begin with a survey of current and past employees about their perceptions of the strengths and weaknesses of the organization. This survey might reveal that improvements are needed in the culture of the organization, improvements in communication or feedback, better expressions of administrative concern for employee well-being, or an overall more positive work environment. Addressing each of these attributes to improve the ethical culture of the environment could result in the resolution of the problems with less expense and effort than would ignoring the problem or addressing the wrong problem [10].

It is the rare organization that can effortlessly exhibit ethical behavior consistently. The best way for an organization to achieve this goal is by integrating the ethical principles of respect, beneficence, and justice found in its mission, values, and vision into the COP. The components of a typical COP are shown in Box 2.

Successful implementation of an ethics plan results in the integration of ethical principles and practices throughout every action of the organization. The competitive, facilities, financial, human resources, information management, and marketing plans all need to be infused with the organization's ethics. Ethics can be incorporated into these plans by considering how the traditional ethical principles of respect for persons, beneficence, and justice, can be addressed in each area. The management of the implementation of these plans should then ensure that actions in all of these areas reflect the organization's ethics as well.

In the competitive arena, an analysis of the opportunities and threats to an organization can have ethical implications. An example might be staffing levels. If staffing levels are inadequate, an organization might choose to

---

Box 2. Comprehesive organizational plan [10]

- The competitive plan
- The facilities plan
- The financial plan
- The human resources plan
- The information management plan
- The marketing plan

accept this as something beyond their control for economic or practical reasons. Other organizations may seek quick fixes in the form of "locums" or "agency staffing" or new hires without analyzing why the situation has occurred. An ethical organization would go beyond this, not settling for readily apparent causes, but rather studying the situation to find the underlying causes within the organization that have lead to the shortfall.

The facilities plan in the context of emergency services is rarely about brick and mortar. In this context, it constitutes an organizational analysis of the need for the services of an organization and where those services should be located. From an ethical perspective, the ethical dimension of this plan would include performing this function in isolation of any financial considerations. An example would be planning emergency services space and resources designed to meet patient and community resources irrespective of payer mix, rather than having a strategy of intentionally under-resourceing them to discourage use by unfounded patients. The facilities plan would also include establishing relationships with important vendors, and ensuring that those chosen are reputable and known for the quality of their products and services, as well as known for their ethical employment and business practices.

The financial plan can raise numerous ethical issues. From an ethical perspective, it should address the financial needs of the organization while encompassing patient and stakeholder data. For example, while increased funded patient volume is positive, the organization should be committed to increasing admitting volume only when care can be provided safely. Similarly, patients should be discharged or transferred out only when it is in the patient's best interest or the patient's expressed wishes.

Emergency medicine organizations in charitable institutions or institutions serving the poor also have special challenges. The ethical financial plan should be to provide defined basic emergency services needed by the population served, with innovations focused on increasing revenue or donations. The budget should not be balanced on the expense side by creating obstacles to care designed to decrease appropriate use, or to provide evaluation or treatment that does not meet the minimums of the standard of care.

Financial issues internal to the organization are important as well. Are staff being compensated fairly? Is the organization sharing profits or partnership opportunities in an equitable manner? Alternatively, do the organization's financial practices appear to exploit staff, members, or providers?

In negotiating contracts with managed care or other payers, organizations should continue discussions until both parties are satisfied that quality care can be provided for the reimbursement agreed upon. Organizations should not allow negotiations to conclude and later resort to upcoding, understaffing, using poorly qualified providers, or other strategies to gain reimbursement or cut expenses on contracts they feel provide unfair payment. Billing practices should be fair and explained clearly. Clinical practices should reflect that dispositions are made for appropriate care, not profit.

Ethical organizations should be patient focused and care driven in their financial decisions, not resorting to unethical practices to remain viable. Charitable organizations should not use their mission statement or tax status to rationalize questionable behavior. Unethical activities designed to promote an institution with an altruistic mission is still unethical behavior, and should not be promoted or tolerated. The end does not justify the means.

Human resources planning and processes are also critical to the overall ethical performance of the organization. In addition to staffing, the human resources category includes space, equipment, support systems, and the development of internal administrative policies and procedures. Organizations must remember that employees and other associates, including physicians, are more than just a collection of skills and capabilities. Great care must be given to fairness, honest contractual dealings, and due process in dealing with all providers or employees. Promises must be kept to the people in the organization. The people in an organization comprise its culture, more powerful than the administration in regard to the organization's ethics.

Information management planning is another area in which ethics is important. The three broad concerns of information planning are to ensure that effective, accessible systems are in place; that continuous training is offered to employees; and that information systems provide valuable output that can be used to provide real-time benefit to the patients, customers, or members of the organization. Information in health care organizations is particularly subject to ethical concerns. While it is important for employees to have ready access to patient information, these data should be restricted to a "need to know" basis. The ethical organization's model of behavior should reflect this mandate and should supercede the Health Care Insurance Portability and Accountability Act (HIPPA) or other governmental regulations. Such behavior will help increase the overall respect for patient's rights [10,15].

The marketing process differentiates the organization's products and services from those of its competitors. It is an operational manifestation of the organization's goals, connecting the organization's strategies with the operational activities. Marketing includes many components, the most obvious of which is advertising. The ethical organization should ensure that any advertising is truthful and accurate. Advertising or informational materials, and promotional items, should reflect the values, goals, and image of the organization and the concepts behind what the organization stands for.

The marketing plan of an ethical organization does not resort to negative marketing about competitors, but rather focuses on the positive attributes of the organization. Advertising should not be based on unprovoked attacks or comparisons with competitors. Products and services marketed by the organization should be able to pass "the family test," which is commonly described as whether or not organizational leaders could, in good conscience, recommend the same product or services, including physician services, to a family member. If the answer is not clear, then the ethical organization should take immediate efforts to improve the product or service, and it should not be marketed until such time that the answer is clearly "yes" [10,14]. In the case of emergency services organizations, this may mean replacing physicians or other providers who do not meet quality or credentialing standards.

Following review of the COP to identify opportunities, policy development or updating with an ethical perspective should be the next element of an ethics program. All existing policies should be reviewed from an ethical perspective, and if they do not already exist, policies should be written on topics such as informed consent, withholding/withdrawing treatment, advance directives, surrogacy, do not resuscitate (DNR), medical futility, privacy, confidentiality, organ transplant solicitation, research, conflict of interest, impaired providers, and conscientious objectors. Those responsible for policy development should be ready to respond quickly to requests for guidance.

Leadership

There are an abundance of challenges for health care leaders in the quest for organizational ethics, ranging from the changing and competitive environment, to complex missions and organizational structure, and from increasing fragmentation in care delivery or unclear provider vision. Organizational ethics provides guidance for leaders in these difficult situations and fosters standards of ethical conduct [5].

Leaders who understand that stewardship presents the organization's mission as the context for fiscal responsibility will foster values consistent with the organizational purpose. The values-based vision of these leaders is the focal point that reflects consensus on anticipated scenarios within the organization. This strategic vision, combined with the organizational mission, should drive the accomplishment of goals that are translated from the performance of objective measures of progress [5].

Governance provides another opportunity for the practical contribution of organizational ethics to health care leadership. There are significant changes occurring in regard to the role and functions of health care boards. Corporate boards are expanding the fiduciary-advisory role for shareholders, and nonprofit sector boards often extend community involvement and advocacy to include strategic oversight. This can challenge board members to examine their role with an integrative focus on stewardship, decision-making processes, and standards of conduct [5].

Leadership is particularly important to creating an ethical culture, as a 2003 study showed. Staff in organizations who perceived leaders to be committed to ethical behavior reported having seen unethical conduct only 15% of the time, while a 56% rate of misconduct was observed by the staff of organizations whose leaders were perceived to not be committed to infusing ethics into the organization [16,17].

Provider and employee selection

Given the overriding importance of the human element, it is critical that organizations recruit, select, orient, and educate competent and ethical staff. The best way to ensure ethical behavior is to hire the right people. Ideally this should include ethics testing, in the form of a preemployment decision tree, as part of the hiring process. To support ethical behavior, organizations should have a "Code of Ethics," periodic educational workshops, and policies that encourage the reporting and discussion of ethical concerns. This focus makes long-term outcomes better, and enforcement much easier [10].

Recruitment and orientation are the first opportunity for the organization to provide ethics education, and a brief overview of ethical issues and appropriate responses will introduce topics and promote awareness. This early introduction to the organization's ethics can provide a chance to determine if a potential new staff member is a good "fit" into the organization's culture. Culture has a unique relationship to ethics. Culture not only benefits from, it is dependent upon, an ethical management and staff [5,10].

Staff education

In the final analysis, the organization's ethical performance is the sum of collective individual behavior. Ethical behavior begins with education. A foundation in formal bioethics education is essential for those leading the program and providing education or consultation. Ethics education must be ongoing, inclusive, integrated, and organized to avoid fragmentation [14].

Organizations have an obligation to teach ethics to staff and associates at the outset of employment, and on an ongoing basis. Educational organizations in health care have a special obligation to select students who could be predicted to model ethical behavior, and to provide students with the foundation for future study in ethics. Unfortunately, there is currently little research on the reliability and validity of measuring moral reasoning on admission to professional schools in relation to creating ethical providers [18].

This leaves the option of providing effective ethics training during the professional educational process, be it schools of medicine, nursing, or allied health, and any associated internship or residency training. Providers are taught to recognize ethical dilemmas; possess the relevant knowledge of norms, laws, and policies; analyze the situation at hand; and demonstrate the skills to negotiate it. In the clinical education phase, evaluation of ethical performance is also possible.

Content for continuing education in ethics can be based on staff and organizational needs. Values identification is often a good way to start. Explaining the differences in values and ethical approaches, and recognizing the relationship between behaviors and values provides a solid foundation for subsequent training [14,19].

A review of ethics vocabulary is also a good early step to facilitate common understanding. Rights, duties, integrity, humility, kindness, compassion, generosity, community, informed consent, confidentiality, surrogacy, and competency are some examples of words useful in ethics dialog. Particular attention to law, cultural diversity, and gender will ensure a comprehensive educational plan. Topics of importance may include research, financial practices, marketing, and conflict of interest, in addition to clinical topics related to the services offered by the facility, including end of life, treatment refusal, pain management, transplants, and human diversity [14]. Sometimes overlooked is the reality that creating an ethical learning environment, and appropriate role modeling, is critical to the process of educating staff. If this is not done, given the subject matter, all other efforts will be wasted [18].

Ethical decision making/performance

With proper leadership, education of staff, and the development of policies, organizations are positioned to make ethical decisions. This is enhanced by recognition of a formal organizational decision-making processes.

Ethical decision making requires a reliable ethical identification and resolution process. Identification has three steps: recognition of the relevant aspects of the problem, designation of the root problem, and estimation of the cause-and-effect relationships. Resolution also has three steps: clarification of options, determination of the best solution, and implementation of the decision [5].

Ethical behavior entails the development of standards of conduct that will enhance performance improvement throughout the organization. These standards should lead to best practices as benchmarks for ethical behavior at all levels of the organization (Box 3).

Box 3. Ethical Standards of Conflict [5]

Ethics of stewardship
- Developing a virtuous organization that enhances its mission
- Pursuing fiscal responsibility for the community

Ethical decision-making processes
- Identification of the ethical aspects of the problem
- Resolution of the ethical problem

Ethical behavior
- Standards of conduct
- Best practices for ethical behavior

Ethics consultation/committees

Organizations should be prepared to provide consultative services in ethics. Ethics consultation should be assigned to a person or group, such as an ethics committee, with demonstrated competency and skill in this area. Skills required of individuals doing this work are assessment, process, and interpersonal relations.

Traditionally, owing to the emphasis on problem solving in specific clinical cases, the primary focus for ethical issues within health care organizations has been the ethics committee. Whereas the ethics committee absolutely should not be the extent of any organization's efforts in ethics, it is an essential part of any health care organization. Unfortunately, the ethics activities of many organizations are limited to the "institutional ethics committee." Although institutional ethics committees may be responsible for many aspects of the organizational ethics plan, in many institutions the only high-profile activity remains the discussion and disposition of specific individual clinical cases referred to it. This is rarely possible in emergency medicine. A more current, expanded role of clinical ethics consultants and committees should be to move beyond specific "crisis" cases and into a proactive role, attempting to influence the organizational culture to prevent ethical mistakes or misconduct [20].

Depending on the size and mission of the organization, it may also be necessary to constitute a separate conflict of interest committee or subcommittee to supplement the activity of the ethics committee in the area of organizational ethics. In analyzing conflicts of interest, the committee structure should develop and follow clear written policies for oversight and management of all areas of potential institutional conflict. In the case of a service provider, this committee or subcommittee should include both internal and external representatives, and in the case of a membership society, it should include both staff and members, to minimize any potential for subconscious internal bias. Finally, the committee should be charged with pursuing educational efforts to acquaint all staff, members, or other individuals interacting with the organization with the ubiquitous nature of organizational conflicts and strategies for managing these conflicts or minimizing their risk [20].

Ethical issues in health care and emergency medicine

Health care organizations encounter a number of key ethical issues on a regular basis. A study of 4000 nurses identified more than 40 specific types of lapses or potential lapses in organizational ethics [21]. A high level of concern was also found in a nationwide survey of 1500 physician leaders who felt that unethical practices were impacting US health care [22]. A list of representative lapses identified in these surveys is shown in Box 4.

Box 4. Health care organization ethical issues [21,22]

- Organizational economic constraints limiting provision of the highest quality care
- Failure to provide service of a quality consistent with highest professional ethics
- Preferential treatment of persons seen as influential (patients, providers, others)
- Discriminatory treatment of persons
- Employment of incompetent or impaired providers
- Failure to provide honest information about the organization's capabilities to patients or referring providers
- Making disparaging remarks about competitors
- Conflicts of interest: financial, gifts, anti-trust, other
- Willful inaccuracy of records or reports: clinical, financial, billing
- Failure to identify and meet community needs in development of services

---

Conflicts of interest are a major issue in organizational ethics, and should be addressed in detailed policies that are monitored and enforced in an ongoing way. It is common for the emphasis of these policies to be on discouraging or preventing individuals in decision-making roles to make decisions that could benefit them financially in personal investments or payments, possibly at the expense of the organization. While important, this focus is narrow-minded and misses the point of organizational ethics. Conflicts of interest also include situations in which behavior may provide a direct benefit to the organization, with or without an indirect benefit to the persons exhibiting the unethical behavior.

Examples of such behavior might be a decision to cut staffing to a level at which the quality of care is arguably affected, or encouraging systematic upcoding of bills. This behavior may be intended to increase the profitability of the organization. Those responsible for this decision might benefit from the increased profit in the form of bonuses, raises, promotions, or job stability. In many cases a financial benefit may extend to physicians or others who are actually providing the clinical services. Of course, the potential for this sort of potential conflict of interest is inherent in all management decisions, even in public or charitable settings. It is therefore critical for managers in health care organizations to recognize this conflict, and ensure that all decisions are driven first by the values of the organization, and then by financial or other goals.

Another common example in health care organizations involves research, and much work has been done in this area [23]. Many academic medical institutions are centered around a research enterprise, and research success translates into grants and funding that often constitute the majority of the organization's budget. The prestige associated with organizational research success translates into increased clinical referrals and patient volume. Individual job security in the form of academic promotions and tenure are usually directly linked to scientific publications and research as well. The sources of financial conflicts of interest are shown in Box 5.

In the absence of strong institutional ethics, a number of incentives exist for systematic research misconduct. The need to enroll large numbers of patients in clinical trials to achieve statistical significance could encourage the enrollment of subjects who may not be good candidates for the study. Proprietary funding sources for pharmaceuticals and medical devices may encourage the design of studies biased to show positive results from their application. Even in the case of governmental or other nonproprietary funding, researchers may be under tremendous pressure to "publish or perish." The phenomenon of publication bias favoring studies that show positive results could therefore encourage data interpretation that results in more ambitious conclusions.

As in other areas, it is essential that organizations participating in research have well-defined policies and procedures to protect patients and the public against potential or real conflicts of interest. Starting with enrollment of subjects, the consent process must clearly acknowledge the ways in which the institution might profit from positive results. When there are potentially direct investment conflicts, the most stringent approach is to preclude the research from occurring at the organization at all, just as an individual researcher would be prohibited from it. Clear firewalls must be established between decision-making committees responsible for investment, technology transfer, and research [23].

Organizational ethics in the emergency care organization that conducts clinical research dictates that the organization do so in a way that protects the rights of subjects, and that the organizational incentives are such that the results published are accurate and unbiased. Particularly challenging to emergency medicine organizations is the concept of informed consent,

---

Box 5. Potential organizational research financial conflicts of interest [23]

- Royalties from the sale of investigational product
- Any equity interest in a nonpublic sponsor of the research
- Significant ownership or interest in a publicly traded sponsor
- Individuals in the organization have significant financial interest in the sponsor

as much resuscitation research requires waiver of consent by the community or other surrogates for individual patients. Such substitute consent requires the most rigorous possible application of ethical principles in all phases of the design and conduct of experiments [24,25].

Organizations must have policies and audit procedures to ensure that research data are reported accurately. Ethical organizations should create promotions and tenure decisions that reward researchers who conduct studies that are well designed, analyzed, and presented, even if they do not yield positive results and are not published. In creating a culture valuing science over publication, they can promote ethical research behavior while continuing to foster new advances in patient care.

Privacy and confidentiality have been significant ethical tenets since the time of Hippocrates, and are no less so today. Moral codes and legal requirements, most recently HIPPA, require practitioners to guard patient privacy and confidentiality. The practice of emergency medicine, from prehospital locations to the crowded emergency department, presents unique challenges to patient privacy and confidentiality [26].

Patient information on "status boards" in public view, open bays, multi-patient treatment areas, and constant traffic in the ED all contribute to the problem. The physical barriers within the ED can be particularly problematic when patients need treatment for conditions that are embarrassing to them, and may not have anywhere else to go for treatment. Similarly, minors may seek care in the ED to avoid telling their parents about their health problem. In all of these cases, the patient is at the mercy of the ED providers [26].

Health care organizations can and should seek to maximize privacy and confidentially within the context of providing high-quality care in the ED. The JCAHO 2003 standards include requirements that organizations implement policies and procedures, physical barriers, and other measures, with particular attention toward the ED and patients informed of these policies on arrival [26].

Respecting both spirituality and individual religious beliefs is an issue for all health care organizations, but can be a particular challenge in emergency medicine. In an emergency, patients may not be able to choose the hospital they are taken to. This could result in a patient being at a facility with a religious sponsor they are not comfortable with, or a nondenominational facility with less emphasis on religious and spiritual support than the hospital of choice [27].

Patient safety is another area that benefits from organizational ethics, by promotion of quality care that results from a dedication to shared mission. Systems should be geared to prevent, detect, and minimize hazards and the likelihood of error affecting care. This safety culture must be a part of all clinical organizations [5].

When patient safety efforts fail, medical errors occur. Communication of medical errors is sometimes considered another ethical dilemma, but in cases where the error is clear, they should not be. Proactive truth telling is another mark of an ethical organization. Informing patients of medical errors is a clear manifestation of this policy and behavior [28]. These policies have the benefit of allowing for timely and appropriate treatment to correct problems, prevents patients from unnecessary worry, and protects the patient's rights.

Palliative care is another issue that has generated concerns. In our culture, acceptance of death outside of the hospital is often difficult. This results in patients being brought to the emergency department with terminal illnesses in the last days of life. Organizations should ensure that these patients receive palliative care, including adequate pain relief, irrespective of any other concerns. At the same time, no religions or philosophies have ethical precepts that require the provision of futile care. Performance of diagnostic tests or treatments that will not lead to improved comfort or extend life in a manner consistent with the patient's wishes are arguably unethical. Organizations should therefore have clear policies in regard to palliative care, particularly when death is imminent [29].

Physician partnerships with nonphysician health care organizations continue to be a challenge to these organizations. No single model has yet emerged as reliably successful. The pressures of cost containment, declining reimbursements, and evolving needs continue to frustrate the success of these arrangements. Organizational ethics should encourage both sides to initiate due diligence that engages the threefold matrix of stewardship, ethical decision making, and ethical conduct. This behavior should occur as a result of shared mission and desire to improve the delivery of quality patient care. This is generally accomplished when all physicians are clear decision makers in all of the organization's decisions and policies that can affect patient care.

All too often, current models of partnerships encounter difficulties because of their primary focus on legal or financial arrangements in which one partner trumps others in power or prominence, whereas organizational ethics locates fiscal responsibility within the context of a broader mission of stewardship and integrity. A sense of stewardship can enable a partnership to emerge that gives primacy to quality patient care rather than falling into the zero-sum game of economic self-interest. Standards should encourage improved clinical services, increased physician fulfillment, and progressive organizational performance. Over the long term, this should be done by building and maintaining relationships that are based on honesty and trust [5].

Emergency organizations and providers face these and many more ethical challenges, and should have clear policies on how they will be addressed. For organizations developing these policies, reviewing the policies of professional organizations, such as the American College of Emergency Physicians (ACEP), can be illustrative and helpful (Appendix 1) [30,31].

Regardless of the issue, the development and implementation of an organizational ethics program should enhance service excellence both in establishing proper standards of conduct and in fostering best practices. If a culture of stewardship is fostered, there is a clear benefit to provider and patient satisfaction that will improve the organization's overall performance [5,32].

Case studies in organizational ethics in health care

The M.D. Anderson Cancer Center began a core-values project that was neither on the goals outlined by management theory nor cognizant of the pitfalls that might befall such a project in an academic medical center. At the outset, it was determined that a decades-old code of ethics, while updated regularly and used in teaching, was not used in day-to-day decision making or even in ethics consultation. At the conclusion of the project, the Clinical Ethics Committee came to view the Center as a moral community distinguished from other hospitals by the value placed on its core missions.

The M.D. Anderson project began with a Core Values Task Force, with 5 of 12 slots being held by past or current members of the Clinical Ethics Committee. Other members represented administration, public affairs, human resources, academic affairs, and faculty. First, the Task Force reviewed both the literature on core values and the existing individual documents. They then interviewed past and present leaders, particularly those with a reputation for moral or dedicated service. Those interviewed were asked to identify the core values of the institution, and their responses where correlated into a frequency table used to rank and then distill them into the final list.

The five prior organizational documents were consolidated into a Mission, Vision, and Values Statement. Focus groups chosen to represent a cross-section of employees and patients were gathered to review the drafts, looking for words or phrases that might not communicate what was intended. After several drafts, and 9 months, during which the documents were simplified, the Task Force moved into the implementation phase.

In the introduction phase of implementation, the process hit a roadblock that, based on the literature, should not have been unexpected. Although physicians had been involved throughout the process, when implementation was discussed with physician leadership groups, significant skepticism was expressed. Faculty were concerned that the values would be used to impinge upon their academic freedom. They objected to having their evaluations based on values in addition to their own professional competencies. This required that values be omitted from faculty evaluations except for teaching purposes.

After the physician delay of nearly a year, implementation began simultaneously on several fronts. Potential employees were made aware of the values so they could determine whether the job fit their goals. New employees were trained in the values, and all nonphysician employees where evaluated by them. Values are used to design institutional policies, processes, and systems. They have become the cornerstone of strategic planning and decision making at the institution [13].

Other published case studies involving clinical organizations include Montefiore Medical Center [33] and HCA Health Care Corporation [34]. These successful examples of integrating ethics into organizational programs are including situations where the organization may have been challenged initially [33,34]. In the case of HCA, the organization is sufficiently large enough to publish high-quality booklets on "Code of Conduct" for all employees and providers, and a "Leader's Handbook" for organizational leaders, clinical and nonclinical, as an enhancement to the program.

Nonclinical organizations need to set ethical tones as well. In medicine, the role of specialty societies and associations is particularly important in modeling and promoting ethical behavior by staff and members. For example, the ACEP has a comprehensive ethics strategy that incorporates a number of concepts.

The recognized specialty society for US emergency medicine, the ACEP has a comprehensive organizational ethics plan for its members and staff. First, ACEP has mission, vision, and values statements that define what the organization does, including why and how [31]. These documents provide the framework for all other policies of the organization, both internal and external.

A centerpiece of ACEP's values-based policies is a policy for members, the "Code of Ethics for Emergency Physicians," which is displayed as Appendix 1 [30]. By acceptance of membership, members are bound to the Code of Ethics for Emergency Physicians. In it, ACEP outlines principles of ethics for emergency physicians, while providing an overview of ethics in emergency medicine and a compendium of policies that offer guidance in common situations that could challenge members. As a proactive measure, The Principles of Ethics for Emergency Physicians are 10 fundamental obligations that should be embraced by all emergency physicians (Box 6).

Member governance processes are intended to be transparent and open to the greatest extent practicable for a large organization.

Concerning it's actions as an association, ACEP has voluntarily adopted Sarbanes-Oxley auditing standards, and has a values- and vision-driven strategic planning process that determines organizational priorities and creates the organizational budget. Human resources policies and procedures emphasize fairness and due process, and management practices are designed to infuse values and a sense of contribution to the mission into every staff member.

Medical societies have a responsibility to motivate members to adherence to the ethical norms of the organization. To accomplish this end, ACEP has a number of policies that are designed to encourage ethical behavior by its members. Expert witness policies are one example of how organizational

Box 6. Principles of Ethics for Emergency Physicians [30]

The basic professional obligation of beneficent service to humanity is expressed in various physicians' oaths. In addition to this general obligation, emergency physicians assume more specific ethical obligations that arise out of the special features of emergency medical practice. The principles listed below express fundamental moral responsibilities of emergency physicians.

Emergency physicians shall:
1. Embrace patient welfare as their primary professional responsibility.
2. Respond promptly and expertly, without prejudice or partiality, to the need for emergency medical care.
3. Respect the rights and strive to protect the best interests of their patients, particularly the most vulnerable and those unable to make treatment choices due to diminished decision-making capacity.
4. Communicate truthfully with patients and secure their informed consent for treatment, unless the urgency of the patient's condition demands an immediate response.
5. Respect patient privacy and disclose confidential information only with consent of the patient or when required by an overriding duty such as the duty to protect others or to obey the law.
6. Deal fairly and honestly with colleagues and take appropriate action to protect patients from health care providers who are impaired, incompetent, or who engage in fraud or deception.
7. Work cooperatively with others who care for, and about, emergency patients.
8. Engage in continuing study to maintain the knowledge and skills necessary to provide high-quality care for emergency patients.
9. Act as responsible stewards of the health care resources entrusted to them.
10. Support societal efforts to improve public health and safety, reduce the effects of injury and illness, and secure access to emergency and other basic health care for all.

values and ethics influence the members and potentially the environment in which they are implemented.

Specialty society guidelines on the behavior of expert witnesses, such as the policy of the ACEP, should guide member behavior, and when violated, are a common source of ethics complaints [35]. Given the conflict of interest that is inherent in providing testimony for a fee, and evidence that the source of the case influences the opinion, it is critical that organizations model and enforce ethical behavior in this area. Fortunately, the ability for medical organizations to do so was recently upheld in the landmark case of *Austin v. American Association of Neurological Surgeons (AANS)*. In this case, the AANS suspended the membership of a neurosurgeon whom it determined to have given testimony that was not supported by the medical literature. A lower court found in favor of the AANS, and the verdict was upheld on appeal to the US Court of Appeals for the Seventh Circuit. While Dr Austin had maintained that the AANS was exacting "revenge" on him for testifying against another member, in an attempt to discourage members from testifying on behalf of plaintiffs, the courts found that the policies of the AANS merely encouraged telling the truth [36]. The ACEP policy is similar, and serves as one example of how organizational ethics can simultaneously influence events outside of the organization, and the behavior of its members.

Summary

The development and implementation of an organizational ethics program can benefit emergency medicine organizations, including hospital emergency departments, emergency medicine groups, and entities providing business or professional support to the practice of emergency medicine, or advocacy on behalf of emergency patients. While the frequently complex matrix of responsibilities to multiple organizations can complicate this task, the benefits of navigating the challenges far outweigh the costs. In addition, the professional imperative to do so is compelling, and should be embraced by all emergency care providers, particularly emergency physicians.

Organizational ethics is a relatively new, and rapidly developing area within health care ethics. Given the unique challenges of emergency medicine in providing care to "patients without choices," and within the context of multiple organizations, it is also an area of ethics in which emergency physicians should chart a clear leadership role.

Appendix 1. ACEP Code of Ethics for Emergency Physicians?

I. Principles of Ethics for Emergency Physicians
II. Ethics in Emergency Medicine: An Overview

A. Ethical Foundations of Emergency Medicine

1. Moral pluralism
2. Unique duties of emergency physicians

B. The Emergency Physician-Patient Relationship

1. Beneficence
2. Respect for patient autonomy
3. Fairness
4. Respect for privacy
5. Nonmaleficence
6. Patient's responsibilities

C. The Emergency Physician's Relations with Other Professionals

1. Relationships with other physicians
2. Relationships with nurses and paramedical personnel
3. Impaired or incompetent physicians
4. Relationships with business and administration
5. Relationships with trainees
6. Relationships with the legal system as expert witness
7. Relationships with the research community

D. The Emergency Physician's Relationships with Society

1. The emergency physician and society
2. Resource allocation and health care access: problems of justice
3. Central tenets of the emergency physician's relationship with society:
   a. Access to emergency medical care is a fundamental right
   b. Adequate inhospital and outpatient resources must be available to guard patients' interests
   c. Emergency physicians should promote cost effectiveness without compromising quality
   d. The duty to respond to out-of-hospital emergencies and disasters
   e. The duty to oppose violence
   f. The duty to promote the public health

III. A Compendium of ACEP Policy Statements on Ethical Issues (Approved 1997; Revised 2000; Revised 2001; Revised 2002; Revised 2004)

A. ACEP Business Arrangements
B. Advertising and Publicity of Emergency Medical Care
C. Agreements Restricting the Practice of Emergency Medicine
D. Alcohol Abuse and Motor Vehicle Safety

E. Animal Use in Research
F. Antitrust
G. Appropriate Interhospital Patient Transfer
H. Collective Bargaining, Work Stoppages, and Slowdowns
 I. College Board Member and Officer Expert Testimony
 J. Conflict of Interest
K. Delivery of Care to Undocumented Persons
L. Disclosure of Medical Errors
M. Discontinuing Resuscitation in the Out-of-Hospital Setting
N. "Do Not Attempt Resuscitation" (DNAR) in the Out-of-Hospital Setting
O. Emergency Physician Contractual Relationships
P. Emergency Physician Rights and Responsibilities
Q. Emergency Physician Stewardship of Finite Resources
R. Emergency Physicians' Patient Care Responsibilities Outside of the Emergency Department
S. Ethical Issues of Resuscitation
T. Expert Witness Guidelines for the Specialty of Emergency Medicine
U. Filming in the Emergency Department
V. Financial Conflicts of Interest in Biomedical Research
W. Gifts to Emergency Physicians from the Biomedical Industry
X. Hospital, Medical Staff, and Payer Responsibility for Emergency Department Patients
Y. Law Enforcement Information Gathering in the Emergency Department
Z. Managed Care and Emergency Medical Ethics
  AA. Mandatory Reporting of Domestic Violence to Law Enforcement and Clinical Justice Agencies
  BB. Nonbeneficial ("Futile") Emergency Medical Interventions
  CC. Patient Confidentiality
  DD. Positive Promotions
  EE. Responsibilities of Acute Care Hospitals to the Community
  FF. Universal Health Care Coverage
  GG. Use of Patient Restraints

From American College of Emergency Physicians. Expert Witness Guidelines for the Specialty of Emergency Medicine. Available at: http://www.acep.org/webportal/PracticeResources/PolicyStatements/ethics/codethics.htm; with permission.

References

[1] Ladd RE. Patients without choices: the ethics of decision-making in emergency medicine. J Emerg Med 1985;3:149–56.

SUTER

[2] Larkin GL, Fowler RL. Essential ethics for EMS: cardinal virtues and core principles. Emerg Med Clin N Am 2002;20:887–911.
[3] Rajput VJ, Bekes CE. Ethical issues in hospital medicine. Med Clin N Am 2002;86: 869–86.
[4] Lo B. Ethical and policy implications of hospitalist systems. Disease-A-Month 2002;48: 281–90.
[5] Magill G, Prybil L. Stewardship and integrity in health care: a role for organizational ethics. J Bus Ethics 2004;00:1–14.
[6] Angelucci PA. Ethics guidenace through gray. Nurs Manage 2003;34(6):30–3.
[7] Sulmasy DP. On the current state of clinical ethics. Pain Med 2001;2:97–105.
[8] Khushf G. A radical rupture in the paradigm of modern medicine: conflicts of interest, fiduciary obligations, and the scientific ideal. J Med Philos 1998;23(2):98–122.
[9] Spencer EM. A new role for institutional ethics committees: organizational ethics. J Clin Ethics 1997;8(4):372–6.
[10] Oetjen D, Rotarius T. Incorporating ethics into your comprehensive organizational plan. Health Care Manag (Frederick) 2005;24:61–7.
[11] Webley S, More E. Does business ethics pay? Ethics and financial performance. London: The Institute of Business Ethics; 2003.
[12] Collins JC, Porras JI. Built to last: successful habits of visionary companies. New York: Harper Collins Publishers; 1997. p. 70–3.
[13] RD Pentz. Core values: an ethics committee's foray into management theory. HEC Forum 2000;12(3):225–34.
[14] Turner MH. A toolbox for healthcare ethics program development. J Nurs Staff Dev 2003; 19(1):9–15.
[15] Layman E. Health informatics ethical issues. Health Care Manag (Frederick) 2003;22:2–15.
[16] Ethics Resource Center 2003. National business ethics survey. Available at: http://www. ethics.org/nbes2003/2003nbes.summary.html. Accessed January 10, 2005.
[17] Romano M, Perception is everything: An ACEP survey reveals the detail of physicians public fall from grace. Mod Healthcare 2005;35(10):6–7.
[18] Singer PA. Strengthening the role of ethics in medical education. Can Med Assoc J 2003;168:7.
[19] Stirrat GM. Education in ethics. Clin Perinatol 2003;30:1–15.
[20] Committee on Bioethics, American Academy of Pediatrics. Institutional ethics committees. Pediatrics 2001;107:205–9.
[21] Cooper RW, Frank GL, Hansen MM, et al. Key ethical issues encountered in healthcare organizations—The perceptions of staff nurses and nurse leaders. JONA 2004;34:149–56.
[22] Adams D. Physician executives worry about lapses in medical ethics. Am Med News 2005; 48:11.
[23] Holmes DR, Firth B, James A. Conflict of interest. Am Heart J 2004;147:228–37.
[24] Lotjonen S. Medical research in clinical emergency settings in Europe. J Med Ethics 2002;28: 183–7.
[25] Bigatello LM, George E, Hurford WE. Ethical considerations for research in critically ill patients. Crit Care Med 2003;31(3 Suppl):S178–81.
[26] Moskop JC, Marco CA, Larkin GL, et al. From Hippocrates to HIPAA: privacy and confidentiality in emergency medicine. Part I: Conceptual, moral, and legal foundations. Ann Emerg Med 2005;45(1):53–9.
[27] McCord G, Gilchrist VJ, Grossman SD. Discussing spirituality with patients: a rational and ethical approach. Ann Fam Med 2004;2(4):356–61.
[28] Hevia A, Hobgood C. Medical error during residency: to tell or not to tell. Ann Emerg Med 2003;42:565–70.
[29] Aulisio MP, Chaitin E, Arnold RM. Ethics and palliative care consultation in the intensive care unit. Crit Care Clin 2004;20:505–23.

[30] American College of Emergency Physicians. Code of ethics for emergency physicians. Originally approved June 1997 and reaffirmed October 2001. Replaced "Ethics Manual" approved January 1991. Available at: http://www.acep.org. Accessed January 11, 2005.

[31] American College of Emergency Physicians. College manual. Available at: www.acep.org. Accessed January 10, 2005.

[32] Dewolf Bosek MS. Ethics in practice. JONAS Healthc Law Ethics Regul 2005;7:4–9.

[33] Foreman S. Montefiore Medical Center in the Bronx, NY: improving health in an urban community. Acad Med 2004;79:1154–61.

[34] Yuspeh A, Worthley J, Grnat P, et al. Above reproach: developing a comprehensive ethics and compliance program. Front Health Serv Manage 1999;16(2):3–38.

[35] American College of Emergency Physicians. Expert witness guidelines for the specialty of emergency medicine. Approved August 2000. Originally approved June 1990. Available at: http://www.acep.org. Accessed January 11, 2005.

[36] Healy GB, Healy LH. Honesty is the only policy: physician expert witnesses in the 21st century. J Am Coll Surg 2004;199:741–5.

ELSEVIER
SAUNDERS

Emerg Med Clin N Am
24 (2006) 605–618

EMERGENCY
MEDICINE
CLINICS OF
NORTH AMERICA

Informed Consent and Refusal of Treatment: Challenges for Emergency Physicians

John C. Moskop, PhD

Department of Medical Humanitites, The Brody School of Medicine at East Carolina University, 600 Moye Boulevard, Greenville, NC 27834, USA

Since its introduction into case law almost half a century ago, the doctrine of informed consent and its corollary, refusal of treatment, have assumed a prominent place in American medicine, bioethics, and health law [1]. Informed consent is now generally recognized as a fundamental moral and legal right of patients, and that recognition has enabled patients to play a more active role in making decisions about their health care [2]. Due to the distinctive features of the hospital emergency department and its patients, emergency physicians confront special challenges in respecting patient rights to informed consent to treatment. After a brief review of the doctrine of informed consent and of its significance in the emergency department, this article will examine three specific challenges for informed consent and refusal of treatment in emergency medicine: (1) assessing patient decision-making capacity, (2) performing procedures on the newly dead, and (3) making treatment decisions for patients in legal custody. This article will focus on issues of informed consent to treatment in the emergency department. See the article by Shahan and Kelen elsewhere in this issue for a discussion about consent issues in emergency medicine research.

Informed consent: the basics

In a previous *Emergency Medicine Clinics of North America* article, the author reviewed the foundations and essential features of informed consent and also pointed out exceptions to the consent requirement [3]. As noted in that article, informed consent fosters fundamental moral values of patient well-being and patient autonomy. Informed consent promotes patient

E-mail address: moskopj@mail.ecu.edu

well-being by allowing patients to choose among treatment options based on an informed assessment of how those options will satisfy their values and desires. Informed consent respects patient autonomy by giving patients the final authority to decide what medical treatments they will receive.

To achieve its moral goals of enhancing patient well-being and respecting patient autonomy, an effective informed consent must exhibit three essential features. First, the patient must have sufficient mental capacity, or competence, to make the treatment decision at hand. Second, the patient must be given sufficient information about the choice to enable him or her to make an informed decision. Third, the patient must be permitted to make the decision freely, without coercion or duress.

Despite its acknowledged importance, informed consent is not always required for medical treatment. There are, instead, several generally recognized exceptions to the consent requirement. The best known of these are the exception for emergency treatment and the exception for patients who lack the capacity to consent. When the patient lacks decision-making capacity, consent is required from a surrogate acting on the patient's behalf. Other instances in which informed consent is not required include situations in which patients waive their right to consent and situations when treatment is mandated to protect the public health. Some, but not all, commentators also recognize an exception called "therapeutic privilege," in which a physician may withhold information about treatment alternatives if the physician judges that disclosing the information would in itself seriously harm the patient.

Informed consent in emergency medicine

What is the specific role and significance of informed consent in emergency medicine? A naive observer might jump to the conclusion that obtaining informed consent is not a significant responsibility of emergency physicians. The argument for such a conclusion could proceed as follows: (1) Emergency care is an exception to the consent requirement; (2) emergency physicians provide emergency care; and, therefore, (3) emergency physicians need not obtain informed consent. The flaws in this argument will be obvious to emergency physicians. First, much of the care provided in the emergency department is not emergency care, but nonurgent care for chronic or minor medical problems [4]. Second, even if the patient's problem is urgent or emergent, it may not require immediate treatment. If there is enough time to discuss the treatment options with the patient and obtain informed consent, then the emergency exception does not apply.

A persuasive case can be made that informed consent is more rather than less important in emergency medicine than in many other medical specialties. Like surgery, emergency medicine is a procedure-oriented specialty, and invasive procedures typically require an explicit consent process with appropriate documentation. Unlike some primary care physicians with long-term physician–patient relationships, emergency physicians very often treat patients with whom they have had no previous acquaintance or relationship. Therefore, emergency physicians cannot rely on prior understanding of a patient's values and preferences and must engage in an explicit process of sharing information and eliciting patient choices.

Finally, many patients do not themselves choose the emergency department as the venue for their care, but are transported to the emergency department by others when care is needed. Many others seek care in the emergency department because they have no ready alternative source of care. Since these emergency department patients have little or no control over the locus of their health care or their care providers, it is all the more important to demonstrate respect for their personal autonomy in one way that remains available—by providing appropriate information and obtaining their informed consent to treatment [5].

The challenge of capacity assessment

As noted above, one of the three essential elements of a morally and legally valid informed consent to treatment is the patient's possession of decision-making capacity, or competence. Though the terms "decision-making capacity" and "competence" are often used interchangeably, it is important to recognize that assessing a patient's ability to make a particular treatment decision is a clinical judgment typically made by the treating physician. The terms "competence" and "incompetence" are also used to refer to judicial determinations that a person is or is not able to make legally effective decisions in other domains. To avoid confusion, the remainder of this article will use the term "decision-making capacity" for medical treatment choices.

Decision-making capacity is based on the following four functional abilities: (1) the ability to understand information relevant to treatment decision-making; (2) the ability to appreciate the significance of that information for one's own situation; (3) the ability to reason, using relevant information, to engage in a logical process of weighing treatment options; and (4) the ability to express a choice [6].

For many emergency department patients, a brief conversation may enable the physician to establish that the patient possesses these abilities. For others, one look may make it clear that the patient lacks decision-making capacity. For example, an unconscious patient obviously lacks decision-making capacity. For still other patients, those who remain conscious but whose mental status is compromised in some way, the determination of capacity may prove more difficult. Many emergency department patients fall into this third category. Their mental capacity may be compromised by acute physical or mental illness, traumatic brain injury, severe pain, substance abuse, dementia, delirium, or mental retardation [7].

Consider, for example, the following scenario: Mr. Adams is brought to the emergency department late one night by the local police. He has a two-inch-long gash across his forehead. The police report that he was cut in a fight over cigarettes outside the local shelter for the homeless. Mr. Adams is awake, alert, and responds appropriately to simple questions. There is an odor of alcohol on his breath, but he refuses a blood alcohol test. Dr. Brown, the emergency physician on duty, examines the laceration and finds it to be superficial, but in need of several sutures to prevent infection and a disfiguring scar. When she explains this to Mr. Adams, however, he responds that he does not want stitches and demands to be allowed to leave the hospital. Dr. Brown presses him for a reason why he does not want the stitches, but his only reply is that he does not like hospitals and does not trust her.

This situation poses an obvious challenge for Dr. Brown. If she judges that Mr. Adams has decision-making capacity for this treatment decision, she will be obligated to respect his refusal of treatment. If, however, she concludes that he lacks decision-making capacity, she may override his refusal and provide necessary treatment, or seek consent for treatment from a surrogate decision-maker. How should she proceed?

This case illustrates a number of the difficulties emergency physicians may confront in determining patient decision-making capacity. Dr. Brown might, for example, be tempted to conclude that the odor of alcohol on Mr. Adams' breath is good evidence of intoxication and that an intoxicated patient lacks the capacity to make treatment choices. There is, however, also evidence that Mr. Adams is not intoxicated: He is awake, alert, and able to answer questions appropriately. Dr. Brown might think that, if only she could do a blood alcohol test, she could establish whether Mr. Adams is intoxicated. However, even if the test were performed and the level exceeded the legal limit, that result would not determine that Mr. Adams lacked capacity. Intoxication can, of course, impair mental function, as can mental illness, mental retardation, dementia, severe pain, and various other conditions, but none of these conditions automatically renders a patient incapable of making treatment decisions. Patients with these impairing conditions are more likely to lack decision-making capacity than patients without them, and so their presence is relevant to judgments about capacity, but whether a patient actually lacks capacity will depend on how the condition affects the patient's actual cognitive functions. Patients with identical blood alcohol levels may, for example, exhibit very different levels of cognitive functioning. In a pilot study of patients with a different medical condition, investigators used three cognitive function tests to assess the decision-making capacity of 25 consecutive patients presenting to the emergency department with an acute myocardial infarction [8]. Five of these patients (20%) scored abnormally low on all three tests, suggesting that they may lack capacity to consent to treatment or research.

Turning her attention to Mr. Adams' actual functioning, Dr. Brown might then reason as follows: Mr. Adams is expressing a clear choice about treatment. His ability to do this implies that he has some understanding of the treatment options and some reason for preferring one over others. Therefore, he has decision-making capacity and his refusal of treatment should be honored. The flaw in this reasoning will be apparent to most readers: The ability to express a treatment preference may imply some understanding and some kind of reasoning, but not necessarily an adequate level of either. Suppose, for example, Dr. Brown asks Mr. Adams why he does not trust her, and he replies, "Because I recognize you. I know that you are Jane Cooper, my life-long enemy." Such a reply would provide strong evidence that Mr. Adams has a very imperfect understanding of the situation and lacks decision-making capacity.

Emergency physicians like Dr. Brown must, therefore, attend carefully to their patients' actual mental functioning to determine their decision-making capacity. Dr. Brown's immediate response to this recommendation might be to inquire what mental function test she should administer to Mr. Adams and how she should apply its results to determine his decision-making capacity. Unfortunately, however, there is no single, simple measure of patient decision-making capacity. Tests like the mini-mental status exam can provide basic information about a patient's orientation, memory, and attention [9]. If a patient is disoriented, lacks simple memory skills, and cannot attend to simple questions, he or she will also lack the ability to make most treatment decisions. Possession of these basic abilities, however, does not imply that the patient has the capacity to make a particular treatment decision, since that capacity requires that the patient understand specific information about the decision at hand and use that information to reach a treatment decision. To assess these abilities, physicians must gather more specific information about the patient's decision-making process.

Grisso, Appelbaum, and Hill-Fotouhi [10] have developed an interview instrument, the MacArthur Competence Assessment Tool-Treatment, designed to assess patient decision-making capacity in a systematic way. Their interview process begins with disclosure of specific information about the treatment choice, then assesses the patient's understanding of the information, appreciation of the situation, reasoning supporting the decision, and expression of choice. Though it requires time to adapt to each particular situation and 15 to 20 minutes to administer, this tool may be helpful in situations where the patient's decision-making capacity is ambiguous.

It is important to note that, since decision-making capacity is not a global determination, but is specific to a particular decision-making task, a patient may have the capacity to make simple treatment decisions, but not more complex decisions. Dr. Brown might, for example, conclude that Mr. Adams has sufficient capacity to make a decision about treatment for his forehead laceration. Mr. Adams might not, however, have capacity to make a much more complex treatment decision, as, for example, surgical versus medical management of acute coronary disease.

In the scenario described above, Dr. Brown must decide, based on limited information, whether Mr. Adams has sufficient decision-making capacity to refuse treatment for his lacerated forehead. She may desire additional information about his cognitive functioning, but not be able to gather such information without his cooperation. She may nevertheless decide, based on the information she does have, to give Mr. Adams the benefit of the doubt and honor his refusal of treatment. This decision may depend heavily on her assessment that Mr. Adams' refusal of treatment, though not medically optimal, is unlikely to have severe adverse health consequences for him. If, however, the situation were identical except for the fact that Mr. Adams was refusing treatment for acute appendicitis or another potentially life-threatening condition, Dr. Brown may conclude that Mr. Adams lacks decision-making capacity and begin appropriate treatment. Are these different judgments morally justifiable? Should decision-making capacity vary not only with the complexity of the decision, but also with its risks? Leading consent scholars defend this linking of capacity judgments with risks [6,11]. Though they acknowledge the value of autonomy, these scholars argue that physicians may also act to protect patients from serious harm by requiring a higher threshold for capacity when a patient's decision poses substantial risk of harm without significant benefits than when the risk of harm is low.

Emergency physicians often confront complex judgments about their patients' decision-making capacity. In making these judgments, physicians must be aware of medical conditions that impair mental functioning. However, except for the severest conditions like coma, emergency physicians should not equate the presence of an impairing condition with the lack of decision-making capacity. Instead, emergency physicians must assess the patient's actual cognitive functioning. Though simple mental status exams may provide information about basic mental functions, physicians should also investigate the patient's ability to understand and reason about the specific treatment decision at hand. Because the physician is judging capacity for a specific decision, he or she must consider the complexity of that decision and the risks attendant on honoring a particular choice.

In summary, when assessing decision-making capacity, physicians should take seven factors into account:

- Presence of condition(s) impairing mental function;
- Presence of basic mental functioning (awareness, orientation, memory, attention);
- Understanding of specific treatment-related information;
- Appreciation of the significance of the information for the patient's situation;
- Reasoning about treatment alternatives in light of goals and values;
- complexity of the decision-making task; and
- risks of the patient's decision.

The challenge of the newly dead

For more than a decade, debate has raged in the emergency medical literature about the practice of allowing resident physicians, as part of their training, to perform invasive procedures on newly dead patients in the emergency department [12–21]. Consider, for example, the following scenario: An 87-year-old man in cardiac arrest is transported to the emergency department of a teaching hospital. Dr. Doe, the attending emergency physician, supervises resuscitation procedures performed by three resident physicians, including intubation, intravenous medications, and defibrillation. After 30 minutes without response, Dr. Doe directs the resuscitation team to cease their efforts and pronounces the patient dead. As Dr. Doe prepares to leave the treatment room, Dr. Ellis, a junior resident, asks for a moment of his time. Dr. Ellis confides in him that she has had very little experience in endotracheal intubation and feels unsure of her technique. She asks Dr. Doe if she may intubate the patient's body while he observes and instructs her. Dr. Doe is not aware of any departmental or hospital policy on this issue. How should he respond to Dr. Ellis' request?

This situation poses an obvious challenge for Dr. Doe. As an attending physician in an emergency medicine residency program, he has a clear interest in helping Dr. Ellis master this essential procedural skill. However, he may be uncertain whether he should allow the resident to perform this procedure on the patient's body for an educational purpose, especially if he is aware of the controversy surrounding this issue. His decision may turn on a question directly relevant to the topic of this article. Must he obtain the informed consent of a family member or other representative of the patient before allowing the resident to perform the intubation?

In the scenario described above, as in many other emergency department situations, Dr. Doe does not have the luxury of time to consult the medical literature for guidance about how to respond to Dr. Ellis' request. If he did have that opportunity, he would find that opinions and practice on this issue vary widely. A survey of program directors of accredited emergency medicine residency programs conducted in 1998 and 1999, for example, revealed an almost even split between programs in which procedures are performed on the newly dead for teaching purposes (45 programs) and programs that do not employ this practice (51 programs) [22]. Of the 45 programs in which procedures are performed on the newly dead, 34 (76%) reported that they "almost never" obtain consent from family members, and only 3 (7%) "almost always" obtain consent.

How, then, should Dr. Doe evaluate the moral propriety of honoring Dr. Ellis' request? The reason for her request is clear: She wishes to gain proficiency in performing endotracheal intubation. There is little or no dispute about the worthiness of this goal. Society relies on emergency physicians to perform life-saving interventions with proficiency, and patients benefit from physicians' skillful performance of emergency procedures when the need for them arises. The social value of providing emergency physicians with excellent procedural skills cannot, however, by itself justify any method used to obtain those skills. Moral analysis of the practice of performing procedures on newly dead patients for educational purposes must, therefore, also examine other reasons for and against this practice, including potential interests of the patient and family, and alternative methods for gaining procedural skills.

In addition to emphasizing the social value of the use of newly dead in teaching procedures, proponents of this practice defend it on the grounds that the procedures performed are brief, nonmutilating, and cannot harm the patient, because he or she is already dead [18]. It is, of course, true that these procedures cannot cause pain or suffering, or compromise the health of a person who is already dead, but they can violate wishes or interests the patient may have had regarding what would happen to his or her body after death. For example, the patient might have been a member of a religious faith that prohibits manipulation of dead bodies [23]. Several authors suggest that patients be given the opportunity to express their wishes about this use of their bodies after death in an advance directive [14,24,25], but it will likely be difficult to enlist the broad social support necessary for widespread completion of advance directives of this nature.

In addition to potential interests of the patient, family members have moral and legal interests and rights regarding the body of a loved one. Sometimes called "quasi-property rights," these include rights to decide about the disposition of the body, to authorize an autopsy, and to grant permission for removal of organs and tissues for transplantation or research [17,20]. Like procedures on the newly dead, autopsies and organ donation are clearly socially valuable practices. Arguing by analogy, then, if these postmortem practices rightfully require consent from family members, so also should performing procedures on the newly dead.

Proponents of allowing procedures on the newly dead argue that requesting consent from family members may be emotionally distressing to them and that most will refuse, thereby foreclosing this teaching opportunity. Several empirical studies have investigated this issue. In two survey studies of emergency department patients and their family members, 74% and 75% of respondents indicated that they would consent to procedures on the newly dead [26,27]. In two other emergency department studies, investigators requested actual consent from family members for postmortem procedures on a newly deceased relative; 59% consented to retrograde tracheal intubation [28] and 39% consented to cricothyrotomy, a more invasive procedure [29]. These studies offer some support for claims that families can tolerate requests for consent to procedures on the newly dead and will often give their consent.

Several medical associations have adopted policy statements on this issue in recent years, including the American Heart Association's Emergency Cardiac Care Committee in 2000 [30], the American Medical Association's

Council on Ethical and Judicial Affairs in 2001 [31], and the Society for Academic Emergency Medicine in 2004 [32]. The policy statements of the American Heart Association and the American Medical Association recommend that institutions develop policies addressing this issue, and all three policies state that informed consent should be obtained from family members for these procedures.

How, then, should Dr. Doe respond to the resident's request? The most defensible course of action, though it may not be the most expedient, would be to speak to the patient's family, explaining what would be done to the body of their relative and why, and requesting their consent. If the family refuses this request, Dr. Doe might seek other ways to help Dr. Ellis gain this proficiency. If the residency program has access to a high-fidelity manikin for intubation practice, for example, he might offer to help her use that tool to improve her skills.

The challenge of prisoner care

At the end of 2003, federal and state prisons and local jails and lockups in the United States held more than 2 million prisoners [33]. Drug convictions have increased the number of prison inmates with HIV infection and AIDS, and stricter sentencing laws have increased the number of older inmates with chronic and progressive illnesses [34]. When prisoners suffer an acute illness or injury, or any health problem that exceeds the correctional institution's health care capacity, they are frequently transported to hospital emergency departments for treatment.

During their incarceration, prisoners lose a variety of basic rights and freedoms, such as freedom of movement and freedom of association. Prisoners do not lose all their rights, however. The US Supreme Court has noted that prisoners "retain those rights that are not inconsistent with [their] status as a prisoner or with the legitimate penological objectives of the corrections system" [35]. In particular, the Supreme Court has ruled that depriving a prisoner of "adequate" medical care constitutes "cruel and inhuman" punishment [36]. Therefore, prisoners retain a constitutional right to health care. Do they also retain rights to informed consent and refusal of treatment? Consider the following scenario: Dr. Ford is an emergency physician on duty in the emergency department one evening. Two police officers arrive with a man in custody. They inform Dr. Ford that the man is a rape suspect and ask him to collect physical evidence from the suspect using a standard protocol, including combing and plucking of pubic hairs. Dr. Ford contacts the chief of service, who tells him that there is an informal agreement between the emergency department and the police department to perform this service. Should Dr. Ford comply with this request? If so, must he obtain the detainee's informed consent to carry out this protocol?

Dr. Ford faces an obvious challenge in deciding how to respond to this situation. He is being asked to assist the police in a law-enforcement activity.

He may question whether this activity is consistent with his professional obligation to do no harm without a compensating benefit, since the evidence he collects may help to convict the prisoner. He may recognize, however, that society has ascribed to physicians a number of other responsibilities associated with law enforcement, including responsibilities to report various injuries caused by acts of violence. He may also recognize that pathologists, psychiatrists, and other physicians sometimes serve law-enforcement goals as forensic medicine specialists. He may regret that the emergency department has entered into an informal agreement with the local police department to provide this service, but since it has, he may feel some responsibility to the institution to comply with this request.

Suppose Dr. Ford is unsure how to proceed, and so decides to consult the emergency medicine literature for guidance on this topic. If so, he will find that, unlike the prior issue of practicing procedures on the newly dead, the published literature offers very little guidance on this topic. A Medline search conducted in March 2005 combining "emergency medicine" and "prisoners" resulted in a grand total of two articles, a 1995 article on medical devices made into weapons by prisoners [37], and a 1985 review article on prisoners in the emergency department [38]. The review article, by Lessenger, asserts that prisoners retain the right to refuse medical treatment. Since that review article appeared, several United States appellate court decisions have reached varying conclusions about prisoners' rights to refuse medical treatment [39].

In *Commissioner of Corrections v Myers* (1979), the Supreme Judicial Court of Massachusetts upheld the authority of prison officials to override prisoner Kenneth Myers' refusal of hemodialysis [40]. Acknowledging both Myers' interests in privacy and bodily integrity and the state's interest in the preservation of life, the court argued that the balance was tipped in favor of forced treatment "by the state's interest in upholding orderly prison administration, particularly the maintenance of proper discipline and supervision of inmates, and the elimination of a serious threat to prison order and security which the state's failure to prevent a death would present" [40].

Three court decisions address inmate refusal of psychotropic medications. In *Washington v Harper* (1990), the US Supreme Court upheld a prison's authority to override inmate Walter Harper's refusal of medication for his bipolar disorder [41]. The court found that prison authorities may restrict prisoners' constitutional rights to satisfy "legitimate penological interests," such as maintaining control in the prison environment and protecting other inmates and prison staff from a dangerous prisoner. In *Riggins v Nevada* (1992), the US Supreme Court again confronted the issue of a prisoner's refusal of antipsychotic medication [42]. Daniel Riggins refused antipsychotic medication while he was being detained for trial. The court ruled that the state could not force Riggins to take the medications if, as he claimed, they would adversely affect his mental state and his ability to participate in his trial. In *Louisiana v Perry* (1992), the Louisiana Supreme

Court rejected the state's attempt to administer antipsychotic medications to death row inmate Michael Perry over his objection [42]. The state sought to force these medications on Perry to render him competent for execution.

Finally, in *Thor v Superior Court* (1993), the Supreme Court of California considered a refusal of food and medication by Daniel Thor, a prisoner with quadriplegia [43]. The court held that, in the absence of significant concerns about prison security or public safety, Thor had the same right to refuse unwanted life-sustaining treatment as did patients outside a prison setting.

Though these court decisions do not directly address treatment of prisoners in the emergency department, they do suggest that prisoners' rights to refuse treatment may be limited by "legitimate penological interests," such as prison security. Dr. Ford, however, may reason that, as an independent professional, he is not bound to serve the interests of the state over those of his individual patient, and so he may decide to carry out the rape-suspect evidence-collection protocol only if the detainee gives his informed consent to this action. To obtain a valid consent, Dr. Ford must inform the "patient" about the procedure, assess his decision-making capacity, and determine that the consent is voluntary. That is, Dr. Ford must determine that the prisoner knows that he may refuse and that the physician will honor his refusal of this procedure.

In a related context, that of participation in biomedical research on human subjects, the National Commission for the Protection of Human Subjects reached the conclusion that, because of their coercive environment, prisoners could not make voluntary choices about participation in research [44]. Acting on the commission's recommendations, the US Department of Health, Education, and Welfare in 1978 adopted regulations strictly limiting the types of research in which prisoners may be involved [45].

Now consider a slightly different scenario: Dr. Ford is on duty once again in the emergency department. Prison officials arrive with an inmate from a nearby state prison. The patient is a 25-year-old male serving a long sentence for a serious crime. He reported to the prison infirmary with a complaint of pain and a discharge during urination. The prison physician decided to send the prisoner to the hospital for definitive diagnosis and therapy. Urinalysis reveals a common sexually transmitted infection. Dr. Ford informs the patient of this diagnosis and recommends antibiotic treatment. To Dr. Ford's surprise, the patient refuses treatment. When Dr. Ford asks why he doesn't want this treatment, the prisoner responds confidentially that he is enjoying a little time away from the prison and hints that he might change his mind about treatment after a day or two in the hospital. Dr. Ford wonders how he should respond, and what information about the patient he should share with prison officials.

This case poses difficult questions of informed consent, confidentiality, and the use of health care resources. The patient appears to be basing his decision on the goal of temporarily avoiding the confinement and monotony of prison life, an understandable desire for a long-term prison inmate.

Should Dr. Ford undermine, assist, or remain neutral in the prisoner's endeavor? How should he interpret his responsibilities to this patient, to the prison system, and perhaps to society? Does the prisoner in this situation have the same rights to refuse treatment and to medical confidentiality as any other emergency department patient? Although emergency physicians may have developed practical answers to these questions, there is little or no evidence in the medical literature of a systematic attempt to address them. Thus, the emergency care of prisoners, and the broader topic of relations between emergency physicians on the one hand and law enforcement and correctional officials on the other is a topic ripe for moral analysis.

References

[1] Faden RR, Beauchamp TL, King NMP. A history and theory of informed consent. New York: Oxford University Press; 1986.

[2] Making healthcare decisions: a report on the ethical and legal applications of informed consent in the patient–practioner relationship. Volume 1: report. Washington (DC): President's Commission for the Study of Ethical Problems in Medicine and Biomedical and Behavioral Research; 1982.

[3] Moskop JC. Informed consent in the emergency department. Emerg Med Clin North Am 1999;17(2):327–40.

[4] Young GP, Wagner MB, Kellermann AL, et al. Ambulatory visits to hospital emergency departments. JAMA 1996;276(6):460–5.

[5] Ladd RE. Patients without choices: the ethics of decision making in emergency medicine. J Emerg Med 1985;3:149–56.

[6] Grisso T, Appelbaum PS. Abilities related to competence. In: Assessing competence to consent to treatment. New York: Oxford University Press; 1998. p. 31–60.

[7] Larkin GL, Marco CA, Abbott JT. Emergency determination of decision-making capacity: balancing autonomy and beneficence in the emergency department. Acad Emerg Med 2001; 8(3):282–4.

[8] Smithline HA, Mader TJ, Crenshaw BJ. Do patients with acute medical conditions have the capacity to give informed consent to emergency medicine research? Acad Emerg Med 1999; 6(8):776–80.

[9] Folstein MF, Folstein SE, McHugh PR. "Mini-mental state." A practical method for grading the cognitive state of patients for the clinician. J Psychiatr Res 1975;12(3):189–98.

[10] Grisso T, Appelbaum PS, Hill-Fotouhi C. The MacCAT-T: a clinical tool to assess patients' capacities to make treatment decisions. Psychiatr Serv 1997;48(11):1415–9.

[11] Buchanan AE, Brock DW. Competence and incompetence. In: Deciding for others: the ethics of surrogate decision making. Cambridge, UK: Cambridge University Press, 1989. p. 17–86.

[12] Iserson KV. Using a cadaver to practice and teach. Commentary. Hastings Cent Rep 1986; 16(3):28–9.

[13] Culver CM. Using a cadaver to practice and teach. Commentary. Hastings Cent Rep 1986; 16(3):29.

[14] Orlowski JP, Kanoti GA, Mehlman MJ. The ethics of using newly dead patients for teaching and practicing intubation techniques. N Engl J Med 1988;319(7):439–41.

[15] Iserson KV. Post mortem procedures in the emergency department: using the recently dead to practice and teach. J Med Ethics 1993;19(2):92–8.

[16] Burns JP, Reardon FE, Truog RD. Using newly deceased patients to teach resuscitation procedures. New Engl J Med 1994;331(24):1652–5.

[17] Goldblatt AD. Don't ask, don't tell: practicing minimally invasive resuscitation techniques on the newly dead. Ann Emerg Med 1995;25(1):86–90.

[18] Iserson KV. Law versus life: the ethical imperative to practice and teach using the newly dead emergency department patient. Ann Emerg Med 1995;25(1):91–4.

[19] Moore GP. Ethics seminars: the practice of medical procedures on newly dead patients—is consent warranted? Acad Emerg Med 2001;8(4):389–92.

[20] Berger JT, Rosner F, Cassell EJ. Ethics of practicing medical procedures on newly dead and nearly dead patients. J Gen Intern Med 2002;17:774–8.

[21] Schmidt TA, Abbott JT, Gelderman JM, et al. Ethics seminars: the ethical debate on practicing procedures on the newly dead. Acad Emerg Med 2004;11(9):962–6.

[22] Fourre MW. The performance of procedures on the recently deceased. Acad Emerg Med 2002;9(6):595–8.

[23] May WF. Religious justifications for donating body parts. Hastings Cent Rep 1985;15(1): 38–42.

[24] Finegold L. Using newly deceased patients in teaching procedures [correspondence]. N Engl J Med 1995;332(21):1446.

[25] Playe SJ. Insertion of femoral-vein catheters for practice during cardiopulmonary resuscitation [correspondence]. N Engl J Med 2000;342(18):1368.

[26] Manifold CA, Storrow A, Rodgers K. Patient and family attitudes regarding the practice of procedures on the newly deceased. Acad Emerg Med 1999;6(2):110–5.

[27] Alden AW, Ward KLM, Moore GP. Should postmortem procedures be practiced on recently deceased patients? A survey of relatives' attitudes. Acad Emerg Med 1999;6(7): 749–52.

[28] McNamara RM, Monti S, Kelly JJ. Requesting consent for an invasive procedure in newly deceased adults. JAMA 1995;273(4):310–2.

[29] Olsen J, Spilger S, Windisch T. Feasibility of obtaining family consent for teaching cricothyrotomy on the newly dead in the emergency department. Ann Emerg Med 1995;25(5): 660–5.

[30] Abramson N, de Vos R, Fallat ME, et al. Ethics in emergency cardiac care. Ann Emerg Med 2001;37(Suppl):S196–200.

[31] Council on Ethical and Judicial Affairs, American Medical Association. Performing procedures on the newly deceased for training purposes. Policy E-8.181, issued December 2001. Available at: http://www.ama-assn.org/ama/pub/category/8509.html. Accessed March 23, 2005.

[32] Society for Academic Emergency Medicine. Performing invasive procedures for teaching purposes on newly deceased patients [position statement]. Approved January 2004. Available at: http://www.saem.org/newsltr/2004/mar-apr/statemnt.pdf. Accessed March 23, 2005.

[33] Bureau of Justice Statistics, US Department of Justice. Prison statistics. Summary findings. Available at: http://www.wjp.usdoj.gov/bjs/prisons.htm. Accessed March 22, 2005.

[34] Dubler NN. The collison of confinement and care: end-of-life care in prisons and jails. J Law Med Ethics 1998;26(2):149–56.

[35] Pell v Procunier, 417 US 817, 822 (1974).

[36] Estelle v Gamble, 429 US 97 (1976).

[37] Hayden JW, Laney C, Kellermann AL. Medical devices made into weapons by prisoners: an unrecognized risk. Ann Emerg Med 1995;26(6):739–42.

[38] Lessenger JE. Prisoners in the emergency department. Ann Emerg Med 1985;14(2):179–83.

[39] Parker FR Jr, Paine CJ. Informed consent and the refusal of medical treatment in the correctional setting. J Law Med Ethics 1999;27(3):240–51.

[40] Commissioner of Corrections v Myers, 379 Mass. 255, 399 NW 2d 452 (1979).

[41] Washington v Harper, 494 US 210 (1990).

[42] Riggins v Nevada, 504 US 127 (1992).

[43] Thor v Superior Court, 5 Cal. 4th 725, 855 P.2d 375, 21 Cal. Rptr. 2d 357 (1993).

[44] Report and recommendations. Research involving prisoners. Bethesda (MD): National Commission for the Protection of Human Subjects of Biomedical and Behavioral Research; 1976.

[45] Subpart C—additional protections pertaining to biomedical and behavioral research involving prisoners as subjects. US Department of Health, Education, and Welfare, 43 Fed Reg 53655 (Nov. 16, 1978).

ELSEVIER
SAUNDERS

Emerg Med Clin N Am
24 (2006) 619–631

EMERGENCY
MEDICINE
CLINICS OF
NORTH AMERICA

Ethical Dilemmas in the Care of Minors in the Emergency Department

Jill M. Baren, MD, MBE, FACEP, FAAP[a,b,c,*]

[a]Department of Emergency Medicine and Pediatrics, University of Pennsylvania
School of Medicine, Philadelphia, PA 19104, USA
[b]Department of Emergency Medicine, Hospital of the University of Pennsylvania,
Ground Floor Silverstein, HUP, 3400 Spruce Street, Philadelphia,
PA 19104, USA
[c]Division of Emergency Medicine, The Children's Hospital of Philadelphia,
Philadelphia, PA 19104, USA

A minor is an individual under the age of majority, which is defined as age 18 years in all but four states [1]. Minors commonly present to the emergency department for medical care and may present accompanied by parents or caretakers or on their own without legal guardians. A 1991 study in Michigan documented that approximately 3% of the visits by minors to emergency departments were unaccompanied [2]. More recently, this number has been estimated to be even higher by the American Academy of Pediatrics, Committee on Pediatric Emergency Medicine [3]. Minors seek care in the emergency department for a variety of reasons, which often involve complex psychosocial issues, such as sexually transmitted disease or undiagnosed pregnancy.

Adolescents in particular are considered relatively disenfranchised from the health care system, more often uninsured, and without a consistent source of primary care. Additionally, adolescence is increasingly understood as a critical development period, in which teens have the greatest morbidity and mortality from often preventable, risk-taking behaviors. Adolescents account for 10% to 15% of all pediatric emergency department visits and greater than 5% of adult emergency department visits [4]. Adolescents using the emergency department are overrepresented relative to their proportion of the population, at an age in which visits to primary care physicians are declining [4]. An analysis of the 1997 Commonwealth Fund Survey of the Health of Adolescent Girls found that 4.6% of adolescents, or 1.5 million individuals,

* Department of Emergency Medicine, Hospital of the University of Pennsylvania,
Ground Floor Silverstein, HUP, 3400 Spruce Street, Philadelphia, PA 19104, USA.
  E-mail address: jbaren@mail.med.upenn.edu

0733-8627/06/$ - see front matter © 2006 Elsevier Inc. All rights reserved.
doi:10.1016/j.emc.2006.05.002   *emed.theclinics.com*

identified the emergency department as their only source of health care [5]. For these reasons, emergency physicians must be knowledgeable about medical and psychosocial issues related to care of minors, especially adolescents.

Fundamentals of treating minors

The basic ethical issues considered in a physician-patient relationship are similar for adults and minors; some of these issues, such as consent, privacy, and confidentiality, require special consideration when the patient is a minor. These concepts are discussed subsequently as they pertain to the treatment of minors. The overall approach to the emergency care of a minor must take into account the physical, mental, behavioral, and emotional differences that exist between children and adults and between children of different ages, intellect, and developmental stages.

In all patient-physician interactions, the history is a crucial part of the emergency department visit. The emergency physician should perform a thorough psychosocial assessment of a minor seeking care for all but the most straightforward chief complaints. Often, physical complaints are found to have underlying psychosocial causes when investigated further. Several authors have recommended structured approaches to the psychosocial interview of teens [6,7]. These approaches have gained widespread acceptance among practitioners who routinely provide medical or psychosocial care to adolescents and are more commonly known as the HEADSS or SHADSSS interviews. HEADSS and SHADSSS focus on the adolescent's life at school and at home; on outside activities; and on issues of depression, substance abuse, sexuality, and safety. In general, the interview begins with the least threatening topics and moves to more sensitive issues as it progresses [7]. Table 1 summarizes HEADSS and SHADSS interview components.

Privacy and confidentiality

Several studies have identified reasons why adolescents choose the emergency department for their health care needs. The emergency department

Table 1
Components of HEADSS and SHADSSS adolescent psychosocial assessment

HEADSS	SHADSSS
Home	School
Education	Home
Activities	Activities
Drug use and abuse	Depression/self-esteem
Sexual behavior	Substance abuse
Suicidality and depression	Sexuality
	Safety

Data from Refs. [6,7].

provides relative anonymity, affords privacy, and under many circumstances offers confidential care where minors often can be treated without parental consent [4]. Confidentiality is considered one of the most important factors from the provider's and patient's perspective in treatment of adolescents [4,8]. The following discussion focuses on these two concepts.

The provision of confidential treatment of minors in the emergency department is endorsed by the American Medical Association and many medical societies, including the American College of Obstetricians and Gynecologists and the American Academy of Pediatrics [9–11]. The American College of Emergency Physicians also recognizes the importance of confidentiality in patient care, but refers to confidentiality and the care of minors as a "problem area" [12,13].

Adolescents are more likely to seek medical care and provide an accurate history if confidentiality is respected [14,15]. Adolescents should be offered the opportunity to speak privately with emergency department providers. Parents or guardians should be asked to leave the patient's room for the entire medical interview and examination if the adolescent prefers or alternatively when sensitive areas of the history are being obtained. This request must be preceded with a discussion of the availability and limits of confidentiality with adolescents and their guardians present. It should be stated clearly that the only times confidentiality may be breeched are in cases of potential injury to self (suicidality) or others (homicidality) or abuse.

Adolescence is characterized by remarkable physical and emotional changes [14]. Teens may be extremely sensitive about undergoing a physical examination. It should never be assumed that it is acceptable for parents or others to remain in the room when a physical examination is being performed. The patient should be queried about this, and their preferences should be respected. Younger adolescents may desire support persons to be present, especially during genital examinations, and this should respected as well. The key point is to allow the adolescent to have some control over the situation. In all cases, examinations should be conducted in a private room with curtains fully drawn and the doors fully closed.

There are many instances when upholding confidentiality is in the best interest of an adolescent patient and enables the emergency physician to provide the best care for the patient. In other instances, particularly in the case of younger adolescents, it may be beneficial to involve parents or guardians in the care. In still other situations, inclusion of a parent or guardian is essential to ensuring the best care for the minor. One common example is when there is a new diagnosis of pregnancy in a young adolescent. The emergency physician should try to work with the teen to determine how to discuss the diagnosis with a parent or guardian. If the adolescent does not wish to make this disclosure, the physician may offer to do so after gaining permission from the adolescent. Involving a social worker to help with the discussion and follow-up also is useful.

When the emergency department visit is concluded, there still may be confidentiality issues to consider. A plan for relaying follow-up test results should be established before discharge to prevent an unintended break of confidentiality by leaving messages on answering machines or with caretakers who were unaware of the emergency department visit in the first place [16]. This may involve the use of mobile phones or pagers or asking the teen to call at a particular time. Issues related to payment for emergency services also may lead to an unexpected breach of confidentiality. Some minors present the family insurance card when they seek care in the emergency department; they should be informed that their parents or caretakers may learn of the visit when an itemized bill is sent to the insured party.

Despite the best attempts to respect and preserve confidentiality during the medical care of minors, it is difficult to extend that protection to written medical records. Although the same basic framework regarding confidentiality of care applies to the documentation of that care, disclosure of medical records may be subject to legal requirements that attempt to balance the interests of adolescents with the interests of their parents [17]. The laws vary from state to state on this issue. In some states, minors have the right to decide whether to release medical records that pertain to the specific care that they may consent for (see further discussion subsequently). In other states, parents may be able to seek a court order to force the release of records. What may happen in a practical sense is that a hospital may release records to an authorizing parent without seeking the permission of the minor. It is imperative that emergency physicians be aware of this possibility and know their specific state laws on this issue.

Consent

Informed consent for medical care is a basic requirement that should be met from the outset of almost all physician-patient relationships. Informed consent may be performed easily when the patient is a mature, competent adult. Potential legal and ethical conflicts arise when the patient is a minor. In general, minors are not legally permitted to give consent for their own care based on their level emotional maturity and cognitive development. Consent for minors is obtained through parents or legal guardians with the presumption that those individuals would use a "best interest standard" when making decisions. Parental consent is generally expected when a minor seeks medical care, but there are numerous exceptions to this requirement. Consent is considered to be implied in the emergency treatment of a minor. It is assumed that the patient is not legally competent to give consent for himself or herself, and that the situation constitutes an emergency, although the criteria for defining an emergency are neither uniform nor universal. Although it is obvious that lifesaving care should be instituted without consent, treatment that may lessen pain or prevent disability in the near or distant future also may be considered to fall under the realm of emergency care [3,18,19].

There are many other situations for which minors may seek and be granted health care without parental consent, such as testing and treatment for sexually transmitted diseases including human immunodeficiency virus (HIV), contraceptive services, substance abuse treatment, and mental health evaluation and treatment [1,3,18,20,21]. These also vary according to state with respect to the provision of confidential care for these situations. Specific consent regulations for all 50 states can be found in the 2003 Guttmacher report on public policy [1]. Another group of minors who may give their own consent for medical care are known as *emancipated minors*. Emancipated minors possess characteristics that show some degree of independence [3,16,18–21]. Emancipated minors include minors who are married, serving in the military, living apart from parents with financial independence, pregnant, or parents themselves. The definition of emancipation varies from state to state. Individual state government websites are excellent resources for this information. Finally, another category of minors permitted to consent to their own medical care are mature minors [3]. Mature minors are generally 14 years old or older and are considered to have the capacity to understand the risks, benefits, and treatment options of their medical condition and to be able to give consent for evaluation and treatment of the condition [22]. In deciding whether or not a minor qualifies as a mature minor, the emergency physician should consider the acuity and severity of the illness and the risks and benefits of treatment.

Special situations

Drug and alcohol testing

Parents may bring minors to the emergency department requesting drug or alcohol testing. There are some situations in which emergency department testing for these substances is appropriate, such as when the goal is referral for treatment for substance abuse. It is expected that under these circumstances, the adolescent would give informed consent for the testing to be performed. Involuntary testing in an adolescent who is capable of providing informed consent is not approved or recommended by the American Academy of Pediatrics [23]. There is no obligation on the part of an emergency department to screen for drug or alcohol use in a minor based on parental request. In the author's emergency department, such requests are not honored; drug and alcohol testing are only prompted by medical, behavioral, or psychiatric emergency conditions. Parents should be given a referral to a primary care physician for a more in-depth assessment of the adolescent's situation when such requests occur. Testing may be performed without the minor's consent when prompt identification of a specific drug could be lifesaving. Occasionally, drug testing is performed in the emergency department when mandated by law in criminal investigations [24]. In this latter instance, the specimens collected must follow a "chain of custody" standard initiated by law enforcement officials, to be admissible as evidence in courtroom proceedings.

Sexually transmitted diseases

Numerous issues need to be considered in the care of a patient whose chief complaint raises the likely diagnosis of a sexually transmitted disease [25]. These issues include privacy, when and how to involve a parent or other support person, the possibility of sexual abuse, the potential need for treatment of a partner, and referral for HIV testing. The possibility of sexual abuse prevents the maintenance of confidentiality. It is also possible that adolescents in this situation may never have had a pelvic examination and may not be aware of what this examination entails. It is often beneficial to have a supportive parent present for the pelvic examination, especially if it is the first such examination. For an adolescent who initially does not wish to have her parent present for the pelvic examination, the physician should take the time to discuss the issue further in the hope of providing the patient with as much support as possible.

The issue of emergency department follow-up is also a major concern. When a teen is diagnosed with a sexually transmitted disease, it is vital to make every attempt to arrange for testing and treatment of his or her partner or partners. Physicians should encourage the teen to be honest with a partner about the need to seek care, or physicians may offer to contact the patient's partner with the patient's permission. Any teen diagnosed with a sexually transmitted disease in the emergency department should be considered for referral to a primary care or anonymous site for HIV testing.

Pregnancy

When it is determined that a minor is pregnant, she has emancipated minor status and may provide consent for her own medical care. There are several, frequently conflicting issues to consider in the case of pregnancy in minors: (1) the diagnosis of pregnancy, (2) how it should be communicated to the adolescent, and (3) the need for further emergent care owing to a pregnancy-related complication. Legal support exists for the private discussion of pregnancy with a minor, which is strongly encouraged, especially if confidentiality was agreed on at the beginning of the visit. Although the inclusion of a parent in discussions related to the diagnosis of pregnancy is often in conflict with the promise of confidentiality, the involvement of a parent or caretaker is generally believed to be beneficial. The emergency physician first must discuss with and have agreement from the minor regarding the specific information to be shared.

Many adolescents do not want their parents to know they are sexually active. They may fear that this will cause disappointment, frustration, or anger and may lead to punishment or abuse by the parent. It is imperative that the physician be sensitive to these possibilities and work to identify a mature, responsible support person who can be included in care [26]. If harm or abuse of the minor is suspected in the wake of a pregnancy disclosure, this information should be kept confidential. Social workers, if available, may help clarify the situation and to arrange a disposition that ensures the safety of the patient.

Sexual abuse or assault

Physicians are legally and ethically mandated to report all cases of suspected abuse of minors [17,22,27]. This mandate should be explained to minors in clear understandable terms. Alleged sexual abuse or assault should be evaluated with a complete history, physical examination, and supporting diagnostic tests. Documentation should be thorough and include direct quotations from the patient. If the patient presents within 72 hours of an alleged assault, specimens should be collected via a rape kit to maintain the evidentiary standard for prosecution. When a prepubertal minor presents with alleged sexual abuse to an emergency department that is not accustomed to caring for such a patient, the best treatment is expedient referral to a center with specialty services for this type of evaluation and care.

End-of-life issues in minors

Each year in the United States, approximately 53,000 children die as a result of congenital conditions, acquired illness, or trauma [28]. Of these, the most likely deaths to occur in an emergency department are traumatic deaths. Almost 17,000 children die each year from traumatic injuries [28]. A vast array of ethical issues surrounds the process of resuscitation in children. In the early stages of resuscitation, when little to no data are available, the emergency physician should be concerned primarily with the restoration of circulation and life of the patient. As additional data are gathered, medical decision making can be broadened to include new information, such as the underlying condition of the patient and the likelihood of survival. An important but often overlooked part of the resuscitation process is the need for lessening the guilt of survivors and providing a sense of closure. This involves developing important skills for incorporating into resuscitation protocols recognition of futility, procedures for stopping resuscitation, and communicating with families.

When a child is dying as a result of a chronic illness, such as cancer, muscular dystrophy, cystic fibrosis, or other previously diagnosed condition, the goals of care may be unclear on presentation to the emergency department and may cause difficulty for the staff. Advance directives are a mechanism for a patient to formulate and communicate health care preferences. Advance directives were not intended to be written by or used for children, at least from a legal perspective. For most children who come to the emergency department, the goal is to save lives; however, in some children, all the best curative efforts do not succeed. Often, when given the opportunity, chronically ill children speak at length about their feelings and what they know. If a child does wish to discontinue life-prolonging therapies, the child's experienced-based knowledge allows one to consider them informed and appropriate decision makers. Many children who have lived with life-threatening illnesses or the sequelae of injuries do have this expertise, perhaps with a stronger base in reality than the adults around them.

Many health care providers have never confronted the death or dying of a child. Physicians, nurses, social workers, chaplains, and others may lack the skills to engage in these conversations. A belief that children do not or should not die often results in an extremely aggressive pursuit of a highly improbable or impossible cure. As with end-of-life decisions in adults, providers must weigh the burdens against the benefits to the child. Even in the emergency department, this information must be conveyed accurately and comprehensively to children and families.

For certain children, the goals of care must shift from cure to comfort. Dying children often have a high symptom burden, and when they come to the emergency department, palliative care must be considered [29]. Fears and lack of information often result in children's pain being undertreated [30,31]. In most cases, optimal pain management does not interfere with an assessment of level of consciousness. The American Academy of Pediatrics, the Canadian Pediatric Society, and the American Pain Society have developed guidelines for the management of pain and stress in neonates, children, and adolescents [30,31].

Abnormal bereavement for survivors can be precipitated by the mishandling of events surrounding a child's death. To facilitate a family's recovery, the following postmortem activities have been suggested: (1) News of a patient's death should be delivered by a physician. (2) Parents should be offered the option and even encouraged to view the body to help them accept the child's death. (3) The child's clothing should be returned even if it first needs to be used as part of the investigation of the cause of death. (4) A physical memento, such as a lock of hair or a mold or print of the child's hand should be provided. (5) A follow-up phone call from the emergency physician or other staff member to offer support to the family should be strongly considered [32]. These activities can be time-consuming, but could be accomplished by a few dedicated individuals. Although the impact of such practices on bereavement and long-term coping by survivors has not been studied, they may at least contribute significantly to the perception that the emergency department, the hospital, and its providers are caring entities.

Minors as human research subjects

Children are viewed as an especially vulnerable population in the context of human research. The Declaration of Helsinki in 1964 was the first document to account explicitly for the protection of children in research [33]. In 1979, the Belmont Report closely followed suit and made recommendations that highly influenced current federal regulations for research with children [34]. These regulations are described in four categories as outlined in Table 2 and are collectively known as Subpart D of the federal regulations [35]. Subpart D provides guidance for investigators and institutional review boards in determining the risk of a child's participation in research.

The effectiveness of the regulations has been under scrutiny because of the difficulty in determining what constitutes actual risk. The definition of risk may not be the same in children as in adults. The perspective of a child may include concerns not usually attributed to adults, such as discomfort, fright, separation from parents, and effect of study interventions on growth and development [36]. There also has been controversy surrounding the terms *parental permission* and *consent*, which are commonly used interchangeably, but which have distinctly different meanings [22]. Because only a competent person of legal age may give consent, parents cannot give consent, but rather give "permission" on behalf of their children [22]. Assent is another important concept for emergency researchers to become familiar with. Assent is the active affirmation of participation by the research subject. Assent should be obtained from any child who is competent

Table 2
Four categories of federal regulations for research with children

Category	Degree of risk/prospect of benefit	Necessary conditions to be met
45 CFR 46.404	No greater than minimal risk	A, B, C
45 CFR 46.405	Greater than minimal risk/prospect of direct benefit	A, B, C, D, E
45 CFR 46.406	Greater than minimal risk/no prospect of direct benefit	A, B, C, F, G, H
45 CFR 46.407	Research not otherwise available	A, B, C, I, J

A—IRB approval

B—Child's assent

C—Informed consent for at least 1 parent or guardian

D—Risk is justified by anticipated benefit to subject

E—Anticipated benefit is at least as favorable as available alternatives

F—Risk represents only a minor increase over minimal risk

G—Study is likely to yield generalizable knowledge about child's disorder or condition, which is vital to understanding or ameliorating that disorder or condition

H—Intervention or procedure that child experiences is reasonably the same as those in child's actual or expected medical, dental, psychological, social, or education situation

I—IRB believes research presents a reasonable opportunity to further the understanding, alleviation, or prevention of a serious problem affecting the health or welfare of children

J—Approval from Secretary of DHHS after consultation with panel of experts in pertinent fields and after opportunity for public review and comment

Abbreviations: DHHS, Department of Health and Human Services; IRB, institutional review board.

From Burns JP. Research in children. Crit Care Med 2003;31:S131–6; with permission.

to understand, and this is defined by the American Academy of Pediatrics as the intellectual age of 7 years [22]. It may be waived in studies in which the child's participation may be of such benefit that the child's welfare would be compromised by failing to obtain assent [22].

In 2004, the Institute of Medicine issued a report entitled, "The Ethical Conduct of Clinical Research Involving Children," which was based on the recommendations of a 14-member expert panel [37]. The panel affirmed that the federal regulations were in general appropriate for children, and identified that the main problems were insufficient government guidance on interpretation, compliance, and variability in investigator and institutional review board interpretations. The report offers suggestions that are worth reviewing before designing and performing clinical research that includes children.

Case presentation

A 15-year-old boy with progressive muscular dystrophy presents with intractable pain secondary to extremity contractures. He has no cognitive deficits and has had normal intellectual development. The patient is fully alert but nonambulatory. He is ventilator dependent with a tracheotomy and is able to communicate verbally. He does not have any fever or signs of infection, but complains repeatedly of severe pain. His parents request admission because pain medication has not been effective at home. They are guarded in discussing their son's prognosis. From the patient's neurologist, the emergency physician learns that the patient has been deteriorating rapidly with worsening cardiomyopathy. He is expected to die within several months. Although several discussions have taken place with the patient and his family, no formal "do not attempt resuscitation" order has been written. The neurologist describes the family as "difficult" and recommends the patient be discharged home with pain medication. The patient asks his parents to leave during the interview, then expresses that he does not want his parents to speak for him and requests that all medical decisions be directed toward him. He specifically states that if he has a cardiopulmonary arrest, he does not want to be resuscitated.

The immediate priority for this patient is the relief of his pain and suffering. Because there is no apparent life-threatening issue, discussions about other treatment options and goals of care can occur after the patient is made comfortable. Because of his status as a minor, the patient's parents are officially his legal decision makers. Presumably, they are acting in his best interest, but this should be fully explored. The patient also may be considered a mature minor because he is expected at his age to be able to understand his condition and should be included in all decisions about his care. The fact that he has been dealing with his chronic illness makes him more likely to have an accurate understanding of his situation. The issue of creating a do not attempt resuscitation order should be revisited with this patient by his continuing care physician. The emergency physician should reassure the patient that his pain and other symptoms will be treated immediately and that he will be involved in medical decision making. The results of this discussion should be relayed to the neurologist, and appropriate arrangements should be made for continued pain relief. The patient's parents also must take part in this discussion to facilitate a better understanding of their child's wishes and of his medical prognosis.

Summary

Many important ethical issues surround the care of minors in the emergency department. As a rule, minors are considered to lack capacity for medical decision making, and standard surrogate decision makers are parents and other legal guardians. There are exceptions, however, that allow the minor to give consent for his or her own medical care; these vary considerably from state to state. For these reasons, it is imperative for an emergency physician to be aware of the laws in his or her practice location. Treatment of an emergency condition in a minor also may proceed without consent. In addition to complying with established legal policies, emergency physicians have a duty to respect confidentiality and privacy in minors when indicated. An understanding of these issues in the care of a minor may help avoid improper administrative procedures and may improve care and patient satisfaction.

References

[1] Boonstra H, Nash E. Minors and the right to consent to health care. Guttmacher Rep Public Policy 2000;3:4–8.
[2] Treloar DJ, Peterson E, Randall J, et al. Use of emergency services by unaccompanied minors. Ann Emerg Med 1991;20:297–301.
[3] American Academy of Pediatrics, Committee on Pediatric Emergency Medicine. Consent for emergency medical services for children and adolescents. Pediatrics 2003;111:703–6.
[4] Ziv A, Boulet JR, Slap GB. Emergency department utilization by adolescents in the United States. Pediatrics 1998;101:987–94.
[5] Wilson KM, Klein JD. Adolescents who use the emergency department as their usual source of care. Arch Pediatr Adolesc Med 2000;154:361–5.
[6] Clark LR, Ginsburg KR. How to talk to your teenage patients. Contemp Adolesc Gynecol 1995;winter:23–7.
[7] Cohen E, Mackenzie RG, Yates GL. HEADSS, a psychosocial risk assessment instrument: implications for designing effective intervention programs for runaway youth. J Adol Health 1991;12:539–44.
[8] Melzer-Lange M, Lye PS. Adolescent health care in a pediatric emergency department. Ann Emerg Med 1996;27:633–7.
[9] AMA Council on Scientific Affairs. Confidential health services for adolescents. JAMA 1993;269:1420–4.
[10] American College of Obstetricians and Gynecologists. ACOG statement of policy: confidentiality in adolescent health care. Washington (DC): American College of Obstetricians and Gynecologists; 1988.

[11] American Academy of Pediatrics. Guidelines for health supervision III. Elk Grove Village (IL): American Academy of Pediatrics; 1997.

[12] American College of Emergency Physicians. Patient confidentiality. Ann Emerg Med 1994; 24:1209.

[13] Larkin GL, Moskop J, Sanders A, et al. The emergency physician and patient confidentiality: a review. Ann Emerg Med 1994;24:1161–7.

[14] Schmidt MR, White LK. Internists and adolescent medicine. Arch Intern Med 2002;162: 1550–6.

[15] Ford CA, Millstein SG, Halpern-Felsher BL, et al. Influence of physician confidentiality assurances on adolescents' willingness to disclose information and seek future health care: a randomized controlled trial. JAMA 1997;278:1029–34.

[16] Tsai AK, Schafermeyer RW, Kalifon D, et al. Evaluation and treatment of minors: reference on consent. Ann Emerg Med 1993;22:1211–7.

[17] Society for Adolescent Medicine. Confidential health care for adolescents. Position paper of the Society for Adolescent Medicine. J Adolesc Health 1997;21:408–15.

[18] Kassutto Z, Vaught W. Informed decision making and refusal of treatment. Clin Pediatr Emerg Med 2003;4:285–91.

[19] Guertler AT. The clinical practice of emergency medicine. Emerg Med Clin N Am 1997;15: 303–13.

[20] Jacobstein CR, Baren JM. Emergency department treatment of minors. Emerg Med Clin N Am 1999;17:341–52.

[21] Kuther TL. Medical decision-making and minors: issues of consent and assent. Adolescence 2003;38:343–58.

[22] American Academy of Pediatrics, Committee on Bioethics. Informed consent, parental permission, and assent in pediatric practice. Pediatrics 1995;95:314–7.

[23] American Academy of Pediatrics, Committee on Substance Abuse. Testing for drugs of abuse in children and adolescents. Pediatrics 1996;98:305–7.

[24] English A. Treating adolescents: legal and ethical considerations. Med Clin N Am 1990;74: 1097–112.

[25] American Academy of Pediatrics, Committee on Adolescence. Sexually transmitted diseases. Pediatrics 1994;94:568–72.

[26] American Academy of Pediatrics, Committee on Adolescence. Counseling the adolescent about pregnancy options. Pediatrics 1998;101:938–40.

[27] American Academy of Pediatrics, Committee on Child Abuse and Neglect. Guidelines for the evaluation of sexual abuse of children. Pediatrics 1991;87:254–60.

[28] Children's International Project on Palliative/Hospice Services (ChIPPS) Administrative/ Policy Workgroup of the National Hospice and Palliative Care Organization. A call for change: recommendations to improve the care of children living with life-threatening conditions. National Hospice and Palliative Care Organization. Available at: www.nhpco,org. Accessed May 3, 2002.

[29] Wolfe J, Grier HE, Klar N, et al. Symptoms and suffering at the end of life in children with cancer. N Engl J Med 2000;342:326–33.

[30] American Academy of Pediatrics and Canadian Paediatric Society. Prevention and management of pain and stress in the neonate. Pediatrics 2000;105:454–61.

[31] American Academy of Pediatrics and American Pain Society. The assessment and management of acute pain in infants, children, and adolescents. Pediatrics 2001;108:793–7.

[32] Aherns WR, Hart RG. Emergency physicians' experience with pediatric death. Am J Emerg Med 1997;15:642–3.

[33] World Medical Association Declaration of Helsinki. Ethical principles for medical research involving human subjects. Available at: http://www.wma.net/e/policy/. Accessed June 25, 2005.

[34] Belmont report. Available at: http://www.hhs.gov/ohrp/humansubjects/guidance/45cfr46.htm. Accessed June 23, 2005.

[35] 45 CFR 46 Subpart D: Additional DHHS protections for children involved as subjects in research. Available at: http://www.hhs.gov/ohrp/humansubjects/guidance/45cfr46.htm. Accessed June 30, 2005.
[36] Burns JP. Research in children. Crit Care Med 2003;31:S131–6.
[37] Chesney RW. Children as clinical research subjects. J Pediatr 2005;146:579–80.

ELSEVIER
SAUNDERS

Emerg Med Clin N Am
24 (2006) 633–656

EMERGENCY
MEDICINE
CLINICS OF
NORTH AMERICA

Privacy and Confidentiality in Emergency Medicine: Obligations and Challenges

Joel Martin Geiderman, MD[a,b,*],
John C. Moskop, PhD[c], Arthur R. Derse, MD, JD[d,e]

[a]*Ruth and Harry Roman Emergency Department, Department of Emergency Medicine,
Cedars-Sinai Medical Center, Los Angeles, CA 90048, USA*
[b]*Cedars-Sinai Center for Health Care Ethics, Burns and Allen Research Institute,
Los Angeles, CA 90048, USA*
[c]*Department of Medical Humanities, The Brody School of Medicine at East Carolina
University, Bioethics Center, University Health Systems of Eastern Carolina,
600 Moye Boulevard, Greenville, NC 27834, USA*
[d]*Center for the Study of Bioethics, Medical College of Wisconsin, 8701 Watertown Plank
Road, Milwaukee, WI 53226-0509, USA*
[e]*Department of Emergency Medicine, Medical College of Wisconsin, 8701 Watertown Plank
Road, Milwaukee, WI 53226-0509, USA*

Consider the following scenarios:

You have been asked to participate on a team that will design your new emergency department to accommodate an ever-increasing patient load. Space is limited. As you embark on your assignment, what are the considerations that must be given to privacy and confidentiality? How do you balance the need to take care of the most patients in the most efficient manner with the patients' right to confidentiality and privacy?

A member of your Board of Trustees with a daughter who is an aspiring actress on television has just landed a guest appearance on *ER*. The trustee would like to know if his daughter can observe several of your shifts in the emergency department to prepare for the role. What is your response?

You receive a call from a pharmacist and discover that a prescription you have written for hydrocodone has been altered from 6 pills to 60. When you try to call this patient to discuss this with him, you are told that he is an airline pilot and he is out of town. What is the proper course of action?

---

* Corresponding author. Cedars-Sinai Medical Center, 8700 Beverly Boulevard, Los Angeles, CA 90048, USA.
E-mail address: Geiderman@cshs.org (J.M. Geiderman).

0733-8627/06/$ - see front matter © 2006 Elsevier Inc. All rights reserved.
doi:10.1016/j.emc.2006.05.005   *emed.theclinics.com*

A distraught and overwrought mother calls your emergency department in search of her 21-year-old daughter who resides at home but hasn't returned at the usual time. The patient is unconscious from a suspected overdose at a rave party and is under your care. What should you tell this mother?

Your Chair inquires about a patient you saw the other night who is the Chair's next-door neighbor. How much information should you share?

Respect for privacy and confidentiality have been professional responsibilities of physicians throughout recorded history [1]. References to these are found in the Hippocratic Oath, religious texts, and virtually all modern Codes of Ethics [2]. The federal Health Insurance Portability and Accountability Act (HIPAA) privacy rules implemented in 2003 focused significant attention on privacy and confidentiality, but these are hardly new concepts or expectations. These duties are affirmed not only in the United States, but also internationally. Virtually all physicians are taught from the time they enter medical school that there is a sacred duty to "protect the patient's secrets" [3].

Despite these obligations, there are daily challenges to protecting privacy and confidentiality in the unique setting of the emergency department. The brief scenarios at the beginning of this article illustrate a few of the dilemmas that arise hundreds, if not thousands, of times a day in US emergency departments. To meet these challenges as they arise, the emergency clinician must have a firm understanding of the moral and legal underpinnings of the duties to protect privacy and confidentiality. In addition, it is important to understand the limits of these duties. This article focuses on these issues, examines some of the challenges that are presented in the emergency department, offers practical advice, and suggests solutions to common problems.

Privacy versus confidentiality

This article addresses issues of privacy and confidentiality. Although the concepts of privacy and confidentiality are closely related, and the two terms are often used interchangeably, several differences between them are worth noting. *Privacy* is the broader of the two concepts; it has at least four primary uses—physical seclusion, protection of personal information ("informational privacy"), protection of one's personal identity, and the ability to make choices without interference [4]. In relationship to the notion of physical seclusion, privacy is the right to a zone of personal space, and access to that space is controlled by the person who holds the right to it. Related to this right is the human instinct for modesty—the desire to protect one's intimate body parts (defined differently in various cultures) from being exposed against one's will, consent, or knowledge.

The concept of *confidentiality* is narrower in scope; it refers to the protection of personal information and, in the context of medicine, the duty not to disclose information that has been conveyed to the health care professional without the patient's approval. Confidentiality is synonymous with informational privacy. This article addresses issues of the physical privacy of patients and of the confidentiality of patients' personal information. Decisional privacy, the ability to make and act on one's personal choices (related to the bioethical principle of autonomy), is also an important concept in emergency medicine; it is addressed elsewhere in this issue in the article by Dr. Moskop entitled "Informed Consent and Refusal of Treatment: Challenges for Emergency Physicians."

Foundations

Moral foundations and limits of privacy and confidentiality

The concept of human dignity has a long history in philosophy and ethics [5]. Simply stated, to respect human dignity is to recognize that human beings have special, intrinsic moral worth, and one should act with careful consideration for their interests, goals, and choices. Among the basic interests of individuals are control over one's physical environment, including protection from unwanted intrusion by others into one's personal space, and control over one's personal information, including protection of that information from unwanted disclosure to others. By protecting these basic human interests in physical privacy and confidentiality, physicians show respect for the dignity, autonomy, and well-being of their patients. The nearly universal recognition in medical oaths and codes of ethics of duties to protect patient privacy and confidentiality is a powerful indicator of the moral significance of these concepts.

Without a significant measure of control over their physical environment and their personal information, human beings would be severely hampered in their ability to make and act on important life decisions, such as the ability to make decisions about medical treatment for a major illness. By protecting physical privacy and confidentiality, physicians enable their patients to exercise meaningful personal autonomy.

Finally, open communication between patients and physicians is essential to an effective therapeutic relationship. Physicians need to know about patient health behaviors and symptoms and need to conduct intimate physical examinations to formulate accurate diagnoses and to provide effective therapy. To disclose sensitive and potentially embarrassing personal information and to permit intimate physical examination, patients must trust that their physicians will keep that information confidential and protect them from any unnecessary or inappropriate bodily exposure. The etymology of the English term *confidentiality* suggests this expectation because it is derived from the Latin word *confidere,* "to trust" [6]. By protecting physical privacy and confidentiality, physicians establish a relationship of trust that promotes effective therapy and maximizes patient well-being. This relationship of trust also encourages patients to seek health care, without fear or apprehension, when they need it.

Privacy and confidentiality are important moral values in health care, but they are not always the most important values. Instead, moral principles, practical exigencies, and legal rules typically recognize and dictate that, in specific circumstances, privacy or confidentiality may be overridden by even more important moral considerations. Protecting physical privacy and confidentiality are best understood as *prima facie* duties, that is, duties that must be honored unless there exists a stronger conflicting moral duty [7]. Duties that may conflict with respect for privacy or confidentiality include duties to act expeditiously to provide benefit and protect the patient from harm, to protect third parties, and to obey the law. When *prima facie* duties conflict in a particular situation, physicians may confront difficult moral judgments about which duty should take precedence; this results in the classic ethical dilemma. To reach a conclusion and resolve the dilemma, physicians must consider the reasons for and against alternative courses of action, such as the magnitude and probability of benefits and harms expected from the different alternatives, and choose the best overall course of action.

Religious foundations of privacy and confidentiality

Privacy is a paramount value in the Jewish tradition. In the Torah, Bilaam, an enemy prophet of the ancient Jewish people, on seeing a Jewish encampment from a hilltop perch declared, "How goodly are your tents, O Jacob!" (Numbers 24:5). The Talmud explains that the tents of the Jewish people are goodly because they are carefully arranged so that no looks into his neighbor's dwelling [8]. Jewish law asks people to avert their gaze if they see someone engaging in a private activity, even an innocent activity that is not being concealed. The Talmud is replete with even a construction code of sorts that includes specifications on how windows should be placed and how walls between neighbors should be built. Neighbors were to be as careful as possible not to look at each other's activities in their common courtyard.

The Old Testament Book of Genesis calls attention to the human instinct for modesty in some of its earliest verses (Genesis 3:10). Adam and Eve discovered their nakedness in the Garden of Eden and sought to shield themselves even from God. Orthodox Judaism also demands a strict dress code that emphasizes modesty.

Confidentiality is emphasized in Jewish law as well, as exemplified by laws that forbid gossip and by the biblical admonition, "Thou shalt not go up and down as a talebearer among the people." Nondisclosure of private facts is also a requirement (described in numerous commentaries and regulations) as in the proscriptions against disclosing judicial deliberations or reading someone else's mail.

Christianity also emphasizes these values [9], as does Islam, which places a particularly high priority on modesty. Any tradition that respects life, liberty, and personal integrity should place a high value on privacy and confidentiality and should respect and honor modesty.

Legal rights and limits of privacy and confidentiality

Federal constitutional law

The US Constitution does not explicitly mention a right to privacy. Late in the nineteenth century, however, an influential and oft-cited law review article by Warren and Brandeis [10] argued that inherent in the Constitution was a fundamental right of privacy, a right to be left alone in one's person and property. The US Supreme Court eventually recognized the concept of the right of privacy in the mid-twentieth century, when the court inferred a right of privacy from the "penumbra" of other rights in the constitution (the 1st, 3rd, 4th, 5th, 9th, and 14th amendments) protecting persons and property from government intrusion [11]. This right of privacy was seen as limiting the ability of government to regulate medical choices, including reproduction. In this regard, the evolution of the constitutional right of privacy was curtailed late in the twentieth century when the court looked not to this right, but instead looked to the liberty interest of the 14th Amendment's due process clause to delineate the ability to refuse medical interventions [12].

In 1998, in *Wilson v Lane* [13], the Supreme Court ruled that a lawsuit for invasion of privacy could be brought against reporters who accompanied police into a suspect's home during the filming of a television show. This ruling could be relevant to intrusion cases involving commercial filming activities in emergency departments.

*State confidentiality and privacy laws and legal
sanctions for breach or disclosure*

Because of their special role as patient fiduciaries, physicians possess highly personal information that their patients have entrusted to them. Physicians who disclose confidential information without permission to unauthorized individuals may be liable for the tort of breach of confidentiality. This tort is recognized as a breach of the special fiduciary role that physicians assume in caring for patients. Physicians have been held liable for breaches of confidentiality for unauthorized disclosure of patient information [14].

Not all disclosure of health care information is subsumed under the physician-patient relationship. If an unauthorized individual breaks into a physician's confidential files and obtains patient information, that individual would not be held liable for breach of confidentiality because the patient information was never given in confidence to that individual. Instead, the individual could be liable for the tort of invasion of privacy.

State common law and statutes have long recognized a tort of invasion of privacy [15]. The form of the tort of invasion of privacy that applies to medical privacy is that of intrusion on seclusion. One who intentionally intrudes on the private affairs or concerns of another may be liable for invasion of privacy, if the intrusion would be highly offensive to a reasonable person

[16]. This tort may apply to situations such as filming a patient without the patient's permission.

Additionally, state statutes restrict access to medical records to individuals who need access to treat the patient and individuals who may need access for health care quality improvement or for regulatory purposes. These laws typically provide civil penalties for unauthorized access. State statutes also may give a higher degree of protection to certain kinds of medical information; examples include HIV test results, genetic test results, and mental health records.

There are also state regulations administered by licensing boards that judge breach of confidentiality as a professional violation subject to medical administrative sanctions. State laws have recognized confidentiality of information obtained in the medical encounter to be so important as to make an exception so that such information may be privileged, and a defendant may prevent a physician from testifying about the information in a court of law, the so-called testimonial privilege.

Federal statutory law—HIPAA

New federal privacy regulations authorized by HIPAA went into effect April 14, 2003. These regulations apply to all US practitioners and health care institutions that electronically transmit statutorily defined protected health information (PHI) [17]. They apply to virtually all US emergency physicians because of the electronically based modern emergency practice environment that includes patient registration, medical records, and billing systems.

PHI is defined as individually identifiable health information that is transmitted by or maintained in any other form or medium, and that relates to past, present, or future physical or mental health or conditions of an individual; the provision of health care to an individual; or the payment for the provision of health care [17]. PHI includes names and any information that identifies or reasonably could be believed to identify an individual, including unique identifying numbers, such as Social Security numbers, medical record numbers, and health plan numbers [18]. Items considered PHI are listed in Box 1.

HIPAA requires practitioners and institutions to adopt and implement privacy policies and procedures, and to notify individual patients of their privacy rights, including information on how their information is used or disclosed [19]. Generally, HIPAA requires patient permission for information disclosure, although patient consent is not required for disclosure of personal health information for purposes of treatment, payment, and health care operations. HIPAA also provides exceptions to the requirement for patient consent for disclosures that are legally required, such as judicial or administrative proceedings, or as required by abuse, neglect, or domestic violence reporting; public health purposes; research; and worker's compensation proceedings.

Box 1. Protected health information

a. Names
b. All geographic subdivisions smaller than a state, including street address, city, county, precinct, zip code and equivalent geocodes except for the initial 3 digits of a zip code if, according to current census data, the geographic unit formed by combining all zip codes with the same three initial digits contains more than 20,000 people, and the initial three digits of a zip code for all geographic units containing 20,000 or fewer people are changed to 000
c. All elements of dates (except year) for dates directly related to an individual, including birth date, admission date, discharge date, date of death, and all ages over 89 and all elements of dates (including year) indicative of such age except that such ages and elements may be aggregated into a single category of age 90 or older
d. Telephone numbers
e. Fax numbers
f. Electronic mail addresses
g. Social Security numbers
h. Medical record numbers
i. Health plan beneficiary numbers
j. Account numbers
k. Certificate/license numbers
l. Vehicle identifiers and serial numbers, including license plate numbers
m. Device identifiers and serial numbers
n. Web Universal Resource Locator (URL)
o. Internet protocol address number
p. Biometric identifiers, including finger or voice prints
q. Full-face photographic images and any comparable images
r. Any other unique identifying number, characteristic or code

From Department of Health and Human Services. 45 CFR (Code of Federal Regulations), 164.514 (a) (b). Standards for Privacy of Individually Identifiable Health Information, 2002.

For violations of HIPAA, sanctions for disclosures made in error range from $100 for each violation to a maximum of $25,000 per year. Criminal penalties for intentional or malicious disclosure range from $5000 to $250,000 and from 1 to 10 years imprisonment [20].

The practical effect of HIPAA in the emergency department has been to eliminate patient names and identifiers from easily viewed areas, such as patient wall rosters and status boards; to require passwords and the ability to audit access to patient information systems; and to require patient permission for disclosure of information to individuals who call to seek information about the patient. HIPAA regulations allow disclosure without patient consent when an emergency exists or the patient lacks decision-making capacity, and the physician determines that sharing information with a family member or other individual is in the best interest of the patient [21]. The HIPAA regulations are the most extensive and uniform standards affecting the privacy practices of emergency physicians, and they are expected to continue to influence the way emergency physicians use and transmit confidential patient information.

Legal limits of privacy—state statutes and common law

There are limits to the legal protection of confidentiality, including long-standing exceptions in state laws for the purpose of protecting the public health. This is true for infectious diseases, including sexually transmitted diseases. Patients diagnosed with tuberculosis, meningitis, or gonorrhea may have confidential information disclosed to state public health officials to warn others who may be at risk for these diseases as a result of patient contact.

Other state statutes require physicians to report confidential information to protect patients and the public from violence. Statutes require the reporting of patients who are suspected to be victims of child abuse and require or permit the reporting of domestic and elder abuse. Many states have statutes that require the reporting of gunshot wounds or wounds suspected to be the result of a violent crime.

State laws also provide for some special situations where traditional protections for confidentiality may be suspended, such as employees who submit for physical examinations for worker's compensation claims, where employees may not be able to restrict their employer from finding out information material to the purposes of the examination.

Even the testamentary privilege is not absolute. In some states, defendants cannot assert the testamentary privilege in homicide trials. These states have balanced the need to protect patient confidentiality against the countervailing values of societal protection and criminal punishment for capital crimes.

The duty to protect individuals at risk for infectious disease was extended to a duty to protect individuals from other risks of patients in the landmark Tarasoff case [22]. In this case, a psychiatrist was found liable for not warning a woman who was at risk of harm from the psychiatrist's patient and was ultimately killed by the patient. The court held that the duty of confidentiality ends where public peril begins. The duty to warn, later expanded to the duty to protect, extends to "third parties," individuals who are not the physician's patient. The physician is now recognized to owe a duty to such third parties who may be at risk from the physician's patient. Many state courts have adopted the Tarasoff reasoning. The challenge for the emergency physician is to protect patient confidentiality while balancing the duty to protect the public and to warn and protect third parties at risk.

Clinical considerations and applications

Design

Today, many emergency departments are vestiges of a recent time when emergency medicine did not even exist as a unique specialty. In the 1970s, "emergency rooms" arose out of hospital "receiving wards," where unsophisticated and ill-equipped ambulances or police cars delivered sick and injured patients to large spaces (or wards), separated by curtains, to be cared for by interns with little experience or training. In those days, even much inpatient care was delivered in large wards (multiple bays, sometimes separated by curtains) rather than in semiprivate or private rooms. As a result of this history, the spaces in which emergency department care is being provided in many hospitals in the twenty-first century do not reflect any real planning for current patient needs or any semblance of respect for privacy.

Newly designed emergency departments should address the privacy needs of patients just as elsewhere in the hospital. Because real estate is an expensive or limited commodity in most locations, there may be a temptation to sacrifice privacy to meet other goals, such as maximizing the number of beds or for ancillary needs. Difficult choices may arise in designing emergency departments, and practical solutions should balance all needs as equitably as possible. It would do no good to maximize the number of private rooms if one knows a priori that this would result in other patients being cared for in hallways. A multipatient bay out of public view would be preferable. Even when space is readily available, the nature of emergency department care requires that at least some patients—the most acutely ill—need to be in a space where staff can see them easily. A special problem arises in the triage area, where patients need to give their medical history privately, but the triage nurse also may need to watch for other patients who are arriving. By its nature, the waiting room may compromise confidentiality, especially for well-known individuals; dividing the waiting room into various sections may help mitigate this.

Optimal design includes a maximum number of individual treatment rooms, usually arrayed around a central nurses' station. One effective design uses rooms with three solid walls and a fourth wall comprising sliding glass doors [23]. This design maximizes acoustic and visual privacy (a curtain can be pulled behind the doors for privacy to achieve the latter). Rooms should be large enough to accommodate at least one seated visitor. Trauma bays, which may be designed to treat more than one patient, should have curtains to separate the gurneys and to avoid exposure of an unclad patient to individuals who are not involved in the trauma resuscitation (eg, police, visitors).

Many emergency departments in the United States are experiencing overcrowding, often as a result of inadequate inpatient capacity, especially monitored beds. When overcrowding occurs, there may be no alternative other than to board multiple patients in the same bay or to place patients in hallways, where they may have to wait for long periods. Under these circumstances, movable privacy screens should be deployed as often as possible, especially when performing procedures, such as electrocardiograms [24]. Other measures—some as simple as positioning of gurneys that must be in hallways so as not to face each other—also should be taken to minimize unnecessary exposure.

It may take years, if ever, for institutions to build adequate emergency department and inpatient capacity to relieve the current crowding. The situation is likely to get worse as financially weak hospitals close their emergency departments or entire facilities, and the population grows and ages. Individual physicians can help relieve this problem by being efficient, using resources including time-consuming diagnostic procedures judiciously, and minimizing other wait times when possible.

Observers

In many institutions, students may appropriately observe and learn in the emergency department environment. Observation of and participation in clinical care are essential aspects of medical education. Because the presence of students in the emergency department serves socially valuable educational functions, most institutions consider general consent to treatment in a teaching institution sufficient to constitute consent to treatment and observation by students. Often acknowledgment of this consent is buried somewhere in the "conditions of admission" forms patients sign during registration. Some authors have stated that explicit consent should be obtained from patients for the presence of students [25]. Most patients agree to the participation of students in their own medical care despite potential threats to their privacy [26–30]. When possible, patients should be informed of the identity and role of all caregivers, including residents, interns, and students. Although consideration should be given to patient requests that students not participate in their care, it need not be guaranteed that such requests be honored. Decisions should be based on practicality and reasons for the request.

Others sometimes may request permission to observe care in the emergency department. Some examples of other potential observers include high school students considering health careers, chaplains, pharmaceutical representatives, journalists, and actors. Whether or not these individuals should have access to the treatment area at all is open to question because the potential for breech of privacy is inherent in the design of any emergency department. In general, the greater the potential benefit to society, the more lenient in granting permission one can be. By this standard, permitting actors or pharmaceutical representatives to observe in the emergency department is probably not justified. For observers who do not play a role in medical care, the patient's consent should be obtained. For patients unable to consent, a "reasonable person" test may be used to determine whether it is morally permissible for an observer to be present by asking the question, "Would a (hypothetical) reasonable person object to the presence of the observer?"

Visitors

Visitors may provide important comfort and support to patients in the emergency department. It also should be recognized, however, that certain visitors may be unwelcome to the patient. Emergency physicians should allow visitors into patient care areas only with the permission of the patient, although there is a reasonable assumption of consent when a patient arrives accompanied by a friend or family member. For patients unable to consent, a surrogate ideally should give permission before allowing visitors, although common sense should prevail. Next of kin generally are allowed to see uncommunicative patients by reasonable request and after proper identification. While in the clinical area, visitors should be instructed to remain in the room with (or at the hallway bedside of) the patient they are visiting. Visitors should be restricted from unauthorized areas of the emergency department, where they inappropriately may observe other patients or PHI [24].

Law enforcement

Law enforcement officials at times are appropriately present in clinical areas. They may be present in the emergency department by staff request to provide physical protection to emergency department staff, patients, and visitors from a potentially violent patient or visitor. Law enforcement officials also may transport injured or ill patients to the emergency department from the scene of an accident or crime. They may play a role in the collection of forensic evidence, interviews, or other aspects of investigation of a potential crime. Each of these activities may justify the presence of law enforcement officials in the emergency department, yet also may threaten the privacy of emergency department patients. Unless acting under legal mandates (eg, court orders), law enforcement officials generally should visit or observe emergency department patients only with their permission [31]. Law enforcement activities should not be allowed to interfere with patient care. As with other visitors, law enforcement officials should not be allowed unauthorized access to PHI of other emergency department patients.

Commercial filming and videotaping

The issue of the commercial filming of patients in hospitals has come to the fore as a result of the proliferation of reality television shows that are based on this practice [32–40]. Emergency medicine and its practitioners have been in the vanguard with regard to participation in these programs and efforts to regulate and control them. Controversy exists as to the acceptability of filming patients in the emergency department in critical situations or without their permission, although the preponderance of opinion now seems to be against this practice.

Commercial filming usually, but not always, is for programs that fall into the reality television category, which aim to capture the drama and terror associated with patients who arrive in the emergency department during life-threatening or limb-threatening injuries or illnesses, or with sensational or gory presentations (eg, a limb that has been caught in a cement mixer). Some authors have called into question the appropriateness of even approaching such patients for permission to be filmed [32,40]. Even if the patient does consent, the validity of consent and whether it can be considered informed under such circumstances is suspect. Emergency department patients also may feel obliged to consent and may be subject to coercion by television personnel who are bound by a different sense of duty and ethics than are physicians.

Some producers, with the permission of participating hospitals, have adopted the practice of filming patients before obtaining permission but not broadcasting the film unless the patient subsequently grants permission. Critics of this approach point out that by the time the patient is asked to grant consent (or refuse), their privacy already has been violated by the presence of the film crew within an area where the patient has a "reasonable expectation" of privacy [32]. In addition, there are no assurances that others would not view the film or that it would not otherwise be misused in the future.

Proponents who defend the practice of filming emergency department patients in the foregoing fashion argue that these shows serve an educational role and help demystify medical care [34]. They also argue cynically that privacy and confidentiality are routinely violated in the emergency department, and filming simply can be viewed as an extension of this practice and is acceptable.

In more recent years, medical societies and regulatory bodies have taken positions that recommend sharp curtailment or elimination of commercial filming in emergency departments. The American College of Emergency Physicians (ACEP) policy states that "ACEP discourages the filming of television programs in emergency departments except when patients and staff members can give fully informed consent before their participation" [41]. The Society for Academic Emergency Medicine (SAEM) takes a stronger stand, saying, "Image recording by commercial entities does not provide benefit to the patient and should not occur in either the out-of-the-hospital or emergency department setting" [42]. An American Medical Association (AMA) Code of Ethics opinion also requires prior consent of the patient for filming except when the patient is "permanently or indefinitely incompetent" [43]. A 2004 Joint Commission on Accreditation of Healthcare Organizations standard requires that "consent is obtained for recordings or filming made for purposes other than the identification, diagnosis, or treatment of the patients" [44]. Finally, lawsuits may have a chilling effect on commercial filming in emergency departments, as several hospitals and producers have been sued for invasion of privacy in relationship to such filming.

Mandatory reporting

Mandatory reporting laws require health care providers to report specific confidential information to governmental agencies or authorities. Mandatory reporting laws exist to cover the following types of circumstances: (1) to protect a patient from further harm caused by a perpetrator; (2) to protect members of the general public from harm by a violent/criminal act, an accidental injury, or a communicable disease; (3) to help law enforcement solve crimes or prevent future crimes; or (4) for epidemiologic and statistical purposes.

Mandatory reporting of criminal acts in an attempt to protect other potential victims is noncontroversial in most cases, especially for extremely violent acts or when there is a specific threat. Disclosure to law enforcement officials is permissible under certain circumstances, including in response to legal orders, such as court orders, warrants, or subpoenas, to assist in the identification or location of a suspect, fugitive, witness, or missing person, or when responding to a law enforcement official's request for information about a crime victim. Disclosure also is permissible and sometimes required when a person's death may be the result of criminal activity, when PHI may be evidence of a crime that occurred on hospital property, or when necessary to inform officials about the nature of a crime or the location of victims or the perpetrator [45].

Reporting of infectious diseases and various types of injuries or deaths has historical precedence and in most cases, is noncontroversial. The Centers for Disease Control and Prevention maintains a Public Health Information Network, which contains data regarding national reportable conditions. National reportable infectious conditions are listed in Box 2. States regulate the reporting of certain conditions to public health officials. Although there is some variation in conditions that mandate reporting, certain conditions are commonly recognized as reportable conditions. Examples of widely recognized reportable conditions include traffic crashes, penetrating trauma, residential fires, occupational injuries, suicide, falls, poisoning, and drowning. Although these disclosures may be considered breaches of physician-patient confidentiality, they may honor duties to maintain public health and the safety and protection of other individuals and groups.

Mandatory reporting of certain types of suspected abuse is morally justified and widely accepted in the United States. Examples include elder abuse and child abuse, both of which involve vulnerable individuals who are not in a position to defend themselves. In these cases, adopting a paternal stance (ie, acting *in loco parentis*) rather than honoring autonomy is appropriate and justified to prevent harm.

Laws mandating the reporting of seizures and domestic violence engender more controversy [46–48]. The ethical dilemma in both situations is whether

Box 2. Nationally notifiable infectious diseases

AIDS
Anthrax
Arboviral neuroinvasive and non-neuroinvasive diseases
Botulism
Brucellosis
Chancroid
Chlamydia trachomatis, genital infections
Cholera
Coccidioidomycosis
Cryptosporidiosis
Cyclosporiasis
Diphtheria
Ehrlichiosis
Enterohemorrhagic *Escherichia coli*
Giardiasis
Gonorrhea
Haemophilus influenzae, invasive disease
Hansen's disease (leprosy)
Hantavirus pulmonary syndrome
Hemolytic uremic syndrome, postdiarrheal
Hepatitis, viral, acute
Hepatitis, viral, chronic
HIV infection
Influenza-associated pediatric mortality
Legionellosis
Listeriosis
Lyme disease
Malaria
Measles
Meningococcal disease
Mumps
Pertussis
Plague
Poliomyelitis, paralytic
Psittacosis
Q fever
Rabies
Rocky Mountain spotted fever
Rubella
Rubella, congenital syndrome
Salmonellosis

Severe acute respiratory syndrome–associated coronavirus
(SARS-CoV) disease
Shigellosis
Smallpox
Streptococcal disease, invasive, group A
Streptococcal toxic shock syndrome
Streptococcus pneumoniae, drug-resistant, invasive disease
S pneumoniae, invasive in children <5 years old
Syphilis
Tetanus
Toxic shock syndrome
Trichinellosis (trichinosis)
Tuberculosis
Tularemia
Typhoid fever
Vancomycin-intermediate *Staphylococcus aureus*
Vancomycin-resistant *S aureus*
Varicella (morbidity)
Varicella (deaths only)
Yellow fever

From Centers for Disease Control. Nationally Notifiable Infectious Diseases, United States, 2005. Available at http://www.cdc.gov/epo/dphsi/PHS/infdis2005. htm. Accessed April 16, 2005.

it is acceptable to breach the confidentiality of patients who do not want these conditions reported in an effort to prevent harm to them or other members of society. Proponents of reporting domestic violence, which is mandatory in a few states, believe that it is justified to stop this scourge and to protect vulnerable victims—either the one in question or a potential different future victim. Proponents who argue for mandatory reporting of seizures do so to limit the dangers of someone having an automobile accident as the result of a seizure, causing serious injuries or death to themselves or others. An argument in common against reporting in both of these situations is that they may discourage people from seeking care when they need it or not being open and honest about their conditions if they do [46]. In the case of domestic violence, victims may fear or actually experience retaliation from abusers. Other unwanted consequences could be family separation, loss of a job, deportation, or other outcomes that may be less acceptable than solutions that could be worked out without police involvement. In the case of seizures, critics of mandatory reporting argue that the risk of having an accident above baseline is minimal, and that the loss of driving privileges that can follow reporting can have severe consequences on someone's life, such as compromised ability to work, loss of independence, social isolation, limited participation in the community, and diminished self-worth [48]. At present, there is no consensus in the ethics community over these two issues. The ACEP has issued a policy statement opposing mandatory reporting laws for domestic violence.

Duty to warn

As previously stated, physicians have a duty to warn individuals or groups when information indicates that they are at significant risk of harm posed by a patient. This duty to warn has been upheld in multiple cases by US courts. National policies including those written by the AMA and ACEP and language in HIPAA also recognize that disclosure of PHI may be appropriate in cases in which there is a potential threat to the public or to an individual [49–52]. This may include disclosure to individuals or law enforcement officials [53]. Based on the authors' collective experience, this duty to warn seldom applies in the emergency department setting, however. A rare example is the patient described in this article's introduction, the airline pilot who had altered his prescription for a controlled substance. In this case, involving law enforcement is morally justified.

Communication

Requests for information

Emergency physicians frequently receive requests for patient information. Such requests may be from interested parties by telephone, e-mail, or in person. Such inquiries for patient information raise important questions regarding confidentiality. The most important task in such situations is to obtain permission from the patient to disclose information. If patients are agreeable to such disclosures, physicians are permitted to release information. Ideally, the identity of the inquiring individual should be confirmed. Institutions should maintain policies for responding to inquiries, including mechanisms for obtaining patient consent for release of information and for ascertaining the identity of the caller (eg, by returning a telephone call) [54,55]. Unless the caller's identity is established, and the patient or a surrogate gives consent for release of information, telephone inquiries for individual patient information generally should not be honored. Occasionally, the limited release of information over the telephone may be justified (eg, relatives may be entitled to basic information about loved ones who are unable to communicate, when travel to the emergency department is not possible). In these cases, the "patient's best interest" standard should be applied. Even in such unusual circumstances, efforts should be made to identify the caller and to release only essential information.

Requests for patient information from the media may be encountered. Generally, media requests should be handled by the hospital's public relations department, who should divulge information only with patient permission. Some institutions confirm that a particular patient has been transported to the hospital and may provide information about the patient's general condition (eg, "critical," "stable"). Patient permission for release of this information should be obtained when possible. Inquiries by law enforcement officials should be handled in accordance with legal requirements.

Communication among health care providers

Communication within the emergency department, although essential, increases the risk of breaches of patient confidentiality. This increased risk often begins in the waiting room, where patients may be interviewed by the triage nurse within auditory range of others, or when waiting patients or family members are called by name to be brought back to the treatment area. Confidentiality also may be compromised accidentally when patients are discussed by name in open spaces in the emergency department or when caregivers are on the telephone. Care must be taken to avoid this accidental compromise of confidentiality. It is also important that charts and other written materials are not left out in the open, where visitors can see them. White grease boards, or "status boards," that display the names of patients and their chief complaints to keep track of them, previously a common staple in emergency departments, are no longer allowable. In many departments, these have been replaced by computerized tracking systems that serve the same purpose. These tracking systems need to be situated so as not to be visible to the public and should have log-on and time-out features.

Communication with health care providers outside of the emergency department, when necessary, is permitted and even essential. An obvious example would be conversations with the patient's physician, consultants, or residents. Such communication should occur in appropriate secure settings and not in open spaces such as hallways, dining areas, stairwells, or elevators [56]. Conveying patient-specific information (or dictating charts) over the telephone should be done in a secure space where the conversation cannot be overheard.

Conveying information that is nonessential or to individuals without a need to know is not permissible. In emergency medicine, there is often an urge to discuss cases involving well-known figures or sensational stories with colleagues, friends, or relatives. Such discussion is legally and morally wrong. It is also important not to discuss the care of hospital employees with supervisors or other employees within the hospital without the patient's permission.

Habitual patient files

It is a long-standing and common practice for emergency departments to keep files of patients who are suspected of seeking drugs—most often opiates or benzodiazepines—for nontherapeutic purposes, including recreation, abuse, or resale [57]. Such files have been termed *habitual patient files* (HPFs). Less appropriate and in some cases pejorative terms for these files include "frequent flyer files," "repeater files," "turkey files," "kook books," and "special needs files." Despite the facts that some think it is unwise to maintain such files, and their efficacy in altering patient behavior has never been established, their common use mandates an examination of the confidentiality issues arising from their existence.

In the event that a decision is made to establish and maintain an HPF in a particular department (a decision that should be made or sanctioned by the Chair and others in authority), emergency physicians should be familiar with state and federal laws that regulate their use. It is recommended further that a hospital or other health care attorney with expertise in confidentiality issues should be consulted to ensure that a particular process conforms to these laws.

HPFs are permissible and may be justified if the goals of using them include protecting patients from harm as the result of drug abuse, preventing the inappropriate use of valuable emergency department resources, or protecting society from harms caused by the resale of ill-gotten drugs or the actions of intoxicated individuals [24]. HPFs also may contain specific treatment plans, usually worked out in advance with managing physicians, for patients with chronic pain conditions. Such plans may contain instructions as to which drugs are permissible or not permissible to use or have other details of "contracts" worked out with patients and their pain managers.

Under HIPAA and other regulations, it is permissible for physicians to share PHI with other physicians for the purposes of treatment. Other members of the health care team also may be permitted access to patient information on a need-to-know basis. In general, such sharing should occur within a single institution. PHI should not be shared between institutions via the telephone or other means. Inappropriate release of information contained in HPFs could result in fines or other penalties.

HPFs should be kept in a secure location, preferably locked, and should be viewed in private. Access should be limited to authorized personnel who have a need to know, and browsing of the file should not be permitted. One of the authors has previously described an electronic HPF (stored on a server) with password protection and the ability to access the files from many sites within a single department [57].

Electronic communication devices

Telephone answering machines, fax machines, personal computers, e-mail, personal digital assistants, and cell phones all present challenges to confidentiality. Telephone messages regarding culture results, addenda, or other information should not be left on answering machines, which may be accessed by others. The patient should be asked to call back and should be able to identify himself or herself with appropriate information when calling back. Also, to ensure adequate privacy and that a patient feels comfortable conversing, speaker phones should not be used by either party unless mutually agreed on during the call.

Fax machines also pose risks. A fax should be sent only when one is reasonably sure that it will be received in a secure location by an authorized party. Departmental fax machines that receive faxes also must be kept in a secure location. If reports are periodically automatically faxed or e-mailed to patients' private physicians, databases must be maintained to be sure contact information is kept up to date.

When information containing PHI is sent via a personal computer, personal digital assistant, or e-mail, it must be encrypted if it passes beyond a secure firewall. All devices should be set to require a password to log on and should time-out when not in use.

Cell phones offer busy emergency physicians the ability to communicate more efficiently and can reduce the amount of walking during a busy shift. Care must be taken, however, not to discuss patients by name when not in a private location. Cell phones with concealed digital cameras in them present risks to privacy and confidentiality. Use of these devices by patients or staff to record a patient's images or information about them, especially covertly, is unethical. It may be useful to post signs forbidding the use of these devices for these purposes in the emergency department waiting room and treatment areas.

Research and education

Research

Research often requires the use of PHI. The use of PHI for research and educational purposes is restricted, however, by HIPAA. If PHI can be deidentified, specific written consent is unnecessary for the use of such information. If the use of PHI is necessary, specific written consent for research use should be obtained. In certain sensitive research areas, such as genetics, a certificate of confidentiality may be a useful tool to relieve researchers from any obligation to release identifying information about research subjects [58]. Various techniques for unlinking research records from identifying information have been used successfully to protect privacy of research subjects [59].

Noncommercial photography

Patient images may serve valid and useful functions in research and education. Images may be used to contribute to documentation, diagnostic tests, treatment, and quality assessment; for education of health professionals and the public; and for research purposes. Each of these uses has different objectives and slightly different standards for consent for use.

Images used for documentation of medical care may contribute directly to patient welfare. Standard institutional measures to protect the medical record from inappropriate access should be sufficient to protect the confidentiality of such images. The use of teleradiology has raised important issues about privacy and security issues. The use of PHI in this setting must conform to HIPAA standards, including appropriate encryption of data and security standards for access to PHI [60].

Patient images also may be used for quality improvement and medical education, such as the practice in some emergency departments of videotaping trauma resuscitations [61–65]. Although such images may be valuable to improving patient care, the patients taped typically do not benefit directly from their own taping and may be unable to consent to the taping. Most institutions consider the use of such images for educational purposes to be acceptable, however, provided that only health professionals directly involved in the practices under analysis and in the quality assessment process have access to these images. The HIPAA privacy rule does not require specific patient authorization for using patient information for quality improvement purposes. Some institutions have chosen to provide general notification of such practices, such as signs posted in the emergency department or information in general patient consent documents.

Several organizations have developed policies to provide guidance regarding the use of patient images. A policy developed by the AMA asserts that "informed consent should be obtained before filming whenever possible. If it is not possible to obtain consent from the patient before filming, then consent must be obtained before the film is used for educational purposes" [66]. This AMA policy allows surrogate consent for the use of a film only in the case of minor children or permanently incompetent adults. This policy does not specify whether patient consent should be written or verbal. A position statement by the SAEM states, "Image recording should undergo a dual consent process. The first addresses privacy issues associated with the actual recording of the image. The second addresses confidentiality issues associated with distribution and use of those images" [67]. The International Committee of Medical Journal Editors has stated that "identifying information should not be published in written descriptions, photographs, or pedigrees unless the information is essential for scientific purposes and the patient (or parent or guardian) gives written informed consent for publication" [68].

Special populations

Emergency physicians often treat patients who are unable to protect their own interests, including children, patients with mental and physical impairments, prisoners, and dying patients. These patients entrust themselves, or are entrusted by others, to the care of emergency physicians, and physicians have a duty to act in their best interests, including safeguarding their privacy and confidentiality.

A limited exception to confidentiality applies to patients who lack decision-making capacity. In caring for these patients, physicians must share information with the patient's legally authorized surrogate to obtain consent for treatment. Emergency physicians also have a responsibility to inform family members of patients who die in the emergency department about the patient's condition and treatment and to report appropriate information about the death to the proper legal authorities. For all of these patients, physicians should guard against disclosure of information to unauthorized persons.

Patients in particular dependency relationships, such as students or prisoners, also merit special protections because they may be unwilling or unable to speak up to protect themselves. This situation may present special problems when these patients are asked for permission to violate their privacy (eg, via photography) or to disclose personal information. Unless there is a compelling reason to do so that is in the patients' own best interest, they should not even be approached for permission.

Addressing the confidentiality requests of adolescent patients can raise difficult questions for emergency physicians. Adolescents may ask that their parents not be informed about their medical condition or treatment. Unless the patient is legally emancipated, however, parental consent for treatment may be required. Many states allow minors to consent to treatment for specific conditions, including pregnancy, sexually transmitted diseases, and substance abuse. In such circumstances, physicians may be required to keep confidentiality, unless they conclude that disclosure is necessary to prevent serious harm to the patient.

Summary

Ensuring and preserving patients' privacy, confidentiality, and modesty are long-standing professional obligations of physicians rooted in tradition, religion, ethics, law, and philosophy. At their core, the philosophical underpinnings of these obligations are the recognition of the dignity and worth of patients as individuals and the inherent right of human beings to control their own affairs. Despite the structural problems in carrying out these duties in the crowded, rushed, and often open environment of the emergency department, emergency personnel should strive to do so.

These duties are not absolute, and physicians and other heath care professionals should understand when it is acceptable, and even desirable, to override them because of conflicting, greater duties. In the final analysis, however, circumstances requiring a breach of confidentiality are rare, and circumstances justifying the invasion of physical privacy are even rarer.

References

[1] Moskop JC, Marco CA, Larkin GL, et al. From hippocrates to HIPAA: privacy and confidentiality in emergency medicine: Part I. conceptual, moral, and legal foundations. Ann Emerg Med 2005;45:53–9.
[2] Spicer SM. Nature and role of codes and other ethics directives. In: Post SG, editor. Encyclopedia of bioethics, vol. 5. 3rd edition. New York: Macmillan Reference USA; 2004. p. 2621–9.

[3] Canadian Medical Association. Code of ethics. Ottowa, Canada: 1998.

[4] Allen AL. Privacy in health care. In: Post SG, editor. Encyclopedia of bioethics, vol. 4. 3rd edition. New York: Macmillan Reference USA; 2004. p. 2120–30.

[5] Hailer M, Ritschl D. The general notion of human dignity and the specific arguments in medical ethics. In: Bayertz K, editor. Sanctity of life and human dignity. Dordrecht (The Netherlands): Kluwer Academic Publishers; 1996. p. 91–106.

[6] Larkin, Moskop, Sanders, et al. The emergency physician and patient confidentiality—a review. Ann Emerg Med 1994;24:1161–7.

[7] Beauchamp TL, Childress JF. Confidentiality. In: Principles of Biomedical Ethics. 5th edition. New York: Oxford University Press; 2001. p. 303–12.

[8] Spitiz E. Jewish and American law on the cutting edge of privacy: computers in the business sector. Los Angeles, CA: University papers. The University of Judaism; 1986.

[9] Horner JS. Confidentiality: Christian virtue or Christian necessity? Nucleus April 1994, p. 2–8. Available at: http://www.cmf.org.uk/literature/content.asp?context = article&id=476. Accessed May 27, 2005.

[10] Warren S, Brandeis L. The right to privacy. Harv Law Rev 1890;4:193–220.

[11] Griswold v Connecticut. 381 US 479 (1965).

[12] Cruzan v Director of Missouri Department of Health, 497 US 261, 110 SCt. 2841, 111 L.Ed.2d 224 (1990).

[13] Wilson v Lane, US 119 SCt. 1692 (1998).

[14] Humphers v First Interstate Bank of Oregon, 298 Or. 706, 696 P.2d 527 (1985).

[15] Keeton WP, Dobbs DB, Keeton RE, et al, editors. Prosser and Keeton on the law of torts. 5th edition. St. Paul (MN): West Publishing; 1984. p. 849–69.

[16] American Law Institute (ALI). Restatement (second) of torts. §652B. Intrusion upon seclusion. 1977.

[17] US Department of Health and Human Services, Office for Civil Rights. Standards for privacy of individually identifiable health information; security standards for the protection of electronic protected health information; general administrative requirements including civil monetary penalties: procedures for investigations, imposition of penalties, and hearings. Regulation text. 45 CFR Parts 160 and 164. December 28, 2000 as amended: May 31, 2002, August 14, 2002, February 20, 2003, and April 17, 2003.

[18] 45 CFR § 160.103.

[19] 45 CFR§ 164.520 (a) and (b).

[20] Pub. Law 104–191, 42 U.S.C. § 1320d-5.

[21] 45 CFR§ 164.510 (b).

[22] Tarasoff v Regents of the Univ of Cal., 17 Cal.3d 425, 131 Cal. Rptr 14, 551 P.2d 334 (1976).

[23] Barlas D, Sama AE, Ward MF, et al. Comparison of the auditory and visual privacy of emergency department treatment areas with curtains versus those with solid wall. Ann Emerg Med 2001;38:135–9.

[24] Moskop JC, Marco CA, Larkin GL, et al. From Hippocrates to HIPAA: privacy and confidentiality in emergency medicine: Part II. challenges in the emergency department. Ann Emerg Med 2005;45:60–7.

[25] Sullivan F. Intruders in the consultation. Fam Pract 1995;12:66–9.

[26] Purdy S, Plasso A, Finkelstein JA, et al. Enrollees' perceptions of participating in the education of medical students at an academically affiliated HMO. Acad Med 2000;75:1003–9.

[27] Devera-Sales A, Paden C, Vinson DC. What do family medicine patients think about medical students' participation in their health care? Acad Med 1999;74:550–2.

[28] Magrane D, Gannon J, Miller CT. Obstetric patients who select and those who refuse medical students' participation in their care. Acad Med 1994;69:1004–6.

[29] Rizk DE, Al-Shebah A, El-Zubeir MA, et al. Women's perceptions of and experiences with medical student involvement in outpatient obstetric and gynecologic care in the United Arab Emirates. Am J Obstet Gynecol 2002;187:1091–100.

[30] Ching SL, Gates EA, Robertson PA. Factors influencing obstetric and gynecologic patients' decisions toward medical student involvement in the outpatient setting. Am J Obstet Gynecol 2000;182:1429–32.

[31] American College of Emergency Physicians. Law enforcement information gathering in the emergency department. ACEP policy statement, approved September 2003. Available at: http://www.acep.org/3,33206,0.html. Accessed February 2, 2004.

[32] Geiderman JM. Fame, rights, and videotape. Ann Emerg Med 2001;37:217–9.

[33] Iserson KV. Response to fame, rights to videotape. Ann Emerg Med 2001;37:219.

[34] Iserson KV. Film: exposing the emergency department. Ann Emerg Med 2001;37:220–1.

[35] Geiderman JM. Response to film: exposing the emergency department. Ann Emerg Med 2001;37:222.

[36] Zibulewsky J. Filming of emergency department patients [letter]. Ann Emerg Med 2001;38:189.

[37] Rodriguez RM, Graham GM, Young JC. Patient and provider attitudes toward commercial television film crews in the emergency department. Acad Emerg Med 2001;38:740–5.

[38] Geiderman JM. In defense of patient privacy [letter]. Ann Emerg Med 2002;39:99.

[39] Geiderman JM, Solomon RC. Filming patients without prior consent [letter]. Acad Emerg Med 2002;9:259–61.

[40] Geiderman JM, Larkin GL. Commercial filming of patient care activities in hospitals. JAMA 2002;288:373–9.

[41] American College of Emergency Physicians. Filming in the emergency department. ACEP policy statement, approved February 2002. Available at: http://www.acep.org/1,5065,0.html. Accessed February 2, 2004.

[42] Society for Academic Emergency Medicine Board of Directors. SAEM position on filming of emergency patients. Acad Emerg Med 2002;9:251.

[43] Council on Ethical and Judicial Affairs, American Medical Association. Filming patients in health care settings. CEJA reports 3-1-01. Available at: http://www.ama-assn.org/ama/upload/mm/369/o3-1-01.pdf. Accessed March 24, 2002.

[44] Joint Commission on Accreditation of Healthcare Organizations. Comprehensive Accreditation Manual for Hospitals: The Official Handbook. Oakbrook Terrace (IL): Joint Commission on Accreditation of Healthcare Organizations; 2004. p. RI-10–11.

[45] 45 CFR § 164.512 (f).

[46] Hyman A, Schillinger D, Lo B. Laws mandating reporting of domestic violence: do they promote patient well-being? JAMA 1995;273:1781–7.

[47] Rodriguez MA, McLoughlin E, Bauer HM, et al. Mandatory reporting of intimate partner violence to police: views of physicians in California. Am J Public Health 1999;89:575–8.

[48] Lee W, Wolfe T, Shreeve S. Reporting epileptic drivers to licensing authorities is unnecessary and counterproductive [editorial]. Ann Emerg Med 2002;39:656–9.

[49] http:www.ama-assn.org/ama/pub/category/4610.htm. Accessed April 14, 2005.

[50] http://acep.org/webportal/PracticeResources/PolicyStatementsByCategory/Ethics/Patient Confidentiality.htm. Accessed June 19, 2006.

[51] Lo B, Dornbrand L, Dubler NN. HIPAA and patient care: the role for professional judgment. JAMA 2005;293:1766–71.

[52] Appelbaum PS. Privacy in psychiatric treatment: threats and responses. Am J Psychiatry 2002;159:1809–18.

[53] 45 CFR § 164.512 (j).

[54] Tammelleo AD. Staying out of trouble on the telephone. RN 1993;October 56:63–4.

[55] Morris MR. Patients' privacy on the line. AJN 1996;96.

[56] Ubel PA, Zell MM, Miller DJ, et al. Elevator talk: observational study of inappropriate comments in a public space. Am J Med 1995;99:190–4.

[57] Geiderman JM. Keeping lists and naming names: habitual patient files for suspected non-therapeutic drug–seeking patients. Ann Emerg Med 2003;41:873–81.

[58] Cooper ZN, Nelson RM, Ross LF. Certificates of confidentiality in research: rationale and usage. Genet Test 2004;8:214–20.
[59] Churches T, Christen P. Some methods for blindfolded record linkage. BMC Med Inform Decis Mak 2004;28:9.
[60] White P. Privacy and security issues in teleradiology. Semin Ultrasound CT MR 2004;25: 391–5.
[61] Ellis DG, Lerner EB, Jehle DV, et al. A multi-state survey of videotaping practices for major trauma resuscitations. J Emerg Med 1999;17:597–604.
[62] Brooks AJ, Phipson M, Potgieter A, et al. Education of the trauma team: video evaluation of compliance with universal barrier precautions in resuscitation. Eur J Surg 1999;165:1125–8.
[63] Olsen JC, Gurr DE, Hughes M. Video analysis of emergency medicine residents performing rapid-sequence intubations. J Emerg Med 2000;18:469–72.
[64] Scheinfeld N. Photographic images, digital imaging, dermatology and the law. Arch Dermatol 2004;140:473–6.
[65] Halsted MJ, Perry LA, Cripe TP, et al. Improving patient care: the use of a digital teaching file to enhance clinicians' access to the intellectual capital of interdepartmental conferences. AJR Am J Roentgenol 2004;182:307–9.
[66] http:/www/ama-assn.org/ama/pub/category/11966.html. Accessed April 18, 2005.
[67] SAEM Board of Directors. SAEM position statement on filming of emergency patients. Acad Emerg Med 2002;9:251.
[68] International Committee of Medical Journal Editors. Style matters: protection of patients' rights to privacy. BMJ 1995;311:1272.

ELSEVIER
SAUNDERS

Emerg Med Clin N Am
24 (2006) 657–669

EMERGENCY
MEDICINE
CLINICS OF
NORTH AMERICA

Research Ethics

Judy B. Shahan, RN, MBA*, Gabor D. Kelen, MD

Department of Emergency Medicine, Johns Hopkins University,
1830 East Monument Street, Suite 6-100, Baltimore, MD 21205, USA

"Most people say that it is the intellect which makes a great scientist. They are wrong: It is character." Albert Einstein

The ethical conduct of research may well have been under question since the very inception of recognizable research activities. However, until the late twentieth century, it was assumed that scientists generally were well intentioned in the conduct of research and that instances of fraud were few. Novice researchers mostly learned from experienced mentors, assimilating the practices and habits of the more seasoned scientist into their own ethical conduct, without the benefit of any standardized or regulated research practices. "This absence of norms … was symptomatic of the neglect of research ethics in the decades leading to the 1980's," according to Caroline Whitbeck in her introduction to a collection of papers on Trustworthy Research [1].

Several notable events over the course of history have helped to shape the current more ethically charged research environment. The Nuremberg Code was developed in response to the Nazi atrocities and resulted in several principles being advanced, including the need for voluntary consent of the human subject, assessment of the societal value of the experiment in relationship to the risks to individuals, and the need for qualified scientist investigators [2]. The Declaration of Helsinki, issued by the World Medical Association, is probably the most influential document governing research worldwide [3]. In addition to emphasizing the basic principles in the conduct of biomedical research, the Declaration highlights an important requirement: patients' participation in research should not put them at a disadvantage with respect to medical care. A circumstance where this is especially apparent is in the conduct of clinical trials, where there may be inherent conflict between the physician's obligations to deliver care that is in the

* Corresponding author.
E-mail address: jshahan@jhmi.edu (J.B. Shahan).

0733-8627/06/$ - see front matter © 2006 Elsevier Inc. All rights reserved.
doi:10.1016/j.emc.2006.05.013
emed.theclinics.com

best interest of the patient versus the scientist's goal of acquiring new knowledge.

During the 1960s and 1970s, several significant events demonstrating compromised human subject rights (including the Tuskegee Syphilis Study [4], the Willowbrook Study [5], and the Jewish Chronic Disease Hospital Case [6]) resulted in congressional hearings and the enactment of the National Research Act of 1974. The National Research Act created the National Commission for the Protection of Human Subjects of Biomedical and Behavioral Research, charged with formulating public policy for all matters involving human subjects. The resulting well-known Belmont Report, codified in the *Federal Register* in 1979, provides the predominant ethical framework for the conduct of human subject experimentation.

The Belmont Report articulated three guiding principles for research: respect for persons, beneficence, and justice. Respect for persons requires that the choices of autonomous individuals be respected and that people who are incapable of making their own choices be protected [7]. This principle underlies the requirement to obtain informed consent from study participants and to maintain confidentiality on their behalf [8]. The principle of beneficence requires that participation in research be associated with a favorable balance of potential benefits and harms while the principle of justice entails an equitable distribution of the burdens and benefits of research. Researchers must not exploit vulnerable people, or exclude without good reason eligible candidates who may benefit form participation in a study [8].

The US federal government became more actively involved in scrutiny of federally funded research in the late 1980s and 1990s as a consequence of the AIDS epidemic and advocacy activities of patients with HIV infection seeking access to clinical trials as a way to augment their medical care. This helped to challenge the view of research as a benefit, and turned the focus on research as a burden. Continued occasional sentinel incidents at major universities, some resulting in the death of research subjects, has caused regulators to continue to tighten controls on research institutions and investigators to provide a safe environment where research is conducted.

Originally incorporated in Massachusetts under the auspices of founding member Public Responsibility in Medicine and Research (PRIM&R), and later incorporated as a nonprofit organization in Maryland, the recently created Association for the Accreditation of Human Research Protection Programs (AAHRPP) [9] is charged to evaluate research organizations in the areas of leadership, institutional review board structure, investigator education in the conduct ethical research, and meeting the concerns of research participants. Through a voluntary process, AAHRPP will certify organizations that have met or even surpassed all federal laws and regulations governing research. Although optional, AAHRPP is rapidly becoming a standard-setting certification body.

Responsible Conduct of Research

The Responsible Conduct of Research (RCR) is composed of several elements, but is really more about the scientist's conscience rather than mere compliance with regulations. It is essentially an ethical code of conduct that scientists must adopt as they prepare for "doing the right thing" in making the variety of choices required in the execution of study protocols. Scientists must learn to distinguish between elements of scientific investigation that are matters of responsibility rather than matters of style, based on the premise of scientific integrity and the demand to do good science. The interwoven elements of RCR include the proper treatment of human and animal subjects, recognition and avoidance of conflicts of interest, management of data to ensure privacy and confidentiality, collaboration, peer review, mentorship, and scientific misconduct.

Because conducting research is a privilege and not a right, scientists are charged with upholding the public's trust. The credibility of science with the general public depends on the maintenance of the highest ethical standards in research. Many scientists feel that the attention devoted to cases of scientific misconduct is disproportionate to their importance and the rate of occurrence. But the seriousness of these events when they do occur, and the perceived limited response on the part of some academic medical centers, have generated public and governmental skepticism about the ability and willingness of the academic community to establish and enforce ethical standards.

Although scientific misconduct became a public issue in 1981 when Congress held the first hearings on the subject, it was not until August of 1989 that regulations were codified in the *Federal Register,* outlining the process for centralizing the oversight of scientific misconduct under the auspices of Office of Research Integrity (ORI) removing the obligation from funding agencies (42 CFR Part 50, Subpart A) [10]. This administrative process became complete in 1993 when the NIH Revitalization Act was signed into law, establishing the ORI as an independent entity within the Department of Health and Human Services. The role, mission, and structure of the ORI is focused on preventing misconduct and promoting research integrity principally through oversight, education, and review of institutional findings and recommendations [11].

Academic institutions that support research activities are required to uphold Public Health Service regulations to ensure that research conducted is done so within defined ethical parameters. Institutions must guarantee that an approved policy and administrative process for responding to allegations of research misconduct is in place and does so by an official assurance, generally indicated by the institutional signature placed on all submitted grant proposals.

Research misconduct is defined in the Code of Federal Regulations as fabrication, falsification, or plagiarism in proposing, performing, or reviewing research, or in reporting research results (42 CFR Part 50, Subpart A) [11].

Scientists have a responsibility to report episodes of misconduct when discovered, as this falls within the tenant of professional self-regulation essential to maintaining the public trust. Oftentimes scientists do not report their own misconduct; instead, allegations are filed by a whistleblower. Institutions investigate the complaint against the respondent, determining any appropriate actions that need to be taken, maintaining confidentiality so that whistleblowers are protected from retribution. If the allegation is not confirmed, a diligent effort is made to restore the reputation of the respondent if at all possible. Falsified allegations in and of themselves constitute an instance of scientific misconduct.

Human subject research

It is generally understood that advances in human health and welfare ultimately depend on research with human participants. At this time, at least 17 federal agencies have regulations for governing human subject research, with the primary focus on the protection of human subjects. Research involving human subjects offers potential benefits to all, yet risk only to those who participate [12]. While it is the responsibility of the researcher to protect the rights of human subjects, it is a responsibility shared among the institution, the principal investigator, and all study personnel.

The primary mechanism for institutional protection of human subjects is by way of the internal review board system. Internal Review Boards (IRBs) operate in compliance with the US Code of Federal Regulations, Department of Health and Human Services (DHHS) Title 45 Part 46 entitled "Protection of Human Subjects," as well as the Food and Drug Administration (FDA) regulations Title 21 Part 50 entitled "Protection of Human Subjects." IRBs must determine that (1) the rights and welfare of the research subjects are protected adequately, (2) the risks to subjects are outweighed by the potential benefits of the research, (3) the selection of subjects is equitable, and (4) informed consent will be obtained and, when appropriate, documented. Periodic reviews of ongoing research, usually at least annually, ensure continued protection of the welfare of human subjects. Additional approved assurance of compliance with the HHS regulations (45 CFR 46.103) [13] for the protection of human subjects from the Office for Human Research Protections (OHRP) is required for those institutions receiving funding from any agency of the US DHHS.

Consent for participation in research studies must be given freely and with full disclosure so that the participant is fully informed of the risks and benefits of study participation. Specifically, for consent to be informed, the provider must explain the potential risks and benefits to the patient, the patient must understand those risks and benefits, and the patient must make a decision that is consistent with his or her life values and goals [14]. Detailed disclosure to ensure informed consent provides many challenges to researchers practicing emergency medicine. In addition to the consent process for standard treatment, disclosure requires an explanation of the research, the research aims, the physician's interests, the uncertainty of a favorable outcome, risks versus benefits, and alternative options for treatment. Further, the potential subject needs to know that treatment will occur with or without participation and that the subject may at any time change his or her mind about participation [12].

The ethical constructs that are basic to informed consent are autonomy, beneficence, and justice. Autonomy means that individuals with the capacity to make decisions have a right to make decisions about their own health care. Given the information they need to decide to participate in a study, individuals should never be pressured to consent to participate. The principle of autonomy also requires that protection be given to potentially vulnerable populations who may be incapable of understanding the information that would allow them to make an informed decision. Children, the extremely elderly, the mentally ill, or those in disenfranchised groups such as prisoners, the homeless, or those with interpretive barriers of language or custom, number among the constituencies of the federally regulated vulnerable populace. Beneficence obligates the researcher to secure the well being of all study participants, balancing risks and benefits. Concern for the research subject must always prevail over the interests of science and society. Justice centers around who will be given the opportunity to participate in studies and who will be excluded. Given the complexity of justice, researchers must attempt at all times to distribute risks and benefits fairly and without bias.

There are circumstances, specifically when life-threatening conditions occur, where individuals lack autonomy and are unable to give informed consent or refuse enrollment. This vulnerable population requires additional protective procedures in the conduct of a research protocol. Requests for exceptions from the informed consent requirements in emergency situations are reviewed closely by institutional IRBs, who must find that the concept of preservation of life is foremost and that the area under study presents as a life-threatening emergency for which current treatment is unproven or unsatisfactory. Known as emergency research circumstances, regulations are promulgated in the Final Rule, published in 1996 in the *Federal Register*, stipulating that the researcher must attempt to contact the legal representative of the patient within a predefined therapeutic window; that prestudy consultation with the community from which the patients will be enrolled will occur; public disclosure about the research must happen before and at the conclusion of the study; and that surveillance of the project is undertaken by an independent data safety management board, including the FDA investigational new drug or device (IND/IDE) process [15].

Privacy and confidentiality

Confidential information is both private and voluntarily imparted in confidence and trust. Confidentiality prevents disclosure of information that was originally disclosed within a confidential relationship. An infringement of a person's right to confidentiality occurs only if the person (or institution) to whom the information was disclosed in confidence fails to protect the information or deliberately discloses it to someone without first-party consent [14].

In contrast, someone who accesses confidential information without authorization violates rights of privacy. Privacy stems from the right to be left alone and the respect for autonomy, allowing an individual to restrict information about him or her or access to his or her body. Once a researcher has collected information (data) about an individual as a consequence of informed consent, the researcher has an obligation to protect the confidentiality of the information collected.

Data can be defined as measurements, observations, or any other primary products of research activities. These provide a factual basis for inference, conclusions, and publications. Integrity of data starts with planning for data collection in the study design period and is ultimately the responsibility of the principal researcher. Because fabrication and falsification of research results are serious forms of scientific misconduct, accurate and unbiased record keeping is essential. Clear and complete records of how data were acquired should allow for the replication of the research process by reviewers and researchers alike, and provide a permanent reference useful to the researcher as analysis, sharing of data, and publication preparations proceed. Requirements for secured storage of data files at the project conclusion vary from institution to institution, but fall within the range of 3 to 7 years.

From a legal perspective, data collected over the course of a study are the property of the institution and not the researcher, but access to the data by the study group should be unencumbered by the institution. Even though products of work by employees of an institution are the property of that institution, researchers do have ownership rights when intellectual property and patentable discoveries are involved. University patent and copyright policies generally allow for the sharing of revenues from licensing, sale, or royalties between the inventor(s) and the institution.

In addition to primary responsibilities outlined above, researchers are further regulated by "HIPAA," the acronym for the federal legislation titled Health Insurance Portability and Accountability Act of 1996, put into place to protect the privacy of an individual's health information (data) and to essentially secure an individual's health information that is sent or stored electronically (as in the case of financial billing information) [16]. An addendum to the legislation, known as the Privacy Rule, was put in place in 2000 to primarily affect health care providers who transmit electronic transactions covered by the HIPAA regulations, health plans and health care clearinghouses, but it has had an impact on the conduct of research that involves data from human subjects. Researchers must now provide supporting documentation that outlines the plan to meet the requirements, conditions, and limitations imposed by the Privacy Rule. Individuals participating in research must provide written authorization for the use of their protected health information (PHI) for study purposes. This authorization is often incorporated within the informed consent document, adding several paragraphs specific to information privacy and security. De-identified health information is not PHI, and thus is not protected by the Privacy Rule. Researchers are granted a waiver of the authorization requirement when using de-identified data for projects such as a limited data set with a data use agreement, preparatory to research, and for research on decedents' information. However, the Rule identifies 18 specific variables considered as potential identifiers, and all must be absent to comply [16].

Privacy also extends to stored tissue samples, which can be any archived human biological materials (blood, DNA, organs, and other tissues). Repositories can be established to collect, store, and distribute human tissue materials for research, and are subject to IRB reviews. According to the Common Rule, research using previously collected samples that contain no personal identifiers to link the sample with the person from whom it came can proceed without the informed consent of subjects [17]. However, for those samples with identifying and clinically relevant information, researchers are faced with deciding whether to recontact subjects to obtain informed consent, which itself presents problems, or to strip all identifying data associated with the samples, which may limit the value of the research results.

Randomized clinical trials (RCTs) present complex data management issues, particularly related to the timely determination that a new intervention has an acceptable risk-benefit profile for enrolled patients. In these cases, independent Data Safety Monitoring Boards (DSMBs) play a significant role in advising researchers about the safety outcomes of the clinical trial as it progresses. In blinded studies this group is the only one not blinded to the actual treatment groups. DSMBs have authority to discontinue RCTs when board members agree that it is unethical to continue, either because the new intervention is harmful, or because it is clearly superior to comparison arms. Statistical monitoring procedures assist the DSMB in repeatedly inspecting outcome data while controlling for false claims for treatment benefit or harm [18]. Rules for stopping trials early either for reasons of benefit or harm are usually predetermined before patient enrollment.

Animal research

Before subjecting humans to experimentation, studies are often conducted on animals to ensure reasonable safety when human trials are entertained. Animals are used for research because of the similarities between the physiological systems of humans and various species of animals, and to date, there are no feasible safe alternatives that would be able to completely replace the use of animals in research. While there are many viable nonanimal research models in use, many require supplementation with animals to provide results that are able to be translated into useful interventions for humans.

The Animal Welfare Act, initially passed by Congress in 1966 and most recently amended in 1985, governs the care and use of research animals [19]. Administered by the US Department of Agriculture (USDA), it outlines stringent standards of care for the treatment of research animals and includes housing, feeding, cleanliness, ventilation, potential pain, and veterinary care. Both private and public institutions are mandated to have Animal Care and Use Committees (IACUC) in place to monitor animal care and charged to establish a research review board to ensure that approved research protocols adhere to the federal guidelines for the appropriate and humane use of animals. Institutions are subject to unannounced USDA inspections and compliance audits. Additionally, the "Guide for the Care and Use of Laboratory Animals" issued by the Public Health Service has set forth detailed animal care standards that must be met in order for institutions and investigators to be eligible to receive National Institutes of Health (NIH) funding. These guidelines apply to species such as rats, mice, and birds, not covered by the USDA regulations. The scientific community advocates the highest quality animal care and treatment not only because animal usage is deemed a privilege, but also because well-treated animals will provide more reliable scientific results. Humane considerations are focused on the avoidance of pain and aggressive medical management to alleviate pain, along with the defined euthanasia polices and practices promulgated by the American Veterinary Medical Association [19].

It is generally accepted, but a largely ignored practice for sponsors to require that scientists look at alternative methods to using animals, and to prove that proposed research protocols cannot be done without the use of animals. Experiments using animal models are also closely scrutinized to determine if the projected results are needed to increase the body of knowledge of the topic under investigation. It is the experience of at least one of the authors (G.D.K.) that these tenets are loosely applied at best, and then so with great bias.

The use of animals in research is not solely for the benefit of human health. Veterinary care continues to advance as a result of biomedical research as evidenced by the fact that animals routinely receive antibiotics, vaccinations, and other treatments that improve upon the quality of animals. Again, this is usually more for the benefit of agribusiness then out of consideration for animal welfare.

Conflict of interest and conflict of commitment

In academia, a researcher's primary duty is to produce objective, fact-based results and ensure the safety of human research subjects. Conflicts of commitment arise when outside activities interfere with obligations to students, colleagues, and the primary missions of the academic institution.

These conflicts are usually tied to an overcommitment of effort, often with the consequence of compromising university policy. Often young faculty overcommit to activities not directly related to academic development as a way of augmenting their salaries. Often this impinges on time that institutions rightly assert should be dedicated to career development. At the other end of the spectrum, more seasoned academicians resist investing their time in mentoring (often with limited funding potential), and instead seek outside activities that would result in additional sources of income. Again, if overdone, institutions do not consider this as fulfilling the scope of an academic position.

Researchers are required to formally report the time they spend on work-related activities, including patient care, research, administrative responsibilities, and teaching, for which their employer (ie, university) provides compensation. This federally mandated system of cost principles outlined in OMB Circular A-21 allows institutions to certify to granting agencies that the effort charged or cost shared to each award has actually been fulfilled [20]. It also provides researchers with an accurate summary of how they are spending their time, useful as a tool for determining appropriate goals for professional development.

Conflicts of interest are generally financial in nature, but it is plausible that interests other than financial could compromise the conduct of research. Examples of nonfinancial interests that may cause conflict include the pressures of career advancement, the drive to publish, the need to secure more projects and funding by enrolling marginally eligible patients, and seeking power and prestige. However, most personal interests do not necessarily result in conflicting circumstances.

Examples of financial situations that represent conflicts of interest are stock ownership in the sponsor of a protocol, receipt of consulting fees from the manufacturer of a study drug or device, or positions on sponsor boards. Conflict often extends when interests are held by family members. Relationships such as these may lead to bias (deliberately or not) in the conduct or interpretation of study results, and could ultimately impact on the safety of human subjects enrolled in biomedical and behavioral research. Even when researchers are truly not influenced by such interests, just the appearance of a conflict of interest may lead the public to believe research is less reliable, a misleading notion that may not be easily remediated even if the potential conflict is resolved.

While institutions are federally mandated to detect and manage financial conflicts, researchers have a professional responsibility to recognize and manage potential conflicts in line with institutional policies and procedures. Conflict of interest committees are charged with reviewing and ruling on actual, potential, or apparent situations that may include royalties and licensing income, equity (stock and ownership interests), income/payments, management or Board of Director positions, and relevant financial interests of family members. Evaluation parameters are used to assess potential risks and focus on the integrity of research data, rights and safety of human subjects, rights of students and trainees involved, availability of research results for use in the public interest, and the very appearance of a conflict of interest. The committee will then make a determination if the conflict of interest can be managed and consequently the research allowed to proceed. Oftentimes one or more conditions will be imposed upon the investigator and can include requiring stock holdings to be liquidated or put into escrow, limitations on the role of the conflicted investigator (eg, preclusion from being a principal investigator), and mandated neutral party oversight of the study conduct. Additionally, terms of public disclosure by the conflicted investigator are required in all publications, presentations, and grant and contract agreements.

Publication, authorship, and academic freedom

Nearly all aspects of publication and authorship are covered only by guidelines and unwritten rules promulgated by professional societies, peer-reviewed journals, and institutions, rather than by any federal regulations. In 1978, a group of medical editors developed the Uniform Requirements for Manuscripts Submitted to Biomedical Journals that were adopted by over 500 journals and are still in place today [21]. Authors are required to transfer copyrights to the journal and textbook publishers and US copyright laws regulate published research articles and chapters. This means that permission must be obtained from the publisher for any reproduction or republishing of the work by even the original author(s).

The published paper is the final record of a finished research project or other scholarly activity [22]. Publications should present some substantive new result or analysis, adding to the body of knowledge already in existence within the public domain. Authorship is the most visible form of credit to participating researchers and is indicative of a substantial contribution to the work being published. Authors agree to take responsibility for a thorough knowledge of the content of the manuscript, being prepared to stand behind their findings. All authors should read and agree to the manuscript before publication, and are now often required to provide a signed attestation to many peer-reviewed journals at the time of submission. Publications should also credit sponsors of the work and acknowledge any requirements outlined in grants or contracts.

Since an authorship track record is used as a measure of success by funding agencies, institutions, and other scientists, there is extraordinary pressure placed on researchers to "publish or perish," making it imperative that authorship assignment is negotiated and dispensed appropriately. Multiple authorship poses additional challenges in that complex relationships between authors can result in diluted or obscured credit or responsibility for the work being described. In academia, authorship is used as a benchmark for measuring creative contributions that warrant consideration for promotion within the faculty professional development process. As such, traditionally awarded authorships solely on the basis of mentorship, senior scientists, or department directorship constitutes honorary authorship, a practice that should be strongly discouraged.

Academic freedom is the right of faculty to independently make all decisions regarding the conduct of research, including dissemination of research data without interference from outside parties, particularly those with a financial or other interest in the data. This freedom is vital for public trust. Generally, this is easily accommodated, and expected for publicly funded endeavors. However, the increasing close links between industry and universities have put strains on this long-held tenet [23].

Because of concerns regarding the integrity of clinical research and increasing private funding and control, the International Committee of Medical Journal Editors (ICMJE), in 2001, revised its Uniform Requirements for Manuscripts Submitted to Biomedical Journals [21,24]. The requirements of the revisions include assurance that the investigators are truly independent of the funding agency, the investigators are fully responsible for research design and conduct, have unfettered access to all data, and most importantly, retain control of all editorial dissemination decisions.

A recent survey of 122 AAMC-member medical schools found that academic institutions routinely engage in industry-sponsored research in contravention to the above requirements of accountability, access to data, and control of publications [25]. In fact, universities and teaching hospitals themselves may have conflicts that undermine the academic process [26]. In one famous case, the University of Toronto was negotiating a large donation with a proprietary company at the same time that one of their faculty scientists was concerned about safety and efficacy of one of their developmental drugs. Based on data generated by a trial sponsored by the proprietary company, the scientist reported the findings at a scientific meeting and to a peer-reviewed journal. The company wished to keep the data confidential and sued. The faculty member was not supported by either her university or teaching hospital. In fact, the institution referred her for research misconduct to the College of Physicians and Surgeons of Ontario. The scientist was ultimately exonerated (J. Cranton, personal communication, December 19, 2001), [27], and the University of Toronto now has appropriate program safeguards in place.

A suggestion to avoid such problems as well as the overwhelming power of industry is to establish an external review panel whose members are acceptable to both parties [26]. In absence of this, universities must establish clear contract policies with industry, and a clear policy regarding academic freedom of their scientists. For their part, individual scientists should understand contractual agreements before entering into them, and negotiate minimal confidentiality periods as possible, and only those with which they are comfortable. It could be considered a breach of ethics (on the part of the scientist) and against the public good to enter into an agreement without assurance of rights conferred by academic freedom.

Summary

Emergency medicine researchers are faced with conducting research in a stringent regulatory environment. These regulations were brought about by unfortunate consequences to subjects, or mistreatment of animals by misguided scientists, and the inattention of many institutions to monitoring their scientific environment. To regain public trust and maintain the integrity of research, it is imperative that scientists become well versed with regulatory guidelines and that compliance become an integral component of study conduct, from inception to conclusion.

References

[1] Whitbeck C. Truth and trustworthiness in research. Sci Eng Ethics 1995;1(4):403–16.
[2] Regulations and Ethical Guidelines. Available at: http://ohsr.od.nih.gov/guidelines/nuremberg.html. Accessed June 27, 2005.
[3] World Medical Association Declaration of Helsinki. Available at: http://www.wma.net/e/policy/pdf/17c.pdf. Accessed June 27, 2005.
[4] The Tuskegee Timeline. Available at: http://www.cdc.gov/nchstp/od/tuskegee/time.htm. Accessed July 5, 2005.
[5] Beecher HK. Ethics and clinical research. N Engl J Med 1966;274(24):1354–60.
[6] Cancer Clinical Trials. Available at: http://www.cancer.gov/clinicaltrials/resources/in-depth-program/page6. Accessed July 5, 2005.
[7] The Belmont Report. Available at: http://www.hhs.gov/ohrp/humansubjects/guidance/belmont.htm. Accessed July 5, 2005.
[8] Levine RJ. Basic concepts and definitions. In: Ethics and regulation of clinical research. 2nd ed. New Haven, CT: Yale University Press; 1988.
[9] Association for the Accreditation of Human Research Protection Programs, Inc. (AAHRPP). Available at: http://www.aahrpp.org/www.aspx. Accessed July 5, 2005.
[10] Office of Research Integrity Policies. Available at: http://ori.hhs.gov/policies/fedreg42cfr50.shtml. Accessed July 5, 2005.
[11] Office of Research Integrity. Available at: http://ori.dhhs.gov/. Accessed July 5, 2005.
[12] SAEM Ethics Committee, et al. Confronting the ethical challenges to informed consent in emergency medicine research. Acad Emerg Med 2004;11:1082–9.
[13] US Code of Federal Regulations Part 46 Protection of Human Subjects. Available at: http://www.hhs.gov/ohrp/humansubjects/guidance/45cfr46.htm. Accessed July 5, 2005.
[14] Beauchamp TL, Childress JF, editors. Professional-patient relationships. In: Principles of biomedical ethics. 5th ed. New York: Oxford University Press, Inc; 2001. p. 303–12.
[15] Brios MH, Runge JW, Lewis RJ. Emergency medicine and the development of the Food and Drug Administration's final rule on informed consent and waiver of informed consent in emergency research circumstances. Acad Emerg Med 1998;5:359–68.
[16] US Department of Health and Human Services, Office for Civil Rights. HIPAA: Medical Privacy - Standards to Protect Privacy of Personal Health Information. Available at: http://www.hhs.gov/ocr/hipaa/. Accessed July 5, 2005.
[17] Meslin EM, Quaid KA. Ethical issues in the collection, storage, and research use of human biological materials. J Lab Clin Med 2004;144:229–34.
[18] DeMets DL, Pocock SJ, Julian DG. The agonizing negative trend in monitoring of clinical trials. Lancet 1999;354:1983–8.
[19] American Veterinary Medical Association. Available at: http://www.avma.org/issues/policy/animal_welfare/policy.asp. Accessed June 16, 2006.
[20] Office of Management and Budget (OMB). Circular A-21. Available at: http://www.whitehouse.gov/omb/circulars/a021/a021.html. Accessed July 5, 2005.

[21] International Committee of Medical Journal Editors. Uniform requirements for manuscripts submitted to biomedical journals: updated October 2001. Available at: http://www.icmje.org. Accessed July 5, 2005.

[22] Gaeta TJ. Authorship: "law" and order. Acad Emerg Med 1999;6:297–301.

[23] Is the university-industrial complex out of control? Nature 2001;409:119.

[24] Davidoff F, DeAngelis CCD, Drazen JM, et al. Sponsorship, authorship, and accountability. N Engl J Med 2001;345:825–7.

[25] Schulman KA, Seils DM, Timbie JW, et al. A national survey of provisions in clinical-trial agreements between medical schools and industry sponsors. N Engl J Med 2002;347:1335–41.

[26] Nathan DG, Weatherall DJ. Academic freedom in clinical research. N Engl J Med 2002;347:1368–71.

[27] Thompson J, Baird P, Downie J. Report of the Committee of Inquiry on the case involving Dr Nancy Olivieri, the Hospital for Sick Children, the University of Toronto, and Apotex Inc. Toronto: Canadian Association of University Teachers; 2001.

ELSEVIER
SAUNDERS

Emerg Med Clin N Am
24 (2006) 671–685

EMERGENCY
MEDICINE
CLINICS OF
NORTH AMERICA

Conflict of Interest in the Physician Interface with the Biomedical Industry

Hal Minnigan, MD, PhD*, Carey D. Chisholm, MD

*Indiana University School of Medicine, Department of Emergency Medicine,
1050 Wishard Boulevard, Room R2200, Indianapolis, IN 46202-2899, USA*

As health care costs continue to escalate, the controversy about relationships between doctors and biomedical industry representatives faces greater scrutiny [1,2]. Prescription expenditures are the fastest rising component of increased health care costs, rising at a rate that far exceeds inflation [3,4]. Americans spend over $200 billion per year on prescription drugs. In 2002, the average price of the 50 drugs most used by senior citizens was about $1500 for a year's supply [5]. Since the average number of pharmaceuticals that a senior takes is six, this amounts to $9000 for the average senior per year, a significant financial burden for an elder living on a fixed income [5]. The Medicare Prescription Drug Benefit (Medicare Part D), set to begin in 2006, is not likely to solve this dilemma for many. The bill specifically prohibits the government from bargaining for the best price for medications. No one knows what the cost of this program will ultimately be, but the original estimate of $400 billion over 10 years was recently increased to $530 billion only weeks after Congress approved the first bill. In all likelihood, the price of the program will erode available funds rapidly, forcing increases in the premiums and cutbacks in other Medicare benefits (including decreased physician reimbursement) to offset prescription prices [6–8].

Studies have shown that over 80% of doctors regularly have contact with pharmaceutical marketing representatives [4,9] and suggest that physician interaction with pharmaceutical marketing representatives is associated with increased prescribing costs [10,11]. Despite an association between physician interaction with pharmaceutical marketing representatives and changes in physician behavior, most doctors deny the influence of industry contacts [12,13]. Industry interactions with individual physicians coincide

---

* Corresponding author.
  E-mail address: hminniga@iupui.edu (H. Minnigan).

0733-8627/06/$ - see front matter © 2006 Elsevier Inc. All rights reserved.
doi:10.1016/j.emc.2006.05.008   *emed.theclinics.com*

with a preference for newer, more expensive medicines that hold no proven clinical advantage, and an accompanying decline in the use of generic drugs [14]. Physician awareness that marketing influences operate at the individual level is less clear, although evidence suggests that the number of gifts that doctors receive correlates with the belief that drug representatives have no effect on prescribing behavior [15,16].

Entanglement with the biomedical industry pervades all sectors of clinical and academic medicine, from individual "detailing" of physicians in the office setting, to funding research at major academic centers. According to estimates, 88,000 pharmaceutical marketing representatives were employed in the United States in 2001. This amounts to an average of one for every five to six physicians [5]. It is not uncommon for doctors to receive multiple, even > 5 visits, in the usual workday from pharmaceutical marketing representatives [17]. At times a tremendous distraction, representatives have gained access to both private offices and examination rooms. Introduced as "observers" or "consultants," these marketing representatives have been allowed to infiltrate clinical settings in exchange for payments to doctors for opportunities to "shadow" or "precept" care interactions. Physicians have allowed representatives to discuss patient care, view medical records, and recommend off-label uses of pharmaceuticals for patients [18].

Gift exchanges often involve commodity trading, such as a "free lunch" (money) for "face time" with doctor-laden audiences. At many of these presentations, physicians identified by industry as key opinion leaders, are paid honorariums to "train up" colleagues on treatment options for common disease processes that favor company-endorsed drugs or devices. Evidence suggests that these presentations are biased and alter the prescription habits of physician attendees [19].

Professional societies and peer-reviewed publications are not immune to marketing influences. Academic societies often rely heavily on revenue from pharmaceutical advertising to support national meetings [20,21]. Meanwhile, the affiliations between authors of clinical practice guidelines and pharmaceutical companies have been revealed, casting aspersions on the integrity of the published consensus recommendations [22]. The US Food and Drug Administration (FDA) appears to be in the midst of controversy with the recent revelation that 10 of the 32 members in the "expert panel" that recommended approval of Vioxx's return to the market have financial ties to pharmaceutical companies involved in marketing cyclo-oxygenase–2 inhibitors, of which Vioxx is one [23]. Journals generate a large amount of revenue from pharmaceutical advertisements, as well as from published symposia and reprints, despite the fact that symposia sponsored by a single company are less likely to have published methods and more likely to have conclusions that favor the drug of interest [24]. Research sponsored by pharmaceutical companies is more likely to favor new drug therapy if funded by industry than if not [25]. It is estimated that 60% of biomedical research and development in the United States is now privately funded, and at least two thirds of academic institutions have financial ties with corporate sponsors. Academic and industry relationships have been roundly criticized for evidence of financial conflicts of interest described as "pervasive and problematic." In a recent review, one fourth of university researchers were noted to have industry funding and one third had personal financial ties to corporate sponsors [26].

Physicians, either through prescribing or research activities, have the greatest influence on what biomedical products are consumed in the marketplace. To maximize revenue, pharmaceutical companies target physicians with proven marketing techniques intended to influence them to prescribe their products [16]. Pharmaceutical marketing representatives employ basic rules of sociologic engagement in their interactions with physicians. This strategy takes advantage of the fact that physicians are generally ignorant of the marketing psychology that underlies these tactics. While this is normal behavior in a market-driven economic mode, health care is different and certainly is not a free market.

The influence of the pharmaceutical industry encompasses virtually all phases of medical education and practice, from individual physician interaction with pharmaceutical representatives, to sponsored continuing medical education and research interactions with academic physicians, and extends even to professional organizations such as the American Heart Association. The advent of direct-to-consumer advertisements has only widened the sphere of influence to include the public. In view of the prevalence of this problem, the authors limit further discussion to the dynamics of the individual physician and the pharmaceutical industry.

The pharmaceutical industry

The pharmaceutical industry is extremely profitable. For example, in 2001, 10 American drug companies in the Fortune 500 ranked above all other corporations in profitability, with an average net return of 18.5% of sales [5, 27]. By 2002, the combined profits for those same 10 companies exceeded the profit margin ($35.9 billion) for the remaining 490 companies [28]. The industry claims that prices are high because it must recoup its heavy research and development costs. As of 1990, 36% of sales revenue was spent on marketing, which is 2.5 times the amount spent on research and development. The category of marketing and administration is the largest single item in the pharmaceutical industry balance sheet. The industry estimates that $800 million is typically spent on research and development of each drug before it comes to market. However, consumer advocacy groups, such as Public Citizen, place this number closer to $100 million [29]. Consider the words of Raymond Gilmartin, president and chief executive officer of Merck: "The price of medicines isn't determined by their research costs. Instead, it is determined by their value in preventing and

treating disease. Whether Merck spends $500 million or $1 billion developing a medicine, it is the doctor, the patient, and those paying for our medicines who will determine its true value" [30].

In 2001, the industry spent over $10 billion to support about 88,000
pharmaceutical marketing representatives [31]. This amounted to over
$10,000 spent on each physician in the United States for marketing. One
might ask why the pharmaceutical industry spends so much on marketing
if the latest drug could sell itself. What prevents the spread of new medications? The answer is that few new pharmaceuticals are truly novel. For
the years 1998 through 2004 over 75% of new medications were not considered by the FDA to be innovative or a significant improvement on existing drugs [32]. There is intense competition to market these "later
generation" drugs despite the fact they are rarely better than older and
less costly alternatives [3]. Drugs are the fastest rising sector of health
care costs, increasing at double-digit rates, which approached 20% in
1999. This increase is far ahead of inflation, and reflects the increased number of total medications most people take, which include the latest to break
on scene. There are clear indications that all phases of drug development,
testing, and trial of safety and efficacy endpoints, are aimed to increase
company profitability.

Case scenario #1

While on an internal medicine rotation, a third-year medical student is
greeted by a pharmaceutical representative during a sponsored lunch. The
student is given a gift of a pocket antibiotic-prescribing guidebook.

Gift giving is at the heart of the personal relationship that pharmaceutical
marketing representatives work to establish with physicians. Gifts are used
to establish rapport, promote specific products, and strengthen company
and specific brand recognition. It is well established that plying most physicians with "food, flattery and friendship" works [10,33]. An examination of
the sociology of gift giving also reveals that gifts invoke the social rule of
reciprocity. The recipient incurs an obligation to repay, in like measure if
possible, favors and gifts [34,35]. Contrary to what might seem to be the
obvious conclusion, feelings of obligation, and propensity of reciprocal behavior are not related to the size of the initial gift. Katz and colleagues [36],
in their monograph on the ethics of gift giving, recount several poignant
examples of reciprocity. The "success secret," according to the world record
holder among car salesman, was to send mass-produced greeting cards to his
customers every month printed with the words "I like you" [35]. When the
owner of a pharmacy gave patrons a $0.50 key chain upon entering the
store, these customers spent an average of 17% more [37]. The Disabled
American Veterans have a 33% response rate to solicitations if an inexpensive unsolicited gift (eg, address labels) is included, compared with an 18%
response rate when no gift is included [35]. The need to reciprocate does not

depend on good will. In fact, those who are mistrusted can gain favors or influence behavior by bestowing an unsolicited gift. The Hare Krishna cult congregated in airports in the 1970s. They preceded their request for a donation with a gift of a flower stating, "This is our gift to you." Social discomfort made it difficult for many people to avoid reciprocating. This tactic helped make the Hare Krishnas wealthy [37].

Physicians also fall victim to self-interested behavior when there are gifts associated with pharmaceutical manufacturers' products. Self-serving bias operates when perceptions of fairness are based on what is in one's own self interest. Well-established social science research shows that this tendency operates below the individual's conscious perception, producing an unintentional bias. Individuals are thus unaware that self interests drive decision making despite a conscious motivation to be impartial. Those who succumb to bias often deny it, further evidence that these forces operate at the level of the unconscious [16].

Gift exchange as a form of social manipulation cannot be overstated in regard to physician interactions with industry. Pharmaceutical marketing representatives choose the scenario for both the initial gift as well as the type of reciprocation. The physician is unconsciously persuaded to support the pharmaceutical marketing representative's products, through prescription writing. For reciprocity to be active, a gift must be associated with a giver, hence the relative paucity of anonymous or unrestricted gifts between pharmaceutical companies and physician groups.

Some providers may believe that detailers also provide an invaluable source of information about new medications. As noted previously, very few of the newly marketed medications constitute a therapeutic "breakthrough." However, the physician should pause to consider the credentials of the message bearer. In the past, most pharmaceutical representatives earned pharmacy or chemistry degrees in college. Now most have degrees in business or marketing. Many studies characterize representative information as inaccurate, misleading, or biased [10,24,38–40]. However, social discomfort with questioning or discrediting a representative who has just provided a gift limits the likelihood that the physician will challenge questionable information. Clearly, an advisory to practitioners to use less-biased resources in maintaining clinical currency is warranted.

Case scenario #2

A second-year emergency-medicine resident receives an invitation in her mailbox to attend a presentation at an expensive local steakhouse by a renowned expert on treatment of emerging infections in community-acquired pneumonia.

Food is an especially powerful tool to gain attention and reinforce positive social feelings [41]. When used with flattery and gifts, food engenders positive feelings in the recipient quite favorably beyond the message delivered by the giver. The juxtaposition of dining and a complimentary atmosphere fosters good will; recipients are receptive to compliments even when they recognize a transparent agenda [37].

Physicians are surprisingly ignorant of the tactics used by pharmaceutical marketing representatives to effect change in prescriber behaviors. In one study, 85% of medical students felt it was wrong for politicians to accept gifts, but only 46% believed it was improper for a physician to accept a similar gift from a pharmaceutical representative [42]. McKinney and colleagues [43] found that 23% of faculty and 15% of residents believed that judgment could not be influenced regardless of value of the gift received. Those who placed a monetary value cutoff on the size of the gift generally favored $100 as a threshold value below which judgment would not likely be affected. Interestingly, faculty, were more likely than residents to discount the effect of representative contact on personal prescribing habits [43]. In another study, 34% of psychiatry residents in Toronto failed to detect subtle influence of pharmaceutical marketing representatives on their prescribing habits, and 56% felt that gifts from pharmaceutical marketing representatives would not influence their judgment. There was a positive correlation between gifts and attitudes: The more money and gifts received by a physician in training the more likely the physician believed discussions with pharmaceutical marketing representatives had no effect on prescribing [12]. A survey of internal-medicine residents found that attitudes and behaviors were incongruous. Of all the residents who indicated that conference lunches and gift pens were inappropriate, 12% admitted to accepting lunches and 18% admitted to accepting pens. More revealing is the attitude of these residents toward the influence of gifts on prescribing habits. Sixty-one percent said that their prescribing habits were not influenced by pharmaceutical marketing representatives, but only 16% believed that other physicians were unaffected [13]. Taken together, these data suggest that physicians are largely unaware of marketing strategies used to influence their behavior and poorly prepared to disentangle themselves from them. Pharmaceutical companies exploit these blind spots in marketing their products.

Recently some pharmaceutical companies have applied their "expert dinner" tactics to physician extenders through "table talk" persuasive to nurses, physician assistants and nurse practitioners. Armed with even less background knowledge about scientific methodology and bias, such audiences may be even more malleable than physicians. Consider a scenario where an emergency department nurse attends a dinner at an expensive steak restaurant during which the "expert" discusses the benefits of the selective serotonin 5-HT$_3$ receptor blockers for treating nausea. The next time this nurse has a patient with vomiting, she will request in her call to a member of the house staff the proprietary serotonin blocker mentioned by the "expert," instead of the usual generic antiemetic alternatives. The member of the house staff, distracted, pressed by other work, or not wishing to rock the boat, acquiesces and provides the order even though the chosen medication wouldn't routinely be their first-line therapy.

Case scenario #3

A practicing emergency medicine physician is invited to attend a meeting in San Francisco sponsored by the makers of a new medication for heart failure. The physician is paid a $1000 honorarium and is reimbursed for first-class airfare and lodging at a five-star hotel, which includes superb cuisine and a complimentary sightseeing tour. The physician has no particular training or cardiovascular expertise. He is asked to sign an agreement to become a "consultant" to the company and agrees to give feedback about the medication and perhaps a brief formal presentation to his colleagues when he returns home.

Examples of high-profile conflicts of interest that may compromise physicians abound. These include physician self-referral [44–46], physician involvement in health maintenance organizations and hospitals [47], funds directed to physician investigators for participant enrollment [52], and even university-level endorsements for industry-related research [50,51]. However, the most common form of conflict of interest involves the acceptance of gifts by individual physicians [48,49].

The conflict of interest between physicians and the pharmaceutical industry is obvious when examining the influence of marketing on prescribing behavior. It is therefore not surprising that the pharmaceutical industry spends more money on marketing and administration that any single budget item [28]. Likewise it should not come as a surprise to physicians that the industry gets what it pays for—influence over the behavior of doctors. Let's take a closer look at this phenomenon.

Orlowski and Wateska [19] reported the results of their elegant study in 1992. Doctors who had participated in a lavish pharmaceutical-industry–sponsored "conference" on one of two new drugs were questioned as to the potential influence the conference might have on their prescribing choices of these drugs. For drug A, 9 of 10 doctors said the conference "would not influence" their behavior (The remaining doctor believed the conference would "be unlikely to influence" personal behavior.). For drug B, 8 of 10 doctors said the conference "would not influence" their behavior (One of the remaining two doctors responded with "unlikely to influence" and the other responded with "could possibly influence."). Hospital pharmacy records were reviewed to determine the prescribing patterns for these two drugs before the symposia and 17 months afterward (Both medications were intravenous only and used only in the hospital setting.). Notably, the prescription rate for drug A was near constant in the 18 months before the symposium. Afterward, however, the prescribing patterns among drug A conference attendees increased three-fold during the 17-month follow-up period, and began within a few months of the symposium. Results for drug B were similar, with a 2.5-fold increase in the likelihood for drug B prescriptions written by conference attendees compared with baseline [19]. More damaging than the actual prescribing pattern effects was the fact that the physicians studied were unaware of their own change in behavior.

Interaction with industry representatives and acceptance of gifts of nearly all kinds is positively associated with increased prescribing of the company's drugs [10]. Meetings with pharmaceutical marketing representatives, attendance at sponsored symposia, and acceptance of sponsored meals are independently associated with requests to add the company's drug to the formulary [38,53]. Requests to the formularies in these studies were mostly for drugs that offered little therapeutic advantage over existing formulary drugs. Frequency of contact with pharmaceutical marketing representatives and acceptance of free meals predicts a change in prescribing habits. Acceptance of honoraria or attendance at symposia also is an independent predictor of increased prescribing of the company's drug [53]. Reliance on materials distributed by pharmaceutical marketing representatives has been shown to increase prescribing costs [54]. Contact with pharmaceutical marketing representatives after the introduction of a new drug rapidly influences the attitude of physicians toward the drug and their willingness to prescribe it [55].

Public awareness of the lavish gifts that have been bestowed on physicians have led to reforms related to giving and accepting gifts [56,57]. With regard to financial conflicts of interest, professional societies limit the amount of the gift, demonstrating the belief among these societies that larger gifts are more likely to influence judgment [56]. However, as already noted, gift acceptance invokes the social rule of reciprocity and the influence on behavior is independent of the size of the gift [37]. Payments and compensation to physicians were to be only of "modest value," and were supposed to be primarily related to a physician's work. One recent study of industry-sponsored "educational" meals revealed that the cost of the meals was above the per-diem norm for the area (Philadelphia), often exceeding $50 per person [58]. With more regulations emerging, the pharmaceutical industry has responded with new marketing strategies, including the generous "consultant" fees (eg, $1000) for even non-subspecialist level physicians posted after completion of sponsored educational symposia at posh destinations [1,19,59]. The primary objective remains to "train" physicians' rank and file. Targeting both physicians regarded as key opinion leaders and the "timeshare" types (ie, close professional associates), industry creates reliable demands for its products. Increasingly, such attendees sign an agreement to be a company "consultant," which obviates former prohibitions on lavish gifts exchanged between industry and science. Attendance at such sponsored symposia has already been noted above to directly affect prescribing habits and formulary requests for the sponsor's drugs [19].

"Free" samples are the ultimate gift. Neither free, nor truly a gift, has the "hangover" lingered? Yes. Pharmaceutical marketing representatives provide samples to physicians in office practice and to hospitals for three reasons—to increase recognition, increase prescribing, and gain market share for their drug. As Michael Rawlins [60] observes: "No drug company gives away its shareholders' money in an act of disinterested generosity." Physicians must ask honestly if a company would give anything away on an ongoing basis if it didn't increase its bottom line. The cost of "free" samples is ultimately transferred to patients who bear the burden of paying for the samples. Hospitals and clinics that use samples are accomplices in a huge "bait-and-switch" scam for which patients ultimately pay. Hospitals often receive steep discounts for new and expensive drugs, which leads to preferential use of that drug in the hospital. Patients who are started on a drug in the hospital or who receive a sample from their physician in the office are much more likely to stay on the same pharmaceutical after finishing the samples. Patients who are started on such drugs in the hospital always have to pay market price when they are discharged [5]. Acceptance of samples by physicians is also a predictor of positive attitudes toward the pharmaceutical marketing representatives [15] as well as prescribing preferences for the drug [55]. Samples to indigent patients are given on the assumption that they will become insured in the future, and that they are likely to be kept on the "medication that is already working." Inexpensive generic medications are invariably lacking from distributed samples, further testimony that motives have to do with marketing, not altruism. Samples are also misused in a myriad of ways [61]. Many are taken for private use of physicians, nurses, and staff [62]. The costs of these diverted drugs are born by all of us, specifically the patients whom physicians are trying to help.

Direct-to-consumer ads have skyrocketed in the wake of a change in the FDA policy that previously required full disclosure of all side effects during the advertisement. Spending on direct-to-consumer ads of prescription drugs in the United States totaled $3.2 billion in 2003 [63]. Pharmaceutical ads to consumers are now the fastest growing segment of pharmaceutical advertising, almost tripling between 1996 and 2000, with a sevenfold increase in television advertisements [64]. In 2000, rofecoxib was the most heavily advertised drug to consumers and retail sales quadrupled between 1999 and 2000 (Rofecoxib's advertising campaign by Merck was bigger than campaigns for either Pepsi or Budweiser in 2000.) [65]. Drugs that are marketed on television are for conditions whose symptoms are easily identified with (but misunderstood) by consumers—asthma, allergies, and abdominal pain. The literature shows that direct-to-consumer ads drive sales of newer, more expensive products for symptomatic relief of chronic conditions or conditions with huge market potential. Indeed, just 20 prescription drugs account for about 60% of the total industry spending on direct-to-consumer ads. It is known that a physician is more likely to prescribe for patients who specifically ask for a prescription than for patients with similar conditions who don't ask for a prescription [66,67]. Survey data suggest that approximately 40% of visits in which a direct-to-consumer–ad discussion occurs result in a prescription for the advertised drug. In more than half the cases, a physician prescribed a drug partly to accommodate a patient's request [68]. Kravitz and colleagues [69] describe the results of a randomized controlled trial using standardized patients to examine the influence of patient requests for a drug on the prescribing influence of physicians. Their data clearly show that patient requests for either a specific brand or a general medication result in increased prescribing by physicians. Physicians prescribed medication 53% of the time when a specific brand was requested, and 76% of the time when a general request was made compared with 31% if no medication was requested.

As physicians struggle to keep their clinical knowledge base up to date, they often turn to clinical practice guidelines (CPGs) endorsed by professional societies to distill current evidence into useable practice advice. A panel of experts is assembled to review and discuss a topic and conclude with the publication of a set of evidence-based recommendations for treatment. It is assumed that these panelists are independent and will represent scientific synthesis of available evidence. Choudry and colleagues [22] surveyed authors of CPGs and reported a significant relationship between the authors of CPGs and the pharmaceutical industry. The report found that 87% of authors had some form of interaction with the pharmaceutical industry, 58% received financial support, and 38% had been employed or paid as a consultant by a pharmaceutical company. Meanwhile, 59% of authors of CPGs had a relationship with a company whose product was considered or referred to in the guideline they authored and 96% of these relationships predated the development of the guideline. In 11 of 44 cases, a pharmaceutical company sponsored the creation and writing of guidelines. Perhaps most importantly, although all 44 of the guidelines examined had authors with relationships to industry, in only 1 of the 44 guidelines was a declaration made to this effect. Only 7% of authors believed that their industry relationships influenced the recommendations that they promulgated, while 19% of the same group believed that their colleagues' recommendations were influenced by industry ties. Although no direct effect on pharmaceutical prescribing can be demonstrated, the pervasive nature of the ties linking CPG authors to industry raises significant questions about the integrity of the authors' conclusions.

Physicians face marketing pressures in their interface with the biomedical industry. On an individual basis, physicians seem to feel obligated to interact with detailing representatives. Residency program directors and educators often cite the perceived need of preparing graduates for future interaction with representatives as a rationale for permitted contact during training. However, these detailers should be dealt with no differently than a telephone solicitor or door-to-door salesperson who makes a call during dinner hour. There should be no obligation to interact with them. This message is clearly and easily conveyed to trainees. Patient confidentiality and privacy concerns should preclude the presence of detailers in the emergency department care area, as it is impossible not to overhear or see patient data.

Such detailing in the emergency department area creates additional interruptions with the accompanying potential to increase medical error or decrease patient flow efficiency.

In addition to the food and gifts provided by such detailers, these forces are disguised as product information, continuing medication education, research, and, recently, even graduate medical education [70]. Subsidies by the pharmaceutical industry are for one purpose—to influence physician behavior in ways that benefit the company's financial performance. It is naïve to believe that pharmaceutical companies have anything other than their financial interests at heart. If physicians choose to remain ignorant of the data that demonstrates that marketing pressure changes behavior, they cannot justify the trust that society places in their hands. Society bestows special privileges upon physicians and in return expects professional behavior. This demands that physicians place patients' interests before their own. For good reasons, other professions have prohibitions against accepting gifts. Professional sporting referees, judges, journalists, and university professors are not permitted to accept gifts from those affected by their judgment. The most telling prohibition is upon pharmaceutical marketing representatives who are not permitted to accept gifts from those they deal with professionally.

Organizations such as No Free Lunch and Healthy Skepticism have been organized as an attempt to address the lack of awareness of marketing in medical practice from within the medical community. This marketing is literally paid for by patients, and as such it compromises the credibility and ideals of patient care that physicians believe in. From first-hand observations, emergency medical physicians are aware of the tremendous financial vulnerability of the patient populations emergency medicine serves. Medical professional organizations have adopted position statements of various stringencies to address these conflicts [56,71–74]. They generally stop short of prohibiting contact with industry marketing representatives. The evidence, however, suggests that there is not a level of contact that is free from potential for conflict. The authors are aware of at least one academic emergency department that has created a completely "market free" workplace. Emergency physicians teach their colleagues in training to "do the right thing." It is time that the emergency medical profession does the right thing and says "no" to interaction with pharmaceutical marketing representatives and adopts clear-cut policies to protect the integrity of the research community. Such policies should take into account the following five points:

- Physicians have a fundamental duty to represent their patients' best interests.
- This duty includes using the most cost-effective method to diagnose and treat illness.
- Pharmaceuticals constitute the largest component of sharply rising health care expenditures in the United States economy. Pharmaceutical companies have a fiduciary responsibility to shareholders.

- Evidence supports the assertions that profit-driven pharmaceutical companies consciously manipulate the academicians of medical research (nonmarket) and the clinical environment of patients and physicians alike through influencing interactions, prescription writing, and educational venues. This corporate influence draws on basic marketing psychology that is entrenched in cultural norms.
- Acceptance of even "trivial" gifts subject physicians' to associated and measurable biases that may affect clinical judgment, and ultimately the medical care provided to patients. These biases are often subconscious, and are carefully orchestrated by the marketing sector. Patients ultimately bear the costs of pharmaceutical marketing.

Some physicians are insulted when confronted with evidence of conflict of interest. Some believe that acceptance of small gifts is harmless, acknowledging that it is often the norm in many business settings. These attitudes do not address the reality that physicians are personally benefiting while their patients ultimately foot the bill (This differs from being paid for providing care, which benefits the individual patient with a service.). Others convince themselves that they are somehow not vulnerable to well-established forces of social behavior. Physicians should be honest with themselves and their patients. Perhaps physicians find it especially hard to admit to being no different that anyone else when it comes to marketing forces. It is sobering to note that physicians are not immune to influence, and must recognize vulnerability. By understanding this weakness, physicians can better ensure that sound professional judgment is not being undermined. Physicians must not abrogate the public trust. Even if it were possible to conclude that industry interactions do not influence prescription behaviors, the costs of marketing directly passed to society and ultimately to individual patients are undeniable. Emergency medical physicians, perhaps more so than any other group, see day in and day out the financial vulnerability of the patient population. Knowing this, it is disheartening to see the behavior continue. Is this the form of entitlement physicians believe they have earned by selecting medicine as a career? And yes, a pen is only pennies. Those pennies add up into billions of dollars, and that pen is part of the process. The authors hope that as individual members of the profession of medicine, physicians would choose not to contribute to that process. As for those physicians who are educators, they should ask what they wish to mentor and teach to the next generation of physicians.

Acknowledgments

H.J.M. wishes to acknowledge R. Knopp for his mentoring.

References

[1] Appleby J. Sales pitch: drug firms use perks to push pills. USA Today. 2001. Available at: http://www.usatoday.com/news/health/2001-05-16-perks-usat.htm. Accessed July 11, 2006.

[2] Steiger B. Unethical business practices in US health care alarm physician leaders. 2005.

[3] Barents Group LLC, Factors affecting the growth of prescription drug expenditures. Washington (DC): National Institute for Health Care Management Research and Educational Foundation; 1999.

[4] Moynihan R. Who pays for the pizza? Redefining the relationships between doctors and drug companies. 1: entanglement. BMJ 2003;326:1189–92.

[5] Angell M. The truth about drug companies: how they deceive us and what to do about it. 2004.

[6] Medicare prescription drug benefit. Fed Regist 2005;70:4443–92.

[7] Aging EAAo. Summary of medicare part D prescription drug benefit. 2005.

[8] Altman DE. The new Medicare prescription-drug legislation. N Engl J Med 2004;350(1): 9–10.

[9] Lexchin J. Interactions between physicians and the pharmaceutical industry: what does the literature say? CMAJ 1993;149(10):1401–7.

[10] Wazana A. Physicians and the pharmaceutical industry: is a gift ever just a gift? JAMA 2000; 283(3):373–80.

[11] Watkins C, et al. Characteristics of general practitioners who frequently see drug industry representatives: national cross sectional study. BMJ 2003;326(7400):1178–9.

[12] Hodges B. Interactions with the pharmaceutical industry: experiences and attitudes of psychiatry residents, interns and clerks. CMAJ 1995;153(5):553–9.

[13] Steinman MA, Shlipak MG, McPhee SJ. Of principles and pens: attitudes and practices of medicine housestaff toward pharmaceutical industry promotions. Am J Med 2001;110(7): 551–7.

[14] Bower AD, Burkett GL. Family physicians and generic drugs: a study of recognition, information sources, prescribing attitudes, and practices. J Fam Pract 1987;24(6):612–6.

[15] Thomson AN, Craig BJ, Barham PM. Attitudes of general practitioners in New Zealand to pharmaceutical representatives. Br J Gen Pract 1994;44:220.

[16] Dana J, Loewenstein G. A social science perspective on gifts to physicians from industry. JAMA 2003;290(2):252–5.

[17] Chin T. Drug firms score by paying doctors for time. Am Med News 2002.

[18] Peterson M. Suit says company promoted drug in exam rooms. New York Times, 2002.

[19] Orlowski JP, Wateska L. The effects of pharmaceutical firm enticements on physician prescribing patterns. There's no such thing as a free lunch. Chest 1992;102(1):270–3.

[20] Johnson RG. Physician education and the pharmaceutical industry. Chest 2001;119(4): 995–6.

[21] Varkey B. Time for introspection. Chest 2001;119(4):1255–6.

[22] Choudhry NK, Stelfox HT, Detsky AS. Relationships between authors of clinical practice guidelines and the pharmaceutical industry. JAMA 2002;287(5):612–7.

[23] Mercola J. Vioxx Reapproved by FDA Panel Members With Ties to Drug Companies. 2005. Available at: http://www.mercola.com/2005/mar/2/vioxx_fda.htm. Accessed July 10, 2006.

[24] Cho MK, Bero LA. The quality of drug company studies in published symposium proceedings. Ann Intern Med 1996;124:485–9.

[25] Davidson RA. Source of funding and outcome of clinical trials. J Gen Intern Med 1986;1: 155–8.

[26] Bekelman J, Li Y, Gross C. Scope and impact of financial conflicts of interest in biomedical research. JAMA 2003;289:454–65.

[27] The Fortune 500. Fortune Magazine. April 16, 2001.

[28] Watch PCC. Pharmaceutical company yearly earnings reports analyzed by Public Citizen, April 2001. Available at: http://www.citizen.org/documents/rdmyths.pdf. Accessed July 11, 2006.

[29] Rx R&D myths: the Case against the drug industry's R&D scare card. Public Citizen 2001. Available at: http://www.citizen.org/documents/rdmyths.pdf. Accessed July 11, 2006.

[30] Relman AS, Angell M. America's other drug problem: how the drug industry distorts medicine and politics. New Repub 2002;227(25):27–41.

[31] Pharmaceutical Sales Force Strategies—driving ROI through best practice in targeting, management, outsourcing and technologies. Business Insights 2004. Available at: http://www.globalbusinessinsights.com/report.asp?id=rbhc0128. Accessed July 10, 2006.

[32] FDA. Available at: http://www.fda.gov/. Accessed July 10, 2006.

[33] Prescription drug promotion involving payments and gifts: physicians' perspectives. Washington (DC): Office of the Inspector General; 1992. Available at: http://oig.hhs.gov/oei/reports/oei-01-90-00481.pdf. Accessed July 10, 2006.

[34] Levi-Strauss C. The elementary structures of kinship. Boston: Beacon Press; 1969.

[35] Cialdini RB. The psychology of persuasion. New York: Quill William Morrow; 1993.

[36] Katz D, Caplan AL, Merz JF. All gifts large and small: toward an understanding of the ethics of pharmaceutical industry gift-giving. Am J Bioeth 2003;3(3):39–46.

[37] Freidman HH. The effect of a gift-upon-entry on sales: reciprocity in a retail context. Mid-American Journal of Business 1990;5:49–50.

[38] Chren MM, Landefeld CS. Physicians' behavior and their interactions with drug companies. A controlled study of physicians who requested additions to a hospital drug formulary. JAMA 1994;271(9):684–9.

[39] Ziegler MG, Lew P, Singer BC. The accuracy of drug information from pharmaceutical sales representatives. JAMA 1995;273(16):1296–8.

[40] Stryer D, Bero LA. Characteristics of materials distributed by drug companies. An evaluation of appropriateness. J Gen Intern Med 1996;11(10):575–83.

[41] Razran GHS. Conditioned response changes in rating and appraising sociopolitical slogans. Psychol Bull 1940;37:481.

[42] Palmisano P, Edelstein J. Teaching drug promotion abuses to health profession students. J Med Educ 1980;55(5):453–5.

[43] McKinney WP, Schiedermayer DL, Lurie N. Attitudes of internal medicine faculty and residents toward professional interaction with pharmaceutical sales representatives. JAMA 1990;264(13):1693–7.

[44] Hillman BJ, Joseph CA, Mabry MR. Frequency and costs of diagnostic imaging in office practice—a comparison of self-referring and radiologist-referring physicians. N Engl J Med 1990;323(23):1604–8.

[45] Mitchell JM, Scott E. New evidence of the prevalence and scope of physician joint ventures. JAMA 1992;268(1):80–4.

[46] Council on Ethical and Judicial Affairs, American Medical Association. Conflicts of interest. Physician ownership of medical facilities. JAMA 1992;267(17):2366–9.

[47] Hillman AL, Pauly MV, Kerstein JJ. How do financial incentives affect physicians' clinical decisions and the financial performance of health maintenance organizations? N Engl J Med 1989;321(2):86–92.

[48] Advertising, marketing and promotional practices of the pharmaceutical industry. Hearings before the Committee on Labor and Human Resources: US Senate, 101st Congress, 2nd Session, 1990.

[49] Kusserow R. Promotion of prescription drugs through payments and gifts. 1991, Washington (DC): Department of Health and Human Services. Available at: http://oig.hhs.gov/oei/reports/oei-01-90-00480.pdf. Accessed July 10, 2006.

[50] Council on Scientific Affairs and Council on Ethical and Judicial Affairs. Conflicts of interest in medical center/industry research relationships. JAMA 1990;263(20):2790–3.

[51] Blumenthal D. Industrial support of university research in biotechnology. Science 1986; 231(4735):242–6.

[52] Shimm DS, Spece RG Jr. Industry reimbursement for entering patients into clinical trials: legal and ethical issues. Ann Intern Med 1991;115(2):148–51.

[53] Lurie N, Rich EC, Simpson DE. Pharmaceutical representatives in academic medical centers: interaction with faculty and housestaff. J Gen Intern Med 1990;5(3):240–3.

[54] Caudill TS, Johnson MS, Rich EC. Physicians, pharmaceutical sales representatives, and the cost of prescribing. Arch Fam Med 1996;5(4):201–6.

[55] Peay MY, Peay ER. The role of commercial sources in the adoption of a new drug. Soc Sci Med 1988;26(12):1183–9.

[56] American Medical Association. Opinion 8.061. Gifts to physicians from industry, and addendum: Council on Ethical and Judicial Affairs clarification of gifts to physicians from industry. American Medical Association 2005. Available at: http://www.ama-assn.org/ama/pub/category/4001.html. Accessed July 10, 2006.

[57] Phrma code on interactions with healthcare professionals. Washington (DC): Pharmaceutical Research and Manufacturers of America; 2002.

[58] Grande D, Volpp K. Cost and quality of industry-sponsored meals for medical residents. JAMA 2003;290(9):1150–1.

[59] Gianelli D. Revisiting the ethics of industry gifts. Am Med News 1998;9:12–4.

[60] Rawlins MD. Doctors and the drug makers. Lancet 1984;2(8406):814.

[61] Nordenberg T. Selling drug samples lands doctor in prison. FDA Consumer 1998;32(2):39.

[62] Westfall JM, McCabe J, Nicholas RA. Personal use of drug samples by physicians and office staff. JAMA 1997;278(2):141–3.

[63] Prescription Drug Trends. Menlo Park (CA): Kaiser Family Foundation; 2004. fact sheet 3057–03.

[64] Rosenthal MB, Berndt ER, Donohue JM. Promotion of prescription drugs to consumers. N Engl J Med 2002;346(7):498–505.

[65] Prescription drugs and mass media advertising. Washington (DC): The National Institute for Health Care Management; 2001.

[66] Ramsden JD, Quinn FR, Witham M. Doctors are not pressured into giving prescriptions. BMJ 1998;316(7135):938–9.

[67] Mintzes B, Barer ML, Kravitz RL. How does direct-to-consumer advertising (DTCA) affect prescribing? A survey in primary care environments with and without legal DTCA. CMAJ 2003;169(5):405–12.

[68] Weissman JS, Blumenthal D, Silk AJ, et al. Physicians Report On Patient Encounters Involving Direct-To-Consumer Advertising. Health Affairs. 2004. Available at: http://content.healthaffairs.org/cgi/content/abstract/hlthaff.w4.219v1. Accessed July 10, 2006.

[69] Kravitz RL, Epstein RM, Feldman MD. Influence of patients' requests for direct-to-consumer advertised antidepressants: a randomized controlled trial. JAMA 2005;293(16):1995–2002.

[70] Kuehn BM. Pharmaceutical industry funding for residencies sparks controversy. JAMA 2005;293(13):1572–80.

[71] Emergency physicians and the biomedical industry. Society for Academic Emergency Medicine; 1992. Available at: http://www.saem.org/download/industry.pdf. Accessed July 10, 2006.

[72] Guidelines for researchers involved in manufacturer-sponsored trials [position statement]. American Academy of Emergency Medicine, adopted, June 25, 2002. Available at: http://www.aaem.org/positionstatements/researcherguidelines.shtml. Accessed July 10, 2006.

[73] Gifts to emergency physicians from the biomedical industry. American College of Emergency Physicians; 2002. Available at: http://www.acep.org/webportal/PracticeResources/PolicyStatements/ethics/GiftsEPBiomedicalIndustry.htm. Accessed July 10, 2006.

[74] Accreditation Council for Graduate Medical Education. ACGME white paper on the relationship of GME and industry. Available at: www.acgme.org/acWebsite/positionPapers/pp_GMEGuide.pdf. Accessed July 10, 2006.

ELSEVIER
SAUNDERS

Emerg Med Clin N Am
24 (2006) 687–702

EMERGENCY
MEDICINE
CLINICS OF
NORTH AMERICA

Vulnerable Populations: Cultural and Spiritual Direction

Tammie E. Quest, MD[a],*, Nicole M. Franks, MD[b]

[a]Department of Emergency Medicine, Emory University, School of Medicine,
49 Jesse Hill Jr Drive, Atlanta, GA 30303, USA
[b]Department of Emergency Medicine, Emory University, School of Medicine,
Medical Office Tower, 550 Peachtree Street, Atlanta, GA 30308, USA

A 30-year-old Chinese-speaking woman presents to the emergency department with left lower quadrant pain and is diagnosed with an ectopic pregnancy. Through a family translator, the patient is told that the pregnancy is nonviable and at risk of rupture. The patient states that she must go home and discuss the options with her family regarding her condition. She states that she does believe harm will come to her body based on her faith and that her extended family and traditional Chinese medicine practitioner will help make the decision regarding further care. What are the cultural or religious issues of this that complicate this patient's emergency department care?

Key points:

- Proper use of translators
- Spirituality/religion informing health care choices
- Exploration of divergent bioethical models
- Exploration of the explanatory model of disease

Health care has the same responsibility as government services and private industry to make a good faith effort to address issues of culture. *Culture* is a term that may be used interchangeably with spirituality or religion and also encompasses language, cuisine, art, music, traditions, and practices that are not necessarily linked to sacred or nonsacred goals. Culture may also be based on geographical location, chronographical experiences, or political climate. In some instances culture is used interchangeably with race, which describes the physical attributes of a person. For the purposes of this

---

* Corresponding author.
E-mail address: tquest@emory.edu (T.E. Quest).

discussion, culture, spirituality, and religion are the focus of the patient's uniqueness that will be addressed concerning potential conflicts of care in the emergency department.

Patients may become vulnerable as a result of their spiritual, religious, or cultural uniqueness. *Vulnerability* in its strictest sense is defined as "open to attack or damage." Virtually all patients that present to the emergency department for care do so in a vulnerable state, regardless of their background. However, patients from diverse cultures and backgrounds are particularly vulnerable to attack. Awareness of a patient's diverse uniqueness is paramount for emergency physicians because it influences communication, decision making, and development of optimal care management plans. When issues of religion, spirituality, or culture are not addressed, important elements of care may be compromised such as care plan adherence and follow-up. While it is not the intent of the emergency department provider to purposely attack or damage a patient or their family, when patients present with unfamiliar cultural, spiritual, or religious practices that influence their health care, patients may find issues regarding whole patient assessment inadequately considered.

To provide the highest quality care, it is our obligation as emergency physicians to consider the whole patient. This review examines some of the diverse cultural, spiritual, and religious factors that exist and complicate ethical decision making in the emergency department setting. Common diverse factors include (1) language differences; (2) cultural, religious, and spiritual differences between patient and provider; (3) differing explanatory models of disease between patient and provider; and (4) diverse bioethical models of decision making. Managing these diverse factors is complicated by limited time at the bedside and balancing the need of time spent with one patient potentially at the consequence of another. Identification of these diverse factors followed by suggested means to address these factors are examined.

The changing face of America and the emergency department

North America is a melting pot of ethnic groups and the challenges of diversity continue to be a headlining topic in the new millennium. Based on the changing demographics, discordant culture and religious/spiritual frameworks are dominating North American emergency departments. In the United States, the number of immigrants has nearly tripled since 1970, increasing from 9.6 million to 26 million [1]. Racial and ethnic minorities comprise 28% of the US population and in 8 of the 10 largest cities in America, ethnic minorities outnumber whites while the majority of physicians are white.

Despite the fact that the patient population is becoming more diverse, the diversity of emergency physicians lags. The work force is predominantly white male with only 18% nonwhite and 17% women [2]. With respect to academic appointments of underrepresented minorities on US emergency department faculty, the numbers are equally low [3]. The lack of diversity in emergency medicine may persist as underrepresented minority medical students in the United States do not regard emergency medicine as a preferable career choice. Although the majority of the US academic and nonacademic work force in emergency medicine is male and white, initiatives in cultural competency training at the undergraduate and postgraduate levels is thought to be inadequate with calls for more training [4,5].

Emergency department challenges: language, spirituality, culture and decision making

The language gap

Projections indicate that by 2010 there will be at least 69 million Americans who speak a language other than English at home and at least 28.4 million Americans with limited English proficiency (LEP). Many of these patients will visit US emergency departments. Multiple studies have documented that quality of care is compromised and increased medical and nonmedical costs are incurred when LEP patients do not get interpreters when needed. Communication barriers greatly complicate the delivery of health care in general and emergency services in particular. In the emergency setting there is time pressure to obtain basic and critical historical information to potentially institute life-saving care. Under these circumstances emergency department (ED) personnel might use ad hoc, nonprofessionally trained translators to address language barriers. Non-English speakers have been shown to be less satisfied with their care in the ED, less willing to return to the same ED if they had a problem they felt required emergency care, and reported more problems with emergency care [6]. The availability of hospital translation services has been a tremendous improvement of patient-doctor communication for non-English speakers. Despite the availability of hospital interpreters, they are often not used despite a perceived need by patients. The interpreters who are used usually lack formal training (ad hoc translators) in this skill [7,8]. When ad hoc, telephone-, and hospital-based translation services have been compared, hospital-based translators have been shown to be superior [9]. By far, underuse of hospital interpreters makes patients vulnerable to lower quality of care.

Language can be a proxy for culture. Just because one may be competent to translate the words of a language, they may not be as able to translate the culture or the cultural context of words and phrases that may impact delivery of care. For example the importance of thinking and speaking positively is fundamental to the Navajo people. Imagine the delivery of a diagnosis and care management plan as simple as a laceration requiring sutures or as complicated as an aortic dissection to a patient whose cultural and spiritual preference mandates the use of positive language. Both diagnoses require addressing the consequences of infection, improper healing, and the worst case of death. Speaking of these possibilities is thought by the Navajo people to ensure its occurrence. It is recommended that referring to a hypothetical third party and focusing on the positive aspects of the illness as the best form of communication for the Navajo people. Notably, research has shown that patients comprehend and retain information given to them by providers of similar cultural backgrounds [10]. These circumstances further stress the importance of using trained interpreters, and culturally concordant translators when available, to prevent miscommunication with patients so that this vulnerability to inappropriate care would also be eliminated.

Spirituality and religion in the emergency department

Defining spirituality and religion should precede their discussion. Spirituality and religion are often assumed to be synonymous. The two terms are closely related because they embrace divinity and the concept of a higher power, but they are not interchangeable. Religion is viewed as a public, structured, and formal practice of beliefs, whereas spirituality is more of a private, unstructured, and independent practice of beliefs [11]. For consistency in health care research and literature, the agreed on definition of spirituality was decided by a panel of experts assigned by the National Institute of Health Care Research. The panel defines spirituality as "the feelings, thoughts, experiences and behaviors that arise from a search for the sacred" [12]. Sacred was further defined as the individual's perceptions of a higher power, ultimate reality, or ultimate truth. Religion encompasses not only a search for the sacred but also a search for nonsacred goals such as identity and uses prescribed behaviors and practices endorsed by a group of people [12]. One's spirituality may stem from religion but the two concepts are not identical. Physicians in general may not routinely ask about spiritual/religious issues despite the evidence that they might have a positive effect on health particularly when patients have severe, chronic, or terminal disease [12–15].

Awareness of customs or beliefs that are held by various spiritual and religious groups may affect decision making and care management that is unique to the emergency department. The bulk of bioethical concerns of spiritual groups that is applicable in the emergency department focuses on end-of-life communications, consent, and family involvement in decision making. A classic example of a bioethical conflict in the emergency department is the issue of life-saving blood transfusions for Jehovah Witness patients. It is the fundamental belief of this Protestant-based religion that its members will not accept blood transfusions. The conflict arises concerning emergency blood transfusions when the patient is altered and no informed blood refusal advanced directive exists, perhaps even more distressing is the case of the child requiring emergency blood transfusions with parent refusal [16]. In another example, Orthodox Jew, Muslim, Hindu, and Sikh patients' adherence to a policy of privacy and modesty that may easily be overlooked in crowded emergency departments. Preference for health care providers of the same sex and an effort to minimize exposure of body parts is a shared concern of these faiths when staff is limited and patients may have their care initiated in a less private setting, such as an emergency department hallway or a trauma resuscitation suite. Diverse viewpoints of various spiritual and religious groups on issues of communication barriers, decision making, and end-of-life philosophies, all of which are relevant to emergency medicine practice, are examined (Table 1) [17–22a].

Diverse explanatory models of disease

Patients may have different explanatory models of illness, which may affect how the patient views his or her illness [23]. Disease is an objectively measurable pathological condition of the body. In contrast, illness is a feeling of not being normal and healthy. Illness may, in fact, be due to a disease but may also be due to a feeling of psychological or spiritual imbalance. By definition, perceptions of illness are highly culture related while disease usually is not. Thus, it is particularly important for the emergency physician to understand that within some cultures it may be unacceptable for a patient to complain of certain illnesses with particular cultural stigmata. Therefore,

Table 1
Potential Bioethical and Communication Centered Concerns of some Religious/Spiritual Groups

	Protestant*	Catholic	Jewish	Islamic	Asian/Eastern (Confucianism, Buddhism, Taoism)
Communication/Translation					
• May require interpreter familiar with culture				X	X
• Alternatives to Truth telling					X
• Choice of Words Important					X
Decision Making					
• Patient Autonomous (retains final decision) *some Jehovah's Witness may want to rely on spiritual directives	X	X	X		
• Family Oriented Decision Making				X	X
End-of-Life Views					
• Death is an accepted reality and part of the life cycle					X
• Preservation of Life Paramount	X	X	X	X	

patients may present with a constellation of symptoms that are more culturally appropriate, particularly when mental health issues arise [24]. Patients
may also present with culturally common complaints that may be foreign
to the clinician such as "empacho" or an impacted stomach. In the Latin-
American culture, "empacho" is felt to be a result of the adherence of
soft food and difficult-to-digest substances (such as popcorn or chewing
gum) to the stomach wall. Symptoms are anorexia, stomachache, vomiting,
pain with diarrhea, and generalized abdominal fullness. The healer noting
symptoms and checking for abdominal tenderness, feeling knots in the
calves, or rolling a fresh chicken egg over the abdomen makes the diagnosis.
"Empacho" is confirmed if the egg appears to stick to a particular area.
Remedies include rubbing the stomach or back, popping of the skin, and
purgative teas of wormwood (*estafiate*) or camomile (*manzanilla*). Lead
(*azarcón*) or mercury (*greta*) powders are still occasionally given. Administration of heavy metals has been thought to be a treatment and has been
known to present with toxicity [25,26]. In another example, fright or scare
has been used as an explanatory model of causation of diabetes in some
Mexican Americans [27,28].

Diverse models of bioethical decision making

Ethics is a system or code of moral values of a particular religion, person,
profession, or group. In the process of ethical conflict resolution, emergency
providers must answer the following questions: what are the medical indications, what are the patient's preferences, what are the issues surrounding
quality of life, and what special contextual features such as spiritual or cultural factors exist [29] (Table 2)? To deliver the highest quality care, emergency physicians commonly act on several patient-centered assumptions
borne from the core principle-based ethics of autonomy and informed consent, beneficence, nonmaleficence, and justice. An autonomous and rights-
based decision-making model is rooted in the idea that humans have the
right to make their own decisions and that their decisions should be respected to preserve human dignity even when grave consequences are
a result.

Western bioethical decision making is autonomy focused and rights
based. Patient autonomy is set at the highest premium. At the bedside,
emergency physicians typically assume the following: the preservation
of life, unless otherwise expressed by the patient or their decision maker;
that the patient is autonomous and unless impaired may make his or her
own decisions; and that the patient should have full disclosure of the options to evaluate the emergency physician's recommend treatment plan.
For patients from diverse cultures where rights-based decision making
is not the norm, this may be the wrong set of assumptions. Patients
may prefer not to know their disease or prognosis and may prefer that
their families make decisions for them and may view their illness/disease

Table 2
The Four Topics: Case Analysis in Clinical Ethics. *From* Jonsen A. et al. Clinical Ethics: A Practical Approach to Ethical Decisions in Clinical Medicine, 2002. 5th Edition; with permission of the McGraw Hill Companies

Medical Indications	Patient Preference
The Principles of Beneficence and Nonmaleficence	The Principle of Respect for Autonomy
What is the patient's medical problem? History? Diagnosis? Prognosis?	Is the patient mentally capable and legally competent? Is there evidence of incapacity?
Is the problem acute? Chronic? Critical? Emergent? Reversible?	If competent, what is the patient stating about preferences for treatment?
What are the goals of treatment?	Has the patient been informed of benefits and
What are the probabilities of success?	risks, understood this information and
What are the plans in case of therapeutic failure?	given consent?
In sum, how can this patient be benefited by medical and nursing care, and how can harm be avoids?	If incapacitated, who is the appropriate surrogate? Is the surrogate using appropriate standards for decision making?
	Has the patient expressed prior preferences, e.g. Advance Directives?
	Is the patient unwilling or unable to cooperate with medical treatment? If so, why?
	In sum, is the patient's right to choose being respected to the extent possible in ethics and law?

Quality of Life	Contextual Features
The Principles of Beneficence and Nonmaleficence and Respect for Autonomy	The Principles of Loyalty and Fairness
	Are there family issues that might influence treatment decisions?
What are the prospects, with or without treatment, for a return to normal life?	Are there provider (physician and nurses) issues that might influence treatment decisions?
What physical, mental and social deficits is the patient likely to experience if treatment succeeds?	Are there financial and economic factors?
	Are there religious or cultural factors?
Are there biases that might prejudice the provider's evaluation of the patient's quality of life?	Are there limits on confidentiality?
	Are there problems of allocation of resources?
	How does the law affect treatment decisions?
Is the patient's present or future condition such that his or her continued life might be judged undesirable?	Is clinical research or teaching involved?
	Is there any conflict of interest on the part of the providers or the institution?
Is there any plan and rationale to forego treatment?	
Are there plans for comfort and palliative care?	

through a more existential lens [17,30,31]. North American physicians typically embrace shared decision making when patients have diminished autonomy [32]. When patients have decision-making capacity yet prefer to defer decisions to others (eg, family, friends, spiritual healer, or spiritual community), this might be particularly frustrating to both the emergency care provider and the patient when not supported.

The ability to effectively communicate and apply bioethical problem-solving models to resolve challenges depends on the practitioner's ability to be cognizant of potential differences (Table 1). Decision making is generally accepted as an autonomous decision by the patient who is Protestant, Catholic, or Jewish and commonly supported by the emergency provider. These groups practice family involvement in decision making, however the patient retains the final word [20–22]. This is not necessarily the case with Islamic, Chinese, and Aboriginal groups because family involvement is imperative from the beginning, which may make timely administration of care difficult when family members are not readily available [17,19]. Concerning communication barriers, the requirement of interpreters for non–English speaking patients is intuitive for some spiritual or religious groups but is not exclusive of Protestant, Catholic, and Jewish groups as its members may share diverse cultures and languages. Examples of communication barriers have been given illustrating the importance of word choice and alternatives to truth telling when communicating care management plans to the Navajo people. This same concern may be shared with Chinese and other Aboriginal groups (North American Native Indian tribes, Inuit and Metis) [17]. Last of all, end-of-life philosophies are generally based on the group's perception of death. The Protestant, Catholic, Jewish, and Islamic faiths believe that it is their duty to protect life given to them by God. The conflicting issue in this instance is that of withholding or withdrawal of care and the timing of that decision during the patient's care so that suicide is not the end result. Rather than making abrupt decisions, these faith groups weigh the consequences of the patient's condition, financial burden on the family, and overall prognosis when making these decisions that are often assisted by respective religious authorities. The Aboriginal group believes that maintaining life is paramount and is generally accepting of death and less accepting of technological interventions that extend life. The Chinese group also shares a concern with the extension of life as death is regarded as good when most of one's moral duties in life have been fulfilled according to Confucian teachings. Philosophical Taoism also supports the acceptance of death. The review of these topics is by no means comprehensive or serves as an absolute truth for each group. The goal is familiarity with the spectrum of beliefs and attitudes that various spiritual and religious groups draw on to make bioethical decisions and recommendations for incorporation of this information into daily practice. Importantly, it must be recognized that simply because someone is a member of a cultural, spiritual, or religious group, does not always mean that they will adopt that group's customs or practices.

Time at the bedside

Bedside patient-provider interactions must be effectively optimized to provide care for the increasing numbers of patients seeking ED care.

When cultural and spiritual barriers exist, emergency physicians likely spend more time at the bedside but may feel frustrated or unprepared to provide optimal ED care when spiritual, religious, or cultural barriers are present. In one study conducted in an academic setting emergency medicine residents spent an average of 7 minutes and 31 seconds at the bedside assessing history and physical and 76 seconds on discharge instructions. Information on diagnosis, expected course of illness, self-care, use of medications, time-specified follow-up, and symptoms that should prompt return to the ED were not discussed in over one third of the cases. Fewer than one in five patients were asked whether they had questions, and there were no instances in which the provider confirmed patient understanding of the information [33]. Time in and of itself may complicate the assessment of cultural and spiritual concerns of patients as well as the discovery of differing ethical frameworks. Thus, strategies to manage language barriers and cultural and spiritual factors, as well as diverse ethical frameworks must be time efficient.

The response of regulatory agencies and emergency medicine professional societies

Hospital regulators have suggested systemwide organizational standards for addressing language, culture and spiritual factors that impact patient care. In the United States, the Joint Commission on Accreditation of Health care Organizations (JCAHO) standards require that health care facilities be sensitive to the linguistic, cultural, and spiritual needs of patients. Examples of the applicable standards can be found in the Joint Commission's *Comprehensive Accreditation Manual for Hospitals* under patient rights and organizational ethics and patient education [34]. Applicable JCAHO standards include that hospitals must consider a patient's cultural and religious practices, as well as various barriers, including linguistic, in its patient assessments. In Canada, as well as other locations in the West experiencing a large multicultural influx, it has been recognized that language barriers are significant in health care. Most hospitals meet the standard of spiritual or religious counseling regarding patient care by providing chaplain services. JCAHO has instituted a program called Hospitals, Language and Culture to examine how hospitals address the issues of language and culture that impact the quality and safety of patient care. The goal of this study is to make recommendations to hospitals and health care providers concerning competency regarding cultural and language barriers to health care.

In the past 10 years, there have been increasing levels of conversation and action by general and emergency medicine professional societies and educators to reduce ethnic disparities in emergency medicine. There has been a call for increased racial, ethnic, and cultural diversity of emergency medicine

faculty and trainees [3,35–39]. Several of the major organizations for organized emergency medicine have adopted position statements supporting cultural and ethnic and cultural sensitivity training of emergency professionals
as well as held special sessions to educate emergency professionals such as
the American College of Emergency Physicians, the Society for Academic
Emergency Medicine, the Canadian Association of Emergency Physicians,
and the US Council of Residency Directors. The Accreditation Council of
Graduate Medical Education and Emergency Medicine supports that
trainees demonstrate sensitivity and responsiveness to cultural and religious
preferences of patients and colleagues. The Canadian Medical Association
published a series of articles called "Bioethics for Clinicians" to inform
and enhance competency of its physicians regarding the concerns of various
spiritual and religious groups.

Vulnerability and informed consent for research or procedures

Research should be voluntary with the risks, benefits, and burdens carefully explained to potential participants with the ability of the participant to
give his or her expressed consent. Consent for research in the emergency setting may be complicated by the fact that patients present under stress [40–
43]. Patients with diminished autonomy and capacity to participate in the
informed consent process are thought of as "vulnerable." Traditionally, vulnerable populations in research have included children, prisoners, adults
with limited capacity to consent, and non–English speaking patients. The
National Bioethics Advisory Commission (NBAC) highlights subjects circumstances, which are situational, that create diminished autonomy and
therefore make them vulnerable [44]. Exclusion of vulnerable participants
may constitute unethical research if those persons who are vulnerable are
most likely to benefit from the research. The NBAC recommends that investigators not exclude persons from research, but importantly, "change the design so that it does not create situations in which people are unnecessarily
harmed." "Vulnerability, in the context of research, should be understood
to be a condition, intrinsic or situational, of some individuals that put
them at greater risk of being used in ethically inappropriate ways in research. Persons defined here are vulnerable to unethical research either because (1) they have difficulty providing voluntary informed consent arising
from limitations in decision-making capacity, or (2) they are especially at
risk for exploitation. Within the recommendations exists a broad array of
considerations that might obstruct an otherwise competent subject's ability
to give his or her voluntary and informed consent [45]. The responsibility of
ethical research first lies in the hands of the investigator. A global shift in
thinking must occur to incorporate the NBAC model of "situation not clas-
sification" into everyday research design and execution.

Similarly, when patients are undergoing medical procedures that require
consent, similar concerns as described to protect vulnerable populations

apply. Patients need to understand the risks, benefits, and burdens of the procedure to be performed. Several important factors such as language barriers, a patient's cultural or spiritual point of reference that shapes his or her decision-making framework, and his or her preferred substitute surrogates for consent (such as family or advisors) should all be taken into consideration when informed consent for a procedure is pursued.

Case summary

Recommended care for the 30-year-old Chinese-speaking woman diagnosed with an ectopic pregnancy includes termination of pregnancy via medical therapy (eg, methotrexate) or surgical therapy that is usually addressed once the diagnosis is confirmed. There are several cultural and religious issues that may complicate her care in the emergency department. Honoring her wish to discuss options about her care in consultation with her extended family and Chinese traditionalist practitioner poses the risk of not acting in a timely fashion to prevent rupture of the ectopic pregnancy and further harm to the patient. The emergency physician must be cognizant of the religious/spiritual preferences that are the basis for this patient's decision for care and this should be considered when determining decision-making capacity.

To optimize rapid and effective communication, a hospital-authorized translator or translation service should be used. Because the patient has identified important decision makers such as her family and spiritual advisor/traditional herbalist, these people should be included in discussion to the extent that the patient would feel helpful. Prospectively, it should not be assumed that the final decision of the patient would be contrary to the recommened course, despite cultural, religious, or spiritual differences. Although the diagnosis of ectopic pregnancy primarily concerns the mother, issues regarding end of life for the fetus also need to be addressed in this stressful situation. Respectfully communicating with patients and their preferred decision makers, and recognition and understanding of a patient's explanatory model of disease is the recommended approach to caring for vulnerable patients.

Summary

In the emergency department, history taking and physical exams are very directed and time conscious. That said, multidimensional assessments of patients with a focus on culture, religion, and spirituality by emergency physicians are recommended to overcome vulnerabilities to inappropriate care experience by some patient populations. Our ability to invest in the physician-patient relationship is threatened by the mere premise of our practice that requires efficiency of thought, interaction, and time [46]. Although something such as a spiritual assessment of a patient presenting for care in the emergency department may not always be necessary, an attempt to address a patient's spiritual needs deepens the ED beside interview. This for instance may allow physicians to connect with that patient and make the emergency department encounter more comfortable. Several recommendations follow to decrease the vulnerability of culturally and spiritually diverse patient populations in the emergency department (see Box 1).

1. *Be cognizant* that patients present with diverse ethical decision-making models or religious/spiritual preferences and may not hold Western bioethical views and that this should be considered in determining decision-making capacity. Emergency physicians should be willing to explore the patient's/family's diverse views as a basis of understanding via

---

Box 1. Some recommendations for working with culturally, spiritually or religiously diverse patients

1. Be cognizant and be willing to assess divergent bioethical models of decision making
   a. Use of open-ended questioning
   b. Involved the patient's family, caretakers or advisors
2. Use Translators whenever a language barrier exists
   a. Inquire with culturally concordant translators regarding word choice preferences when applicable
   b. In order of preference:
      i. Hospital Translator: Same language and culture as patient
      ii. Hospital Translator: Same language
      iii. Hospital Translator: Phone
      iv. Ad-Hoc (not recommended)
3. Conduct a Brief Spiritual Assessment
   a. Particularly when high stress decision or end-of-life issues
   b. Call the chaplain to the ED for referral
   c. Be willing to involve patient's own trusted clergy/advisors
4. Explore the Patient's Explanatory Model of Illness
   a. Use open-ended questioning
   b. Check if the recommended care plan is acceptable within the patient's model
5. Respect and support cultural, spiritual or religious preferences to the extent possible in the emergency department.

a combination of open-ended and more directed questioning. One might use an open-ended phrase such as, "Can you tell me what is important for you to consider as we try to come to a decision?" When family or other trusted persons are identified as important in the decision-making process, with the patient's permission, these persons should be invited to be a part of the discussion.

2. *Use professional translators whenever a language barrier exists.* To overcome barriers concerning language and culture, the emergency physician should make a concerted effort to involve trained interpreters. To establish consistency, an interpreter trained in a medical translation that is also familiar with the cultural traditions is preferred. If this option is not available, then an interpreter trained in the language only, followed by telephone interpreters and then ad hoc interpreters (hospital staff, family, friends) should be used in that order.

3. *Conduct a brief, bedside spiritual assessment in conjunction with ED chaplain support particularly in times of stress.* The directed questions in the HOPE (Hope, Organized religion, Personal spiritual practice, Effect of medical care) spiritual assessment tool created by Anandarajah and Hight [47] may help the emergency physician acknowledge a patient's spiritual needs in a timely fashion, especially in the event of crisis (see Box 2). Once one or more screening question have been asked, the emergency physician may make the appropriate referral to chaplains for further counseling or employ the use of the chaplain at the bedside to work cooperatively. Anything more than acknowledgment of a patient's spirituality and referral to chaplain services will depend on the emergency physician's comfort with his or her own spiritual beliefs. However, a physician's comfort level with his or her spiritual beliefs should not dictate competency of knowledge on various spiritual and religious practices.

4. *Explore the patient's explanatory model of illness.* Trying to assess why the patient or family/caregiver thinks that they are ill and even what the cultural norm of treatment may be can reveal useful information in the clinical work-up of a patient and the interaction with the patient's family or caregivers. Ask a question as simple as, "Tell me what you think is causing you (your family) to be ill and how you might think it should be treated?"

5. *Respect and support cultural, spiritual, or religious preferences to the extent possible in the emergency department.* With very little effort, one may be able to be supportive of a patient or family by respecting culturally or religiously motivated rights and rituals in the emergency department such as prayer, clothing, bathing rituals, or death rituals. Be prepared to support the emergency department staff in helping respect the patient/family request when no foreseen harm would be incurred.

Box 2. Examples of questions for the HOPE approach to spiritual assessment

H: Sources of hope, meaning, comfort, strength, peace, love and connectionWe have been discussing your support systems. I was wondering, what is there in your life that gives you internal support?
   What are your sources of hope, strength, comfort and peace?
   What do you hold on to during difficult times?
   What sustains you and keeps you going?
   For some people, their religious or spiritual beliefs act as a source of comfort and strength in dealing with life's ups and downs; is this true for you?
   If the answer is "Yes," go on to O and P questions.
   If the answer is "No," consider asking: Was it ever? If the answer is "Yes," ask: What changed?

O: Organized religion
   Do you consider yourself part of an organized religion?
   How important is this to you?
   What aspects of your religion are helpful and not so helpful to you?
   Are you part of a religious or spiritual community? Does it help you? How?

P: Personal spirituality/practices
   Do you have personal spiritual beliefs that are independent of organized religion? What are they?
   Do you believe in God? What kind of relationship do you have with God?
   What aspects of your spirituality or spiritual practices do you find most helpful to you personally? (e.g., prayer, meditation, reading scripture, attending religious services, listening to music, hiking, communing with nature)

E: Effects on medical care and end-of-life issues
   Has being sick (or your current situation) affected your ability to do the things that usually help you spiritually? (Or affected your relationship with God?)
   As a doctor, is there anything that I can do to help you access the resources that usually help you?
   Are you worried about any conflicts between your beliefs and your medical situation/care/decisions?
   Would it be helpful for you to speak to a clinical chaplain/community spiritual leader?
   Are there any specific practices or restrictions I should know about in providing your medical care? (e.g., dietary restrictions, use of blood products)
   If the patient is dying: How do your beliefs affect the kind of medical care you would like me to provide over the next few days/weeks/months?

References

[1] Carmamota SA. Immigrants in the United States -1998. A Snapshot of America's Foreign-born Population. Center for Immigration Studies. 1999. Available at: http://www.cis.org/articles/1999/back199.html. Accessed June 28, 2006.

[2] Augustine JJ, Kellermann AL. The emergency medicine workforce study: more questions than answers. Ann Emerg Med 2002;40(1):16–8.

[3] Heron S, Haley L Jr. Diversity in emergency medicine–a model program. Acad Emerg Med 2001;8(2):192–5.

[4] Flores G, Gee D, Kastner B. The teaching of cultural issues in US and Canadian medical schools. Acad Med 2000;75(5):451–5.

[5] Puchalski CM, Larson DB. Developing curricula in spirituality and medicine [erratum appears in Acad Med 1998;73(10):1038]. Acad Med 1998;73(9):970–4.

[6] Carrasquillo O, Orav EJ, Brennan TA, et al. Impact of language barriers on patient satisfaction in an emergency department. J Gen Intern Med 1999;14(2):82–7.

[7] Baker DW, Hayes R, Fortier JP. Interpreter use and satisfaction with interpersonal aspects of care for Spanish-speaking patients. Med Care 1998;36(10):1461–70.

[8] Baker DW, Parker RM, Williams MV, et al. Use and effectiveness of interpreters in an emergency department. JAMA 1996;275(10):783–8.

[9] Garcia EA, Roy LC, Okada PJ, et al. A comparison of the influence of hospital-trained, ad hoc, and telephone interpreters on perceived satisfaction of limited English-proficient parents presenting to a pediatric emergency department. Pediatr Emerg Care 2004;20(6):373–8.

[10] Flores G, Rabke-Verani J, Pine W, et al. The importance of cultural and linguistic issues in the emergency care of children [review]. Pediatr Emerg Care 2002;18(4):271–84.

[11] Boudreaux ED, O'Hea E, Chasuk R. Spiritual role in healing. An alternative way of thinking. Prim Care 2002;29(2):439–54, viii.

[12] Larson DBSJ, McCullough ME. Scientifc research on spirituality and health: a consensus report. Rockville, MD: National Institute of Healthcare Research; 1997.

[13] Armbruster CA, Chibnall JT, Legett S. Pediatrician beliefs about spirituality and religion in medicine: associations with clinical practice. Pediatrics 2003;111(3):e227–35.

[14] Larson DB, Koenig HG. Is God good for your health? The role of spirituality in medical care. Cleve Clin J Med 2000;67(2)(80):83–4.

[15] Puchalski CM, Dorff RE, Hendi IY. Spirituality, religion, and healing in palliative care. Clin Geriatr Med 2004;20(4):689–714, vi–vii.

[16] Migden DR, Braen GR. The Jehovah's Witness blood refusal card: ethical and medicolegal considerations for emergency physicians. Acad Emerg Med 1998;5(8):815–24.

[17] Bowman KW, Hui EC. Bioethics for clinicians: 20. Chinese bioethics. CMAJ 2000;163(11):1481–5.

[18] Coward H, Sidhu T. Bioethics for clinicians: 19. Hinduism and Sikhism. CMAJ 2000;163(9):1167–70.

[19] Daar AS, al Khitamy AB. Bioethics for clinicians: 21. Islamic bioethics. CMAJ 2001;164(1):60–3.

[20] Goldsand G, Rosenberg ZR, Gordon M. Bioethics for clinicians: 22. Jewish bioethics. CMAJ 2001;164(2):219–22.

[21] Markwell HJ, Brown BF. Bioethics for clinicians: 27. Catholic bioethics. CMAJ 2001;165(2):189–92.

[22] Pauls M, Hutchinson RC. Bioethics for clinicians: 28. Protestant bioethics. CMAJ 2002;166(3):339–43.

[22a] Ellerby JH, McKenzie J, McKay S, Gariepy GJ, Kaufert JM. Bioethics for clinicians: 18. Aboriginal cultures [see comment]. CMAJ 2002;163(7):845–50.

[23] Dein S. Explanatory models of and attitudes towards cancer in different cultures. Lancet Oncol 2004;5(2):119–24.

[24] Dein S. ABC of mental health. Mental health in a multiethnic society. BMJ 1997;315(7106): 473–6.

[25] Baer RD, Garcia de Alba J, Leal RM, et al. Mexican use of lead in the treatment of empacho: community, clinic, and longitudinal patterns. Soc Sci Med 1998;47(9):1263–6.

[26] Weller SC, Pachter LM, Trotter RT 2nd, et al. Empacho in four Latino groups: a study of intra- and inter-cultural variation in beliefs. Med Anthropol 1993;15(2):109–36.

[27] Jezewski MA, Poss J. Mexican Americans' explanatory model of type 2 diabetes. West J Nurs Res 2002;24(8):840–58; discussion 858–67.

[28] McCabe R, Priebe S. Explanatory models of illness in schizophrenia: comparison of four ethnic groups. Br J Psychiatry 2004;185:25–30.

[29] Jonsen A, Siegler M, Winslade W. Clinical Ethics: A Practical Approach to Ethical Decision Making in Clinical Medicine. 5th ed. New York: McGraw-Hill; 2002.

[30] Carrese JA, Rhodes LA. Bridging cultural differences in medical practice. The case of discussing negative information with Navajo patients. J Gen Intern Med 2000;15(2):92–6.

[31] Wright F, Cohen S, Caroselli C. Diverse decisions. How culture affects ethical decision making. Crit Care Nurs Clin North Am 1997;9(1):63–74.

[32] Catalano JT. Ethical decision making in the critical care patient. Crit Care Nurs Clin North Am 1997;9(1):45–52.

[33] Rhodes KV, Vieth T, He T, et al. Resuscitating the physician-patient relationship: emergency department communication in an academic medical center. Ann Emerg Med 2004; 44(3):262–7.

[34] Joint Commission on the Accreditation of Healthcare Organizations. Comprehensive accreditation manual for hospitals: the official handbook. Duluth, MN: 2005

[35] Cone DC, Richardson LD, Todd KH, et al. Health care disparities in emergency medicine. Acad Emerg Med 2003;10(11):1176–83.

[36] Hamilton G, Marco CA. Emergency medicine education and health care disparities. Acad Emerg Med 2003;10(11):1189–92.

[37] James T. SAEM diversity position statement. The SAEM Diversity Interest Group. Acad Emerg Med 2000;7(9):1055.

[38] Martin ML. The value of diversity in academic emergency medicine. Acad Emerg Med 2000; 7(9):1027–31.

[39] Weaver C, Sklar D. Diagnostic dilemmas and cultural diversity in emergency rooms. West J Med 1980;133(4):356–66.

[40] Herlitz J. Consent for research in emergency situations. Resuscitation 2002;53(3):239.

[41] Marco CA, Committee SE. The Society for Academic Emergency Medicine position on informed consent for emergency medicine research. Acad Emerg Med 2004;11(10): 1090–1.

[42] Schmidt TA, Salo D, Hughes JA, et al. Confronting the ethical challenges to informed consent in emergency medicine research. Acad Emerg Med 2004;11(10):1082–9.

[43] Smithline HA, Mader TJ, Crenshaw BJ. Do patients with acute medical conditions have the capacity to give informed consent for emergency medicine research? Acad Emerg Med 1999; 6(8):776–80.

[44] National Bioethics Advisory Commission. Ethical and Policy Issues in Research Involving Human Participants. Report and Recommendations of the National Bioethics Advisory Commission. 2001;(1): 61–94.

[45] Quest T, Marco CA. Ethics seminars: vulnerable populations in emergency medicine research. Acad Emerg Med 2003;10(11):1294–8.

[46] Propp DA. Is spirituality an emergency physician's competency? Acad Emerg Med 2003; 10(10):1098–9.

[47] Anandarajah G, Hight E. Spirituality and medical practice: using the HOPE questions as a practical tool for spiritual assessment. Am Fam Physician 2001;63(1):81–9.

ELSEVIER
SAUNDERS

Emerg Med Clin N Am
24 (2006) 703–714

EMERGENCY
MEDICINE
CLINICS OF
NORTH AMERICA

Ethical and Practical Aspects of Disclosing Adverse Events in the Emergency Department

Samantha L. Stokes, MPH[a],
Albert W. Wu, MD, MPH[a],*,
Peter J. Pronovost, MD, PhD[a,b]

[a]Johns Hopkins Bloomberg School of Public Health, 624 North Broadway,
Baltimore, MD 21205, USA
[b]Center for Innovation in Quality Patient Care, Johns Hopkins Medical Institutions, 901
South Bond Street, Suite 318, Bond Street Wharf, Baltimore MD 21231, USA

Errors and emergency medicine

The emergency department (ED) will never be an error-free environment. All practicing clinicians make mistakes, and any clinician who sees many patients will be involved eventually in an incident where a patient suffers an adverse event caused by medical care error. An adverse event is defined here as an injury to a patient resulting from medical care [1]. An error is defined as an act not completed as intended, or the use of the wrong plan of action to achieve a specific aim [1]. A medical error may or may not result in an adverse event.

The Institute of Medicine report, "To Err is Human," estimates that between 44,000 and 98,000 deaths result annually from medical errors [1]. Errors occur frequently in emergency medicine (EM), as in all of medicine. Although little information is available about the frequency of adverse events caused by errors in the ED, errors that result in a severe harm are much less frequent than errors with less serious consequences. Fordyce and colleagues [2] found that an error in care occurred in 18% of cases in the ED; only 2% of the reported errors had a serious adverse outcome.

Efforts are underway to help reduce the frequency of adverse events caused by errors in medical care. However, how caregivers handle adverse

This work was supported by a grant from MCIC Vermont, Inc.
* Corresponding author.
E-mail address: awu@jhsph.edu (A.W. Wu).

events when they occur is nearly as important as limiting their number. When possible, steps must be taken to limit the harm caused by the incident, initiate an investigation into the causes of the adverse event, and reduce the probability that the incident will recur. Full disclosure must be made to the patient.

Emergency medicine and disclosure

The patient–physician relationship is unique in EM in its duration, intensity, and character. Patients who use ED services usually have little or no choice regarding selection of hospital, and even less choice of medical providers upon arrival. This lack of choice affects the nature of the patient–physician relationship. Most encounters in the ED represent the initial and final meeting between patient and physician. It is rare that an EM physician will develop a longitudinal relationship with a patient or family member. Because of the lack of a long-term personal relationship, engendering a patient's trust is a greater challenge for EM physicians [3]. In addition, the unexpected and emergent nature of the patient's situation heightens stress and emotional upset, making the patient feel more vulnerable and less secure in the EM environment than when interacting with his/her primary caregiver.

In emergency situations, patients may also have less autonomy in decision making when rapid decisions are required. Standards for informed consent may yield to physician judgment of what treatment is acutely needed, which in some cases may be deemed as paternalism [4]. This decreased patient autonomy can increase tension in cases in which the patient is harmed, rather than helped, by medical care. Under different circumstances, patients often are inclined to give the physician the benefit of the doubt when a medical error arises. Insecurity in the ED environment and unfamiliarity with the physician providing medical care can lead to distrust, potentially contributing to a greater likelihood of litigation unfavorable to EM physicians when there is an adverse event.

Because EM physicians operate in a high-risk environment with the potential for distrust between physician and patient, it behooves them to become excellent communicators. Such a strategy may not only improve their relationships with patients and help them be more effective, but may also reduce the probability of being sued. EM physicians have only a short time to interact with their patients and demonstrate that they are candid, capable, and trustworthy. When a medical error occurs in the short EM interaction, good communication becomes even more vital. Patients have high expectations for physician behavior. If the physician appears less than honest and forthright during the communication of the error, this may increase distrust, anger, frustration, and willingness to sue for a perceived wrongdoing [5]. If the physician approaches the discussion with open, honest, and clear communication, and demonstrates a willingness to work with the patient to remedy the error and investigate the cause, there is a greater chance that the patient will trust the physician despite the error [6].

The ethical duty to disclose

Ethical arguments supporting full disclosure of adverse events include fiduciary obligations, autonomy, truth telling, respect for patients, and professional standards. Arguments can be made for and against disclosure of errors that do not cause harm; this will be addressed later. The following discussion of ethics pertains to errors resulting in adverse events, or preventable adverse events.

The role of the fiduciary can be traced back to Roman law, where a second party became the fiduciary of the first party's property when the second party was entrusted with the management and responsibility of the first party's property. The second party, now in the role of the fiduciary, was responsible for making decisions pertaining to the property that would benefit the first party solely. Similarly, when the patient puts him- or herself into the hands of the physician, the physician becomes the patient's fiduciary and is required to act in the best interests of the patient [7].

Part of acting in the patient's best interest is enabling patients to make autonomous decisions about their care. To make an autonomous decision, patients must be informed fully about their condition and the potential consequences of various courses of action [8,9]. In the context of an adverse event, this means presenting the patient with the facts relating to the incident, so that he/she can make decisions about diagnostic and therapeutic options. Disclosure provides patients with the opportunity to understand the basis of recommendations, and to proceed with care under the current physician or to have their care transferred to another physician. Disclosure also allows the patient the option of seeking restitution. If the patient is kept unaware of the details surrounding a preventable adverse event, he/she cannot begin this course of action.

In sum, the physician has the obligation to tell the truth [8–10], which is consistent with the principle of respect for the patient. Truth telling enables the patient to make autonomous decisions and seek remediation, which in turn ensures that a physician will fulfill the role of patient fiduciary.

Professional standards also dictate full disclosure of adverse events. The American College of Physicians [11] ethics manual reads, "...physicians should disclose to patients information about procedural or judgment errors made in the course of care if such information is material to the patient's well-being. Errors do not necessarily constitute improper, negligent, or unethical behavior, but failure to disclose them may." The Joint Commission on the Accreditation of Healthcare Organizations [12] states that, "Patients and when appropriate, their families, are informed about the outcomes of care, including unanticipated outcomes." These and other professional ethics standards have led organizations to develop their own codes for dealing with medical errors. For instance, the Johns Hopkins Hospital's medical error disclosure policy [13] states, "It is the right of the patient to receive information about clinically relevant medical errors. The JHH has an obligation to disclose information regarding these errors to the patient in a prompt, clear and honest manner." Such policies regarding honest and full disclosure reflect the ethical arguments addressed previously: fiduciary obligations, autonomy, truth telling and respect for patients. These policies are also consistent with the core mission of the institution. Additionally, professional standards pertaining to disclosure of adverse events encourage the patient to develop greater trust in the medical profession as a whole.

When organizations take an active role in developing an open disclosure policy, they are also promoting patient safety. An environment in which reporting and disclosing adverse events caused by medical errors are encouraged may allow more dialog surrounding error and may decrease the associated stigma. A culture that promotes the discussion of errors also promotes an increase in error reporting and allows more incident investigations to be initiated. The results of these investigations can then be evaluated, contributing factors identified, and steps taken to prevent the future occurrence of similar events.

Barriers to disclosure

Despite an ethical duty to disclose, and growing consensus that disclosure is in the best interest of the patient, physician, and medical profession, it does not always occur, and may even occur only rarely. Even when it does occur, disclosure is often incomplete; details may be altered [14], or pertinent facts omitted, leaving the patient with only part of the story. This may be done in an attempt to present the involved individuals in a better light, or to obscure responsibility. In either case, the knowledge the patient receives is misleading, limiting the patient's ability to make informed decisions.

Why doesn't full disclosure happen more often? Adverse events are emotionally difficult for physicians [15]. They respond to making a mistake with fear, remorse, guilt, hostility, anger and self-doubt. The prospect of disclosing an adverse event and incurring the patient's reaction is also upsetting, and may discourage a physician from admitting to that error.

In general, it is difficult to admit that one has made a mistake of any kind, particularly in medicine, where the culture shared by patients and providers promotes expectations of flawless performance [16]. Caregiver feelings of guilt, shame, and self-doubt enshroud medical errors [17]. By admitting to a mistake, the physician may lose self-confidence and risk damaging his/her professional relationships and reputation with colleagues and patients.

The fear of lawsuits is a large barrier to disclosure. The idea that "Anything you say can be used against you" is prevalent. Many physicians believe that a full disclosure is tantamount to an admission of guilt and increases the chances of being sued [18,19]. Ironically, research and anecdotes suggest exactly the opposite. If anything, when patients are told what happened in a candid, clear, and honest fashion, they may be less likely to file a lawsuit [19,20]. Lack of clear communication surrounding the adverse event can be pivotal in the patient's decision. Vincent and colleagues [5] found that patients or family members take legal action not only because of the original adverse event, but also because of the poor handling of the incident after it occurred. Sandra Gilbert's [21] memoir, "Wrongful Death," illustrates how the lack of transparency regarding the details of her husband's death, and her need to know the truth, led to the lawsuit she filed. The experience of the Veterans Affairs Medical Center in Lexington, Kentucky, is encouraging [22]. Since 1987, its policy pertaining to adverse events has emphasized the duty of the physician as caregiver to notify the patient (or family) if there was an error in the patient's care. The center's liability claims are moderate, and their payouts are lower than comparable institutions. Also, out of 88 claims filed in a 7-year period, only 8 proceeded to federal court, where 7 were dismissed; the single remaining case, which proceeded to trial, concluded with a favorable verdict found for the center.

Nevertheless, evidence regarding the impact of disclosure is incomplete. Lawsuits may result if people are made aware that they were injured by a previously unsuspected error. On the other hand, those who are aware of an injury may be less likely to sue after full disclosure. The balance between these two types of events has yet to be determined.

Perhaps the most remediable barrier to disclosure is lack of instruction in communication: physicians simply are not trained in how to disclose a medical error and, as a result, have a harder time fulfilling the ethical duty to disclose. The remainder of this article focuses on this barrier and addresses how to approach and conduct the disclosure process. The authors recognize that the journey of training physicians in the art of disclosure has just begun; this is their first attempt to develop recommendations that will continue to evolve over time.

How to disclose

Despite ample support for medical error disclosure, there is very little instruction or training available. There are a few training materials, such as The American Society for Healthcare Risk Management's Patient Safety Curriculum's session on "Adverse Event Disclosure" and its Monograph series on disclosure [23–25]. Recently, Johns Hopkins University developed the training package, "Removing Insult from Injury: Disclosing Adverse Events," in which the disclosure process is explored in a 25-minute instructional video [26]. The video discusses the rationale for disclosure and describes the who, where, when, what, and how of disclosure. It also focuses on specific elements of the discussion, including accepting responsibility and apologizing in a sincere fashion. The elements described in "Removing Insult from Injury" are discussed below, keeping in mind the vicissitudes of the EM environment.

The disclosure process

It is helpful to approach the disclosure process as a special case of breaking bad news [27]. More important is to view the disclosure of an adverse event as a part of the ongoing dialog between the patient and physician about the patient's condition and what is occurring in his/her health care.

Once an error has been recognized, or its effects are noticed, steps should be taken immediately (if possible) to prevent or rectify any harm caused by the error. This process is illustrated in Fig. 1. In cases where harm to the patient has occurred, the patient or, when appropriate, the family, should be notified as soon as possible. An investigation into the cause of the adverse event should be initiated, and strategies implemented to reduce the probability of it recurring. The dialog surrounding the incident does not end with the initial disclosure. Just as patient care continues, the dialog with the patient should continue as more is learned from the incident investigation. The patient's medical care should be adjusted because of the error, and the incident investigation should be seen through until the end, a challenge for EM physicians because follow-up is rarely planned. However, in the case of adverse events, ED physicians should ensure there is adequate follow-up.

In cases where the patient is not harmed (a near miss), disclosure of the error is discretionary. However, the error still should be reported so an investigation can be launched. Much can be learned from errors that do not result in an adverse event. The investigation may turn up system problems related to errors that do result in adverse events. When an error occurs

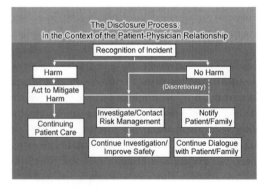

Fig. 1. The disclosure process in the context of the patient–physician relationship. (Courtesy of Johns Hopkins University; with permission.)

that does not cause harm, it should be looked on as an opportunity to improve patient safety through investigation [28].

Although the disclosure of a near miss is discretionary, it is important to keep in mind the needs of the patient. Multiple studies have indicated that patients wish to be notified of all errors pertaining to their care, not just the errors resulting in adverse events [20,29]. An open dialog with a patient regarding all errors (both those resulting in and those not resulting in adverse events) can help maintain the patient's trust and gives the patient full autonomy regarding medical decisions. However, discussion of all errors is not always practical. In many cases, such disclosure would burden both caregivers and patients. Perhaps a more feasible approach to disclosing errors not resulting in harm is to disclose those that slip through all defense mechanisms (ie, those errors that "reach the patient"), even though that concept has yet to be proven valid and reliable. Veterans Affairs now encourages that all events that require a change in a plan be disclosed or a note written about the incident [30].

When should an adverse event be disclosed?

An adverse event should be disclosed as soon as possible after it has been recognized. This initial notification should be viewed as part of routine communication within the patient–physician relationship. However, if there is a serious adverse outcome, then talking to a risk manager or counselor experienced with the disclosure of adverse events, before notifying the patient, can provide the physician with support, and make the disclosure process less painful for all concerned. Many adverse events are identified after the patient has left the ED. Additionally, because of the lack of follow-up that characterizes EM, EM physicians usually learn about errors and adverse events in an arbitrary fashion. For these reasons, EDs will need to establish systems to review cases and to follow up potential adverse events.

Who should disclose the adverse event?

The health care professional whom the patient perceives as being responsible for his/her care should be the person to disclose the error. In the ED, this is generally the supervising attending physician or the physician who cared for the patient. If others were involved in the error, or are in a good position to explain what happened, they may also participate in the initial disclosure. An administrative representative, such as a risk manager, may be useful to the patient later in the disclosure process, but his/her presence at the initial disclosure is not always necessary and may make the patient feel wary. If the patient has left the ED, the treating physician should discuss the case with the department chairman and with risk management to clarify who will call and what will be said.

Where should the disclosure take place?

The disclosure of an adverse event is emotionally difficult for both the patient and the physician, and the location of the disclosure should respect this. Privacy is paramount. The best location for disclosure is a private room or quiet space in the ED, or a physician's office if possible. When these options are not available, the physician should make every effort to conduct the disclosure with as much privacy as possible. The ED poses unique challenges related to crowding and close quarters, without the luxury of family conference rooms. However, the ED director should identify an appropriate area in which to disclose and facilitate confidential discussions, and communicate this to staff.

What should be disclosed?

An initial disclosure should include everything the physician is certain of at the time of the discussion. The story generally emerges over time. If information regarding the error is unknown or unclear, the physician should say so, and should not speculate about what might have occurred. The patient should be assured that as information is obtained through the investigation, it will be shared with him/her. Patients appreciate the honesty and willingness to have an ongoing dialog.

Apology

When asked, patients usually mention three things they want and expect to hear in a disclosure: a description of what happened, an assurance that the problem will be investigated and fixed, and an apology [20,31,32]. Understanding that someone regrets and feels bad about a situation can help a patient to cope better with the incident. Although a full disclosure with a sincere apology conveys respect for the patient and allows for forgiveness to occur, the physician should keep in mind that they do not ensure this. Forgiveness may take a long time, or may never occur. However, without the apology and disclosure there is no groundwork to allow for the process of forgiveness to begin [33].

Physicians should take care to be empathetic in the disclosure discussion, which includes validating the patient's emotions, offering support, and conveying a sense of understanding the patient's situation. Respect for patients can be communicated by listening, but empathy should not be overstrained. The physician cannot know exactly what the patient is feeling or the exact context of his/her emotions. Stating, "I know just how you feel," or something similar may belittle the emotional reaction of the patient [27]. Instead, the physician should say, "I am greatly distressed by what has happened. If you need to discuss anything, I am always available."

In keeping with the physician's role as fiduciary, the apology should be sincere and should acknowledge responsibility. Patients want someone to take responsibility for what happened [31,32] and responsibility must be assigned at some level to enable the harmed patient to engage in the process of justice. In the case of individual responsibility, the physician should say, "I am sorry that I did this." However, situations are often complex, involving multiple system factors and various overlapping responsibilities. In cases such as this, the physician can still accept responsibility on behalf of the health care team or institution by saying, "I am sorry that this happened. We are responsible for this." It is also vital to avoid blaming another individual. When making the disclosure, the physician should take care not to name, blame, or criticize anyone involved in the patient's care or the medical error.

Apologizing is not the same thing as stating guilt. Some evidence suggests that apologizing does not increase the chance of litigation, and, in some cases, an apology has appeared to diffuse anger and avert a claim [34]. Anecdotal evidence also suggests that an apology made in mediation assists in resolving the dispute. In response to the healing power of an apology, and the ethics that dictate it, states have begun to pass legislation that makes an apology inadmissible in a court of law [35].

Advice for conducting disclosure discussions

Every instance of disclosure is in some ways unique, and no guideline can provide all the instruction a physician may need when disclosing an error. However, some basic communication strategies should be kept in mind when conducting disclosure discussions. It is important to try to make the patient feel comfortable in a situation where one is likely to feel powerless. It is helpful for the physician to begin by making eye contact with the patient, and adapting to be as close to the patient's eye level as possible [27]. If the patient is sitting, the physician should sit. If the patient opts to remain standing, the physician should do the same. Physical barriers, such as a desk or hospital bed, between the physician and patient should be avoided because this conveys a sense of aloofness and a lack of identification with the patient.

The initial statement is important; it may be the only thing that the patient remembers. Therefore, as in the case of breaking bad news, the disclosure of a medical error should begin with a forthright statement such as, "I am afraid I have bad news..." It is vital not to make assumptions about what the patient knows. Before discussing details of the adverse event, the extent of the patient's knowledge should be determined. In this way, the physician can align the discussion to where the patient is starting from and engage the patient in a more meaningful disclosure dialog.

The physician should not rush the disclosure, but should pause frequently, so the patient can absorb the information, ask questions, and make comments. Important facts may have to be repeated more than once, and questions asked to ascertain whether or not the patient understands the information.

The patient is likely to be upset to learn there has been an error in his/her care and may react with strong emotions, including anger. The physician should expect this and take care to manage emotional reactions by not becoming defensive or angry when confronted with questions from the patient or family member.

Although all the desired components of the disclosure process should occur (a thorough explanation of what happened, a sincere apology, and an assurance that an investigation will be conducted), there is no particular order or frequency in which these elements must occur. The physician should let the patient direct the disclosure by observing cues: questions asked, body language, emotional reactions, and other commentary (eg, stated previous knowledge). The clinicians conducting the discussion should not focus solely on their own agenda. Allowing the patient to direct the conversation will give the patient a greater comfort level with the physician. The patient should be allowed to complete thoughts and sentences and the physician should not jump in to insert his/her own perspective or feelings. Strong emotional reactions from a patient can make a physician uncomfortable, and in response he/she may pull back or belittle the patient's feelings. Instead of attempting to refute what the patient expresses, the physician should validate those strong reactions and empathize with the patient. By using these skills and techniques, the physician conveys trustworthiness, respect for the patient, and regret and empathy for the patient's current situation, and demonstrates that the best interests of the patient are his/her utmost concern.

After the initial disclosure

The initial notification of the error is only the first step in the disclosure process. The physician or other appropriate person must plan for future contacts with the patient and family, and follow through with those plans. The health care team should clarify which clinician or hospital administrator will be the primary contact person for the family and patient.

Together, the physician and patient should develop a list of priorities and come up with a plan to address them. This process provides the patient, and the physician, with a sense of control of the situation, which can lead to some comfort for both parties. Additionally, the physician should help the patient identify a support network to help cope with the after-effects of the medical error. It is very important for the physician to provide the patient with an easy way to contact him/her with any questions or concerns.

The physician should obtain updates on the patient's ongoing medical condition and ensure that he/she is referred to the appropriate physicians for additional care necessitated by the adverse event. Following through and planning a patient's care is particularly complicated in the ED and not likely to occur in an effective manner without preparation and practice. EM teams should discuss this reality, develop a plan, train caregivers, and if possible, simulate the process.

Summary

Disclosure is difficult in any field of medicine. Environmental factors in the ED that make disclosure even more difficult are the same factors that make a well-conducted disclosure paramount. Communicating an adverse event clearly to the patient or family is in line with the ethical duty to disclose, maintains patient trust, enables patient safety improvements, and may even help avoid a lawsuit. Learning how to disclose and communicate effectively with patients will help make full disclosure more commonplace.

References

[1] Institute of Medicine. To err is human: building a safer health system. Washington, DC: National Academy Press; 2000.

[2] Fordyce J, Blank FSJ, Pekow P, et al. Errors in a busy emergency department. Ann Emerg Med 2003;42:324–33.

[3] Kelly JJ, Njuki F, Lane PL, et al. Design of a questionnaire to measure trust in an emergency department. Acad Emerg Med 2005;12:147–51.

[4] Ladd RE. Patients without choices: the ethics of decision-making in Emergency Medicine. J Emerg Med 1985;3:149–56.

[5] Vincent C, Young M, Phillips A. Why do people sue doctors? A study of patients and relatives taking legal action. Lancet 1994;343(8913):1609–13.

[6] Liebman C, Hyman CS. A mediation skills model to manage and disclose of errors and adverse events to patients. Health Aff 2004;23(4):22–32.

[7] Perkins HS. The physician as fiduciary: the basis for an ethics of patient care. In: Stein JH, editor. Internal medicine, Volume 2. Boston: Little, Brown & Co; 1990. p. 2448–50.

[8] Vogel J, Delgado R. To tell the truth: physicians' duty to disclose medical mistakes. UCLA Law Rev 1980;28(52):52–94.

[9] Wu AW, Cavanaugh TA, McPhee SJ, et al. To tell the truth: ethical and practical issues in disclosing medical mistakes to patients. J Gen Intern Med 1997;12:770–5.

[10] Gallagher SM. Truth telling. Ostomy Wound Manage 1998;44(11):17–9.

[11] American College of Physicians. Ethics manual. 4th edition. Ann Intern Med 1998;128:576–94.

[12] Joint Commission on the Accreditation of Healthcare Organizations. Standard RI.1.1.2. July 1, 2001.

[13] Johns Hopkins Hospital. Interdisciplinary Clinical Practice Manual PAT 026. Medical Error Disclosure. Available at: www.insidehopkinsmedicine.org/icpm; Accessed March 25, 2005.

[14] Finkelstein D, Wu A, Holtzman N, et al. When a physician harms a patient by a medical error: ethical, legal, and risk-management considerations. J Clin Ethics 1997;8(4):330–5.

[15] Wu AW. Medical error: the second victim. The doctor who makes the mistake needs help too. BMJ 2000;320:726–7.

[16] Baylis F. Errors in medicine: nurturing truthfulness. J Clin Ethics 1997;8(4):336–40.

[17] Wears R, Wu A. Dealing with failure: the aftermath of errors and adverse events. Ann Emerg Med 2002;39(3):344–6.

[18] Gallagher TH, Waterman AD, Ebers AG, et al. Patients' and physicians' attitudes regarding the disclosure of medical errors. JAMA 2003;289(8):1001–7.

[19] Witman AB, Park DM, Hardin SB. How do patients want physicians to handle mistakes? A survey of internal medicine patients in an academic setting. Arch Intern Med 1996;156: 2565–9.

[20] Mazor KM, Simon SR, Yood RA, et al. Health plan members' views on disclosure of medical errors. Ann Int Med 2004;140(6):409–18, E419–E423.

[21] Gilbert S. Wrongful death. New York: W.W. Norton; 1995.

[22] Kraman SS, Hamm G. Risk management: extreme honesty may be the best policy. Ann Intern Med 1999;131(12):963–7.

[23] Monographs Task Force of the American Society for Healthcare Risk Management. Disclosure of unanticipated events: the next step in better communication with patients. Chicago: ASHRM; May 2003.

[24] Monographs Task Force of the American Society for Healthcare Risk Management. Disclosure of unanticipated events: creating an effective patient communication policy. Chicago: ASHRM; November 2003.

[25] Monographs Task Force of the American Society for Healthcare Risk Management. Disclosure: what works now & what can work even better. Chicago: ASHRM; February 2004.

[26] Wu AW, Stokes SL. Removing insult from injury: disclosing adverse events. Johns Hopkins University, 2004. Available at: www.jhsph.edu/removinginsultfrominjury.

[27] Buckman R. How to break bad news: a guide for health care professionals. Baltimore, MD: The Johns Hopkins University Press; 1992.

[28] Wu AW. Is there an obligation to disclose near-misses in medical care? In: Sharpe VA, editor. Accountability: patient safety and policy reform. Washington, DC: Georgetown University Press; 2004. p. 135–42.

[29] Hobgood C, Peck CR, Gilbert B, et al. Medical errors-what and when: what do patients want to know? Acad Emerg Med 2002;9:1156–61.

[30] National Ethics Committee of the Veterans Health Administration. Disclosing adverse events to patients. National Center for Ethics in Health Care, Veterans Health Administration, Department of Veteran Affairs; March 2003.

[31] Hingorani M, Wong T, Vafidis G. Patients' and doctors' attitudes to amount of information given after unintended injury during treatment: cross sectional, questionnaire survey. BMJ 1999;318:640–1.

[32] Schwappach DLB, Koeck CM. What makes an error unacceptable? A factorial survey on the disclosure of medical errors. Int J Qual Health Care 2004;16(4):317–26.

[33] Berlinger N. Avoiding cheap grace: medical harm, patient safety, and the culture(s) of forgiveness. Hastings Cent Rep 2003;33(6):28–36.

[34] Zimmerman R. Doctors' new tool to fight lawsuits: saying 'I'm sorry'. Wall Street Journal. May 18, 2005:A1.

[35] Cohen JR. Toward candor after error: the first apology law. Harvard Health Policy Review 2004;5(1):21–4.

ELSEVIER
SAUNDERS

Emerg Med Clin N Am
24 (2006) 715–731

EMERGENCY
MEDICINE
CLINICS OF
NORTH AMERICA

Expert Witness Testimony: The Ethics of Being a Medical Expert Witness

Louise B. Andrew, MD, JD

Coalition and Center for Ethical Medical Testimony, 136 East 8th Street, #230,
Port Angeles, WA 98363, USA

"To put it bluntly, in many professions service as an expert witness is not generally considered honest work. Experts in other fields see lawyers as unprincipled manipulators of their disciplines, and lawyers and experts alike see expert witnesses—those members of other learned professions who will consort with lawyers—as whores. The best that anyone has to say about this system is that it is not as bad as it seems, and that other methods may be worse."—Samuel R. Gross. Expert evidence. Wisconsin Law Review 1991, Vol. 6, p 1125.

Basic issues

Most decisions regarding medical malpractice in the United States are made by judges or juries. Because most lay jurors are not educated in medicine, the courts depend on expert witnesses to help them to understand and decide complex cases. To protect the rights of injured patients and innocent physicians, and to uphold legitimate standards of medical care, it is morally and legally appropriate for physicians with sufficient expertise to testify in medical malpractice and other types of cases.

Similar to much of American jurisprudence, the use of expert witnesses in medical litigation had its origins in English common law. The case of Slater v Baker and Stapleton (1767) established what is called the *professional standard* (also known as the *rule of the profession*), which is that evidence required to ascertain the standard of care against which physicians are to be judged is "the usage and law of surgeons ... the rule of the profession as testified to by surgeons themselves" [1]. In other words, to establish what standard must be met by the profession (of medicine), someone from within the profession itself must be available to give evidence of that standard so that the trier of fact (whoever is making the judgment, either a judge or jury) can

E-mail address: mail@mdmentor.com

be knowledgeably guided in an area outside of the common sphere of knowledge and practice.

As the US legal system has developed, much of the original rule of the profession has been retained in Federal Rule 702, which reads: "If scientific, technical, or other specialized knowledge will assist the trier of fact to understand the evidence or to determine a fact in issue, a witness qualified as an expert by knowledge, skill, experience, training, or education, may testify thereto in the form of an opinion or otherwise" [2].

This rule defines the legally prescribed role of an expert witness: to assist the trier of fact to determine the applicable standard of care. According to the rule, the expert witness is an agent of the court, not of a particular party. This basic obligation of candor to the tribunal, rather than to any participant in the proceeding, underlies the ethical obligations of the expert witness in giving testimony.

The entire system of expert testimony rests on the assumption that expert witnesses are independent of retaining counsel, and that they testify sincerely [3]. The most important obligation of an expert witness is to approach every question with independence and objectivity [3]. As an expert witness, a physician has a clear ethical responsibility to be objective, truthful, and impartial when evaluating a case and to do so, whenever possible, on the basis of generally accepted standards of clinical practice. The appropriate role of an expert witness is that of an *educator,* not an advocate. It is unethical for an expert to overstate his or her opinions or credentials, to misrepresent maloccurrence as malpractice, to offer false testimony, to become an advocate for one party or another, or to testify on any sort of contingency basis.

In the past, there was a "conspiracy of silence" in many professions, including medicine. It was difficult to find physicians willing to testify as to standards of care in the profession, if such testimony would tend to call into the question the care provided by a peer. This situation led to the development of several legal mechanisms and theories designed to reduce or obviate the need for expert testimony to establish negligence, such as the use of stipulated authoritative documents, such as statutes, learned treatises, and policies and *res ipsa loquitur* in lieu of expert testimony [4]. Today it is no longer difficult to find medical experts in any field who are available to testify. Legal journals contain more advertising from medical experts than almost any other kind, and Internet searches yield thousands of medical witnesses, many organized into well-developed referral services. Because it is usual for an emergency physician to earn more per hour as an expert witness than as a practicing clinician, with no "off hours" required and very little overhead, it is predictable that more and more physicians will spend greater amounts of their professional effort pursuing this option.

Traditionally, there has been little awareness of the activities of medical expert witnesses because most testimony occurs behind closed courtroom doors, and most cases are not even transcribed, let alone reported. In the current liability environment, however, this is changing. As defendant physicians have become more open about their litigation experiences, others are becoming aware that sworn testimony by self-designated experts is not always accurate, honest, or informed. There is a dearth of education regarding the proper role of a medical expert witness and little published information regarding what constitutes ethical expert testimony.

In response to member concerns, the American Medical Association (AMA) and most specialty societies have begun to establish policies regarding expert witness testimony to guide their members in providing such service. The typical policy states that to act as an expert witness, at a minimum, a physician should be familiar with the applicable standard of care and be in the active practice of medicine as of the date of the incident. Some societies, including the AMA [5], now require that the member be board certified or prepared in the specialty area involved in the claim. Some societies require a certain number of years in practice or currency of clinical practice as of the time of the incident giving rise to the claim, and all require a willingness to review cases thoroughly and fairly, with a commitment to truth telling and impartiality. All societies state that it is unethical to accept compensation that is contingent on the outcome of the case. The American College of Emergency Physicians (ACEP) Expert Witness Guidelines for the Specialty of Emergency Medicine (Box 1) [6] incorporate all of these components.

Many specialty societies and medical associations are initiating a voluntary program of "affirmation" by members of their willingness to abide by ethics policies and expert witness guidelines promulgated by the association [7]. Increasingly, societies are instituting peer review or disciplinary proceedings that specifically address the problem of allegedly false expert witness testimony. In light of the 1998 AMA policy equating expert witness testimony with the practice of medicine, state medical licensure boards also gingerly have begun to consider the issue of professional discipline for physicians who are dishonest in rendering medical expert testimony.

Qualification as an expert

Legal requirements for qualification as a medical expert witness vary significantly from state to state, and federal court standards are different and to some extent less rigorous than many state statutes and regulations. Federal Rule 702 requires only that an individual be qualified as an expert by virtue of knowledge, skill, experience, training, or education and does not delineate the applicable categories further. Many states do not define their qualifications, but some do require medical licensure, a few require board certification, and several states require a period of years in practice or proximity to the jurisdiction [8].

Although Federal Rule 706 allows judges to appoint expert witnesses, this is as yet rarely done for a variety of reasons, including the question of payment for such services and concern by judges that they might be accused of partiality in their selections. Generally, judges and juries are limited to hearing the

Box 1. Expert witness guidelines for the specialty of emergency medicine

Approved by the American College of Emergency Physicians (ACEP) Board of Directors, August 2000, this statement replaces one with the same title approved by the ACEP Board of Directors, September 1995. This policy statement was originally approved by the ACEP Board of Directors, September 1990.

Expert witnesses are called on to assess the standard of care for emergency physicians in matters of alleged medical malpractice and peer review. Because medical expert witness testimony has demonstrated the potential to set standards of medical care, such testimony will be considered by the ACEP to fall within the realm of the practice of emergency medicine. This testimony would therefore be subject to accountability by appropriate licensing authorities.

Expert witnesses in the specialty of emergency medicine should meet the following criteria:

- Be certified by a recognized certifying body in emergency medicine [1].
- Be in the active clinical practice of emergency medicine for 3 years immediately before the date of the incident [2].
- Be currently licensed in a state, territory, or area constituting legal jurisdiction of the United States as a doctor of medicine or osteopathic medicine.
- Abide by the following guidelines for an expert witness:
  The expert witness should possess current experience and ongoing knowledge in the area in which he or she is asked to testify.
  The expert witness should be willing to submit the transcripts of depositions and testimony to peer review.
  It is unethical for an expert witness to accept compensation that is contingent on the outcome of litigation.
  The expert witness should not provide expert medical testimony that is false, misleading, or without medical foundation. The key to this process is a thorough review of available and appropriate medical records and contemporaneous literature concerning the case being examined.
  After this process is completed, the expert's opinion should reflect the state of medical knowledge at the time of the incident.

The expert witness should review the medical facts in a thorough, fair, and objective manner and should not exclude any relevant information to create a view favoring the plaintiff or the defendant.

Expert witnesses should be chosen on the basis of their experience in the area in which they are providing testimony and not solely on the basis of offices or positions held in medical specialty societies, unless such positions are material to the witness' expertise.

An emergency physician should not engage in advertising or solicit employment as an expert witness where such advertising or solicitation contains representations about the physician's qualifications, experience, or background that are false or deceptive.

Misconduct as an expert, including the provision of false, fraudulent, or misleading testimony, may expose the physician to disciplinary action [2,3].

References

1. American College of Emergency Physicians. ACEP recognized certifying bodies in emergency medicine [policy statement; approved March 1998]. Ann Emerg Med 1998;32:529.
2. American College of Emergency Physicians. Code of ethics for emergency physicians [policy statement; approved June 1997]. Ann Emerg Med 1997;30:365–6.
3. American College of Emergency Physicians. College Manual. American College of Emergency Physicians Website. Available at: http://www.acep.org/1,4853,0.html. Accessed June 28, 2000.

From American College of Emergency Physicians. Expert Witness Guidelines for the Specialty of Emergency Medicine. Available at: http://www.acep.org/web portal/PracticeResources/PolicyStatements/ethics/emexpwitnessguidelines.htm; with permission.

testimony of potential "experts" procured and brought to them by the parties to the case. In the United States, the questions that are posed to the expert for the most part must come from the attorneys representing the party, rather than directly from the judge. (In civil code countries, such as France, judges not only appoint their own experts, but also question them directly.)

When state law does not otherwise specify, the qualification of a witness to serve as an expert is determined by the judge on a case-by-case basis. Judges have broad discretion in making such determinations. Since the 1993 Supreme Court Daubert decision [9], federal court judges and judges in most states are required to assume a "gatekeeping" role in determining whether expert opinions regarding scientific issues should be admitted or excluded from the hearing of the jury. The thrust of Daubert is an attempt to ensure the relevance and reliability of an expert's opinion. Since the Kumho Tire decision [10] in 1999, this gatekeeping role of judges extends to testimony in professional and scientific matters. State courts have their own parallel procedural rules, many of which mimic Daubert.

Expertise in the specialty in which the defendant is practicing should be the *sine qua non* of an ethical expert witness. Yet most juries and some judges do not know what constitutes expertise in a medical specialty. Expertise is appropriately established on the basis of (1) *knowledge* of the field and (2) recent, *relevant experience*. Board preparation and current certification are the "gold standards" (although not the only indicators) of knowledge of the specialty. For several legitimate reasons (eg, grandfathering into a new specialty), some experts are unable to certify in the specialty they practice, but still may be qualified to serve as experts by virtue of continuing medical education and study of the literature in addition to extensive practice. Rural areas may not have board-certified physicians in certain specialties, including emergency medicine, and local experts may not be board certified. Relevant experience is established by a period of active clinical practice beyond training, and particularly by practice during the time frame of the incident giving rise to the case [11].

Although it seems to most physicians that an expert who testifies in a medical malpractice case should be knowledgeable, experienced, trained, or certified in the specialty of the defendant involved in the claim, few states have laws that require this degree of qualification of medical experts. Some require only medical licensure (and some do not even require this). It might be difficult for an attorney to convince a jury that a psychiatrist has expertise in orthopedic surgery, for example, but laxity in statutory qualifications produces a significant vulnerability for certain specialties, such as emergency medicine. Because emergency medicine encompasses clinical problems and procedures crossing traditional specialty lines, physicians from a variety of fields have been allowed to testify as experts in cases involving emergency physicians. By the same token, some emergency physicians have testified as experts in cases involving other specialties, despite limited familiarity with the actual standard of care prevalent in that specialty.

Many physician expert witnesses, including emergency physicians, have testified as to the standard of care of other health care providers, such as nurses, technicians, and therapists, based on their *observation* of the practice of these providers, rather than any specific knowledge, training, or experience. Although a physician could testify knowledgeably about observations of the practice of another type of provider, it is overreaching to assert a working knowledge of the standard of care for a profession to which the physician does not belong.

As a general rule, an expert witness should be a member of the same profession and specialty as the defendant in the case, unless the defendant was clearly practicing outside the confines of his or her specialty during the incident giving rise to the case. This is the law in North Carolina and in California. If state law allows for another type of specialist to act as an expert witness in evaluation of specific practices or procedures that are performed by a defendant, it is appropriate that such procedures, when performed by the testifying expert, must take place at least some of the time in the same or a similar clinical setting as when performed by the defendant in the present claim. A neurosurgeon should not be testifying as to the standard of care of an emergency physician placing burr holes in the cranium in the emergency department unless he or she has done so himself. This is because an operating room cannot be compared with the facilities available in a typical emergency department or medical office, so standards can differ significantly depending on where a procedure is performed.

Objectivity and candor

The expert witness' primary responsibility always must be to the truth. Full discernment of the truth means that before forming any opinion, the physician must be thoroughly knowledgeable about all aspects of the case. Ideally, the prospective witness should know nothing about the case except the individuals involved (to avoid conflict of interest), the broad subject matter (to determine relevant expertise), and filing deadlines before undertaking review of the records. After reviewing provided materials, the expert should request additional records, original documents (eg, x-rays), and any other possibly relevant information that is needed during the evaluation of the case, even if the attorney does not volunteer them. Failure to do so could allow erroneous conclusions to be drawn, for which the witness (not the attorney) would be responsible in any applicable ethics investigation.

Because experts often must be named at a time in the case when all materials are not yet available for review, the initial opinion of an expert must be considered provisional and subject to modification if additional information comes to light during discovery that alters significant parameters of the case. What this means is that an expert, on learning additional information that affects his or her opinion of whether or not the applicable standard of care was met, must be willing to change his or her opinion accordingly, regardless of which side has engaged him or her. This situation may result in withdrawal from the case if the attorney cannot use the expert who no longer can support that side's theory of the case. According to legal ethicist Lubet, "a lawyer with integrity will normally accept a negative opinion, or even appreciate it, since that may help counsel and client formulate a settlement strategy rather than take a losing case to trial" [3].

Standard of care

Analysis and testimony should reflect knowledge of and comparison with concurrently applicable and generally accepted standards of care. The medical expert must be aware of and apply the standard of care that existed *at the time of the incident* giving rise to the claim and regional variations in practice and alternative treatments. The location and capabilities of the facility in which the incident giving rise to the case occurred also must be taken into account.

The legal principle of the medical "standard of care" usually is defined by case law or statute for each jurisdiction and is some version of "that degree of care which would be rendered by a reasonably competent physician practicing under the same or similar circumstances" [12]. Whether because they do not themselves understand it or because it does not suit their purpose, attorneys often do not define this concept clearly for their experts.

As a result, even the general concept of standard of care is not well understood by many expert witnesses [4], although most believe that they understand it and can accurately describe the specific standard applicable in a given case. Legal scholars believe that medical expert testimony as to what constitutes the standard of care is more apt to reflect what experts think that they and their immediate colleagues would do, rather than what most physicians actually do [13]. Research suggests medical expert witnesses share with all physicians the tendency to have selectively optimistic recall of how well they themselves characteristically have handled clinical situations [14]. This means that well-intended expert testimony often tends to overestimate the applicable standard of care to which physicians will be held. As a fundamental principle, it is important to understand that the standard requires only that the physician acted reasonably under the circumstances.

The specific facts in a given patient situation make defining the applicable standard even more difficult for the expert witness. A reader-response feature series in a popular monthly emergency medicine publication [15] continuously illustrates that there is incredibly wide divergence of opinion in what practicing emergency physicians believe to be the standard of care applicable to any given case scenario. Reader opinions in the same case might vary from "there is absolutely no deviation from the standard of care" to "this is the most heinous example of malpractice I have ever seen."

More scholarly research on the topic confirms that there is little agreement among practitioners as to what constitutes the acceptable standard of care and how it might be discerned in legal cases [16]. A symposium based on this issue may be of interest to the dedicated reader [17].

> Even when physicians critique the care of a colleague, they seldom agree on the "standard of care"; finding consensus of opinion is elusive. On many occasions, especially when multiple treatment options are available, ethical experts may have to admit that no true standard of care exists [14].

It may be easier to define what the standard is *not,* than what it is. The legally required standard of medical care is *not* perfect care or care that creates a perfect result. Although presumably such care would meet the standard, in many if not most instances, it would exceed the actual standard that is required under the law. The standard of care also is *not* what a physician would have done in his or her own practice (on a good day), which the physician assumes others also do. It also is not what the physician was taught to do in training, what the textbooks recommend, or even what clinical policies/guidelines say it is (although these may be good indicators of the things that peers believe to represent optimal care, best practices, or recommended practices under the best available evidence). Each of these sources can provide information as to what constitutes good or excellent care for a given condition, but they do not define the legal standard of care.

How then is an ethical expert to determine what the standard actually *is* or was at the time of the incident? At the very least, an expert should consult available written materials, in the form of a brief literature review. Although the attorney may offer to do this for the witness, the physician should bear in mind that the attorney is likely to be selective in the materials that are actually provided to the physician. The physician witness should limit his or her consideration to references that were current and reasonably available to clinicians as of the time of the incident. The physician should look to other then-available materials, such as hospital and clinical policies and guidelines and continuing medical education course materials. The physician should discuss the case (without identifiers) with peers if the opportunity presents itself. The physician should not say that "most practitioners would agree with me that this does (or does not) meet the standard" without objective proof.

Clinical policies and guidelines have been developed by specialties to address many medical conditions, but most have been intentionally worded so as to make it clear that they are "guidelines" and not standards of care (because crafters are well aware that "standards" can and would be used against medical providers judicially). Experienced medical practitioners know that there is rarely a clear-cut standard of care for any condition, given the variability of human clinical presentation and response. The standard is *reasonable* care (or care that would be required of a reasonable, competent physician) under all of the facts and circumstances of the case.

An expert must be aware of the prevailing legal standards in the community where a case is being tried. If the locality rule applies rather than a national standard in a given jurisdiction, the expert has an ethical obligation to be familiar with the local standards that are applicable and to explain how he or she has gained this knowledge. Even if the locality rule is not applicable in the jurisdiction, objectivity and fairness require that regional differences in practice patterns be taken into account in formulating opinions. It is often said in jest in the medical community that "the standard of care is established the first time someone is successfully sued for not doing something" [18]. In states that are moving toward a jury-determined standard of care, local precedents also would have to be taken into account in assessing whether or not the applicable standard has been met.

An ethical witness must be careful in differentiating for the benefit of a jury between a widely used standard of care on the one hand and ideal care that might be provided by the most astute clinician practicing under optimal circumstances on the other. Application of an "ideal" standard (so-called counsel of perfection) may be a particular hazard for clinicians whose only practice experience has been in a tertiary care facility, such as medical school faculty or newly graduated residents, who are testifying in cases involving community facilities with typical practicing clinicians, who have limited backup and equipment.

An expert also must be able to help the jury understand the difference between the type of evaluation or care that is most commonly rendered for a particular condition and an equally acceptable method (the "two schools of thought" or "respectable minority" test) that is not often rendered, but is also medically valid or theoretically sound. The expert also must be able to understand and to delineate clearly for a jury the difference between reasonably competent care and care that would be considered substandard by an average practitioner under any circumstances.

An ethical expert must be careful to evaluate each case as if the end result is not known. Everyone knows that "hindsight is 20/20," yet many attorneys and their witnesses cannot seem to resist applying the taint of an untoward outcome to their analysis of the case. This is understandable in the case of plaintiff attorneys. It is unethical behavior for a physician expert witness.

Representation of one's personal opinion as absolute truth is misleading to a lay jury and is unethical. Personal opinion and preference may be offered during expert testimony, but should be clearly designated as such. An ethical witness recognizes that in most cases differences of opinion between competent medical practitioners exist in the management of any case and acknowledge that the ideal course of events is almost always clearer when viewed retrospectively in light of a less than optimal outcome.

The ACEP is pioneering a new concept in determining the applicable standard of care through its Standard of Care Review Process [19]. A committee meets to review testimony submitted by members in closed malpractice cases. The testimony and all documents are blinded as to the identity of the experts and parties. The purpose of the consideration is to determine whether testimony that has been given under oath accurately reflects the standard of care as ascertained by the review committee. The findings will be published in various places to educate emergency physicians about the opinions of colleagues with respect to the applicable standard of care. The process is intended to serve a needed educational function, and is not disciplinary in nature. The American Academy of Emergency Medicine intends to publicize cases of "remarkable" expert physician testimony [20]. The concept is still in development stages.

Dishonest statement

One of the most invidious aspects of the misunderstood standard of care issue is that some members of the medical community have espoused ludicrous myths promulgated by risk managers and many members of the bar, as if they actually constituted a medical standard of care. The most rampant example of such a myth, regularly regurgitated by expert witnesses, is what is sometimes referred to as the IDWD statement, which is, "If it Isn't Documented, it Wasn't Done."

A physician who states "If it was not documented, it was not done" is either lying or has never practiced medicine. Yet this is a common misstatement made by expert witnesses serving the plaintiff's bar. Although the concept of complete and compulsive documentation may be a useful teaching tool for risk managers, it flies in the face of the reality of practicing medicine and has no place in a deposition or courtroom. Even the most compulsive video docu-dramatist could not possibly document every aspect and element of any one clinical encounter. So to tell a jury that, "If it isn't documented, it wasn't done" is not just an innocent or well-intentioned misstatement of fact, it is a fabrication that can be and often is profoundly destructive. The myth of IDWD plays heavily into the need and desire on the part of the jury to believe that all medical records, similar to all medical care and outcomes, can be perfect if only physicians are careful enough. It is a lie. An ethical expert could not make this utterance at all, let alone under oath.

Ethical Expert: an Educator, *not* an Advocate

Physicians are patient advocates, and for the most part physicians entered the profession because of a desire to help people. Physicians also are naturally competitive with one another. This competitiveness brings physicians successfully into medical training and is nurtured there. Also, physicians hate to be wrong. All of these tendencies are played out in the expert witness arena, where physicians are contacted by one side or the other to analyze a case whose outcome is known and presumably not optimal. If physicians agree to testify, they are providing their expertise to a team whose objective is to win the case, and with all of the time and intensity of preparation for trial it is easy to forget that physicians are not supposed to function as members of this team, but as neutral agents of the court. The most common mistake made by medical expert witnesses is to think of themselves as advocates, rather than educators, and to allow judgment to be clouded by the need to "win" the case. This is not merely a plaintiff witness failing. Many who testify on behalf of defendants have admitted that they do so, at least in part, to "even the playing field" that they perceive between physicians and lawyers. It is easy to fall into an advocacy role (which belongs *solely* to the lawyers in the case and not to the experts), especially when one is aware that the expert on the opposing side already has given in to this temptation. Two wrongs never make a right. This type of competition undermines the justice system at the same time and to the same degree as it demeans the medical profession.

One final responsibility of the expert witness is to differentiate for the jury between malpractice and maloccurrence. Many laypeople do not understand that when an untoward outcome occurs, this does not mean that the standard of care was not met. Plaintiffs predictably do not dispel this misconception, which helps to sway and inflate jury verdicts, particularly in cases with catastrophic outcomes. Typically, defense counsel attempts to refute this perception during cross-examination, but the ethical expert witness sometimes needs to state this specifically to the jury even when it may detract from their theory of liability in the case. All experts have an ethical obligation to educate the jury about the reality of the practice of medicine.

Financial influences

Expert testimony should never be provided solely, or principally, for financial gain. Reasonable compensation for a physician's time used in analysis or testimony in a case is ethically acceptable, but financial remuneration must not be the key motivation behind expert witness work. Compensation for time expended acting as an expert witness should be commensurate with compensation that would be earned during the same amount of time devoted to medical practice and not indexed to the "market rate" for expert testimony [21]. For a physician to earn more through work as an expert witness than as a practicing physician is morally questionable if not unethical, yet testimony suggests that many do. Expert testimony by physicians can be useful to juries, the profession, and society, but exorbitant fees charged for such review and testimony predictably will increase the cost of malpractice defense and threaten liability insurance premiums and availability and ultimately the availability and affordability of health care.

Under no circumstances is it appropriate for an expert's professional remuneration to be contingent on the outcome of a case [22]. Such an arrangement immediately casts doubt on the objectivity of an expert witness. As a general rule, an ethical expert should establish a fee schedule at the beginning of any case and require payment at the time service is rendered (the rendering of an initial opinion) and not at the conclusion of the case, so as to avoid even the appearance of contingency billing and attendant bias. Experts also should recognize and acknowledge that there is an unspoken inherent contingency in every consultation by an attorney because repeat engagement is less likely when an expert is unable to provide the opinion or the testimony sought by that attorney [23].

Unethical expert problem

According to Samuel Gross [24], a law professor expert on expert evidence, "The contempt of lawyers and judges for experts is famous. They regularly describe expert witnesses as prostitutes, people who live by selling services that should not be for sale. They speak of maintaining 'stables' of experts, beasts to be chosen and harnessed at the will of their masters." No other category of witnesses, not even parties, is subject to such vilification. If jurors do feel this way, it is a reflection of what judges and lawyers say and do. Jurors, judges, and lawyers are informed by what they witness daily in their cases and courtrooms.

Acting as an expert witness has become a profession for some individuals. The medical legal case reports are replete with testimony by "hired guns" who earn a significant portion or even most of their professional income from testifying in malpractice cases. Some have not practiced for years, falsify their current level of practice or past experience, or practice just enough to keep their medical licenses or be qualified in their states as expert witnesses. Some have been barred from acting as expert witnesses in certain states, yet continue to testify in other states. Some use past credentials, membership, or participation in professional associations or boards to bolster the impression that they have current clinical expertise. Some witnesses typically testify almost exclusively for either the defense or the plaintiff. Accurate records should be kept by all medical experts of the number of cases that they have reviewed, given depositions in, or given testimony in and the nature of the case and the side that engaged them [25]. If there is a significant imbalance, either the expert is selectively choosing cases, or the bar is selectively choosing experts based on previous testimony. A predominance of testimony for one side or the other tends to cast doubt on the objectivity of the witness because an honest, skilled, and objective witness should be sought out equally by all members of the bar who participate in medical malpractice.

Recourse for victims of unethical witness testimony

The basic flaw in the judicial system's dependence on expert witness testimony is that there is no accountability for statements made by experts under oath. Even if the testimony is successfully impeached (shown to be false) during trial, very little if anything happens to the expert. Rarely, an expert may be disqualified by a judge for behaving unethically on the witness stand (eg, exchanging signals with clients or attorneys during testimony) or on the basis of some obvious falsification of qualifications uncovered through cross-examination during the course of a trial. Some courts have disqualified individual experts as not being sufficiently expert in a given field or based on Daubert considerations (see earlier), which disqualification has some precedential value in other courts. Perjury by a physician on the witness stand is exceedingly unlikely to attract the resources of a prosecutor (although some activism in this area by opposing attorneys and judges is beginning to be publicized) [26].

Counterclaims or other means of legal redress by a defendant against expert witnesses who testify falsely are extremely difficult to mount because of the financial and time commitment involved, and because of the legal presumption that testimony provided under oath and not impeached at trial is truthful testimony that has been provided in the public interest. To be actionable in a civil suit, actual malice must be shown on the part of the expert witness in providing false testimony that is damaging to the defendant physician, and this for all intents and purposes has been found to be a nearly insurmountable standard. There is a developing jurisprudence of liability for expert witnesses in cases brought by *those who engaged them* (so-called litigation support liability), which is beyond the scope of this article, but is worthy of review by individuals who testify extensively [27].

Peer review of expert testimony

Ideally, medical expert testimony would be routinely peer reviewed to ensure it meets the ethical standards of the AMA and other medical professional societies. In some states, expert testimony has been subject to peer review and licensure action by the state medical board under the authority of the state Medical Practice Act. A few states are moving toward requiring a limited state license to testify in the state. Although several states have issued discipline based on falsification of credentials by individuals acting as medical experts [28], only one state to date (North Carolina) has removed the license of a professional expert witness on the basis that unsupportable testimony constituted unprofessional conduct [29]. The Lustgarten ruling is under appeal, and presumably other states are waiting for the final outcome in this case before deciding whether to proceed in any complaints pending in their own states regarding this issue.

Some professional societies [30], including the ACEP, following the lead of the American Association of Neurological Surgeons review the testimony of members acting as expert witnesses on complaint by another member [31]. Sanctions in the event of proven false or unethical testimony are generally limited, however, to those affecting the expert's membership in the society. The AMA does not take action except in the case of state licensure action or conviction of perjury and in expert witness testimony related to tobacco legislation.

The US Supreme Court upheld the right of a professional society to discipline a member for inappropriate expert testimony in the Austin case [32]. The American Association of Neurological Surgeons suspended a member for giving improper expert witness testimony at a medical malpractice trial. Judge Posner speaking for the 7th Ct court of appeals applauded the association for its part in increasing the accountability of experts from its ranks.

This precedent represents an important victory for professional societies that include ethics review of expert witness testimony in their policies and disciplinary procedures. A member who believes that an expert has not acted ethically while giving testimony has standing to request a review of the testimony by the specialty society (if the witness is a member). Not all societies have a mechanism in place to perform this function, however, and it is not without attendant costs and liability to the society. Not all "experts" belong to medical societies. There is an inherent selection bias rightfully noted by plaintiff's bar that members are extremely unlikely to report questionable testimony on behalf of a defense witness. If the expert is from a different specialty than the defendant, as is often the case in emergency medicine, the expert's specialty society has no obligation to a nonmember complainant from another specialty.

Certifying experts and affidavit testimony are no different

Another type of expert witness is emerging in states whose professional liability statutes require some form of precertification of the likely existence of professional negligence before the initiation of a suit. A physician is asked to review the records of the case and submit an affidavit with the case filings. Often a single specialist is asked to opine about the liability of every health care worker whose name appears in the record, including physicians of other specialties and nonphysicians. The affidavit sometimes is prepared by the law firm and submitted to the expert along with the records for initial review and a signed check for the service. A "certifying" expert in some states, notably Illinois, must sign the affidavit, but his or her identity need never be revealed to the parties named in the case. There is no possibility of any type of peer review of this type of expert "testimony" because it cannot even be determined by a defendant that the affiant is a physician, unless that expert also serves as a testifying expert witness in the case [33].

Certifying "experts" may believe that they need not conform to the same standards as an expert who is actually testifying in a case because the risk of a given named defendant making a settlement of the claim is less predictable at this stage of the case. Physicians named as possibly negligent by a certifying expert are forced to defend themselves, however, and have the claim on their records with credentialing agencies and institutions forever, regardless of the outcome. The exact same standards of ethicality in acting as a certifying expert should apply as those that apply to "testifying" experts.

An ethical physician who is asked as an expert to certify a claim for potential negligence would consider carefully whether or not he or she would qualify to serve as a testifying expert witness in the case. Such a physician at a minimum should be familiar with the standard of care for each potential defendant whose care he or she intends to consider, using the criteria outlined previously for "testifying" experts of knowledge and relevant experience in the field of the potential defendant. A physician who makes a certification against a health care provider without such qualification as an expert should be subject to peer review in the same manner as any other expert witness.

Summary

It is appropriate and necessary for qualified, clinically active physicians to serve as expert witnesses in the judicial system. Serving as an expert carries certain moral and ethical obligations, however. A physician who partici-pates in medical legal case evaluation or offers to give expert medical testi-mony first should have a basic understanding of an expert's roles and responsibilities under the law. The expert should have knowledge and cur-rent relevant experience in the specialty or the procedure involved in the case. An ethical expert must exercise due diligence to become educated about every aspect of the case; to analyze all available information carefully informed by the appropriate standard of care; and to give an informed, truthful, nonbiased opinion about the care that the patient received. The ex-pert exists to educate and serve the judge and jury, and it is unethical to ad-vocate for the parties to the case even though this is often requested by legal counsel. Ethical expert medical opinion should never be influenced by what the witness believes the attorney desires or by the remuneration that is of-fered. All physicians offering expert testimony should follow ethical guide-lines established by the AMA and other medical societies and should be willing to undergo peer review. See Box 1 for the expert witness policy adop-ted by the ACEP in 2001.

The hallmark of the ethical expert witness must always be unswerving dedication to truth. Accepting this obligation, and acting accordingly, is the only way in which a physician can serve as an ethical medical expert wit-ness and preserve the justice system, uphold the integrity of the profession, and contribute to the betterment of medicine.

References

[1] 95 Eng. Rep. 860 (K.B. 1767).
[2] FRE 702.
[3] Lubet S. Expert witnesses: ethics and professionalism. Geo J Legal Ethics 1999;12:465.
[4] Sullivan W. Standard of care: does it exist in every malpractice case? ED Legal Letter 2003;
    14:133–44.
[5] Latest AMA policy on expert witness issues as of this writing can be found at http://www.
    ama-assn.org/ama/pub/category/8539.html   and   http://www.ama-assn.org/ama1/pub/
    upload/mm/465/bot8fin.doc.
[6] http://www.acep.org/1,560, 0.html.
[7] ACEP uses the term "ReAffirmation" because members already affirm all ethics policies
    when they join or renew their membership. The statement is available at: http://www.
    acep.org/download.cfm?resource=1024.
[8] See AOA. Policy statement on expert witness, for recent compilation. Available at: http://
    do-online.osteotech.org/pdf/cal_midyr05ressup26ff.pdf.
[9] Daubert v Merrell Dow Pharmaceuticals, 509 US 579 (1993).
[10] Kumho Tire v Carmichael, 526 US 137 (1999).
[11] Although some physicians believe themselves to be eminently qualified to testify after retire-
    ment from clinical practice because of their knowledge of the basic precepts of the specialty
    and the breadth of their experience, what is needed by the courts—education about the pre-
    vailing standards of clinical practice—cannot realistically be known by an individual who no
    longer practices clinically. An ethical expert witness should be actively practicing within his
    or her field at the time of the incident involved in a claim to be aware of the actual applicable
    standard of care in effect as of that date. A retired physician might ethically render an opinion
    about causation, however, as opposed to the prevailing standard of care.

[12] Shilkret v Annapolis Hospital Emergency Association, 349 A 2d 245, 249–250 (Md 1975).

[13] Peters PG. Empirical evidence and malpractice litigation. Wake Forest Law Review 2002; 37:757.

[14] Meadow, Sunstein. Statistics, not experts. Duke Law J 2001;51:630–1.

[15] EP Monthly, Standard of Care Project, ongoing.

[16] Hartz A, Lucas J, Crown T. Physician surveys to assess customary care in medical malpractice cases. J Gen Intern Med 2002;17:546.

[17] Wake Forest Law Review 2002;37, No.3. Available at: http://www.law.wfu.edu/x2065.xml.

[18] The textbook case basis for this quip is Helling v Carey (83Wn.2d 514,519 P.2d 981), a 1974 Washington Supreme Court case in which, based on their understanding and balancing of the risks and benefits, testing for glaucoma in patients younger than 40 years of age was established by the judge as the medical standard of care. Although Helling has been statutorily overturned in Washington and not followed by other states, an emerging jurisprudence in some states allows the jury to determine what the "reasonable" physician should have done, as opposed to the customary or prevailing practice in the community.

[19] http://www.acep.org/1,33422,0.html.

[20] http://www.aaem.org/aaemtestimony/caselisting.html#.

[21] Which is increasing dramatically in recent years and reportedly can reach $600–1000 per hour in some specialties. Baldas. Nonexperts taking the stand. National Law Journal March 21, 2005. Available at: http://www.law.com/jsp/article.jsp?id=1111572309683.

[22] All medical professional ethics codes and legal codes of professional responsibility prohibit this practice.

[23] Moss S. Opinion for sale: confessions of an expert witness. Available at: http://www.legalaffairs.org/issues/March-April-2003/review_marapr03_moss.html#.

[24] Gross SR. Wisconsin Law Review 1991;1113. This is a classic and comprehensive article on this topic.

[25] By FRE 26, providing an accurate record of this history is a requirement for testifying in federal court.

[26] See Year of the expert witness. Available at: http://www.ccemt.org/displaycommon.cfm?an=1&subarticlenbr=78.

[27] See Sullivan W. Expert opinions: defendants aren't the only ones on trial. ED Legal Letter 2004;15:97–108, and Weiss L. Expert witness malpractice actions: emerging trend of aberration. The Practical Litigator 2004;March:27–34.

[28] Maryland, Washington, DC, New York, and on other grounds in Washington state.

[29] Andrew L. Lustgarten appeals suspension by NC Medical Board. Available at: http://www.ccemt.org/displayindustryarticle.cfm?articlenbr=19883.

[30] Such as the American College of Obstetricians and Gynecologists, American College of Surgeons, American College of Radiologists, American Association of Neurology, and American Society of Plastic Surgeons.

[31] ACEP ethics review policies relating to expert witness testimony can be found at: http://www.acep.org/1,4853,0.html.

[32] Donald C. Austin v AANS, 253F3d 967 (2001).

[33] See Grow B. Expert witnesses under examination, and related articles at: http://www.ccemt.org/displayindustryarticle.cfm?articlenbr=19857.

ELSEVIER
SAUNDERS

Emerg Med Clin N Am
24 (2006) 733–747

EMERGENCY
MEDICINE
CLINICS OF
NORTH AMERICA

Ethical Issues in Medical Malpractice

Robert C. Solomon, MD

214 Briar Path, Imperial, PA 15126-9686, USA

The interrelationships between biomedical ethics and the law are perhaps nowhere as starkly apparent as in the realm of medical malpractice. Although ethical and legal conduct and practices are often in harmony, in many areas ethical principles and the issues surrounding medical liability appear to come into conflict. Disclosure of errors; quality improvement activities; the practice of defensive medicine; dealing with patients who wish to leave against medical advice; provision of futile care at the insistence of patients or families; and the various protections of Good Samaritan laws are just a few of these. In addition, the ethical principles governing the conduct of physicians serving as expert witnesses in medical malpractice cases have become a subject of intense interest in recent years.

In our system for adjudicating torts (civil wrongs), medical malpractice is defined by four elements: duty, breach of duty, damages, and causation. Juries are instructed that these four elements must be present for the plaintiff to meet the burden of proof and the defendant to be found guilty of medical malpractice.

A duty on the part of the emergency physician is present when the patient seeks care in the emergency department, thereby establishing a doctor–patient relationship. The emergency physician has an ethical duty to attend such a patient. The Emergency Medical Treatment and Labor Act also establishes a legal duty under federal statute. A breach of that duty (or negligence) occurs when the physician, in evaluating and treating the patient, fails to meet the standard of care; that is, the physician does not provide care in such a manner as would any reasonable physician practicing in a comparable setting in treating a patient with the same or similar clinical presentation. Damages are present when the patient suffers an adverse outcome in relation to the medical condition for which care was sought. Causation requires that the negligent care be shown to be the proximate cause (in some jurisdictions a proximate cause) of the harm suffered by the patient.

E-mail address: rcsmd82@comcast.net

0733-8627/06/$ - see front matter © 2006 Elsevier Inc. All rights reserved.
doi:10.1016/j.emc.2006.05.017   *emed.theclinics.com*

These definitions become important as one considers the reliability of our tort system in adjudicating medical malpractice cases fairly and arriving at verdicts that accurately reflect the facts in evidence at trial. The jury's understanding of standard of care and causation are critically dependent on the physicians who serve as expert witnesses in malpractice cases.

Compensation for medical injury as an ethical obligation

According to John Rawls' [1] theory of justice, an individual's needs that are occasioned by disadvantages relative to others are typically the result of misfortune in the form of what he describes as the "natural lottery" and the "social lottery." Rawls argues for the conferring of benefits to the disadvantaged to even out such inequalities. Others take a less far-reaching view and attempt to distinguish between disadvantages that result from simple misfortune and those that are unfair or undeserved. In this context, setbacks to health are typically matters of misfortune; although they may be ameliorated by measures of benevolence or compassion, there is no obligation based in justice. However, harm to health, as the result of maleficent or negligent conduct, is regarded as unfair, and justice demands compensation through the use of state force [2] (in the current system, the civil courts).

A fundamental requirement of this application of justice to the harms caused by medical malpractice is that all victims of medical malpractice should be compensated fairly, whereas those who have not been harmed or whose harm was not the result of negligence should be excluded. The question of whether our tort system achieves this goal will be examined later.

Quality improvement

Trial attorneys, and even some physicians, assert a simple reason for the alarmingly high (and rising) number of malpractice claims, settlements, and awards, and the total amount of money paid to compensate plaintiffs in medical malpractice cases: there is a lot of malpractice. Although the amount of malpractice is arguable, it does occur, and those harmed by it deserve compensation as a matter of justice. Physicians hold the key to reducing the incidence of medical malpractice, and the cornerstone of their efforts is quality improvement.

Successful quality improvement relies on a system in which physicians can engage in frank discussions of cases in which there were adverse outcomes (or near misses) and focus on errors that could have been avoided. The desired outcome is that they learn from each other's mistakes as well as their own. Physicians who exhibit a pattern of substandard care can be monitored closely, required to obtain remedial education, or even proctored for a period of time. In exceptional cases, physicians whose patient care raises persistent questions about their competence may be referred for possible disciplinary action according to the process prescribed by medical staff bylaws.

In addition, the identification of errors-especially those that occur repeatedly or appear to be part of a pattern, or those that have the potential to cause death or serious harm (sometimes called a sentinel event)-can lead to changes in the patient care system, to reduce the likelihood that such errors will continue to occur.

Unfortunately, there are several obstacles to the success of a quality improvement program. Physicians are often hesitant to be critical of their colleagues, even in a closed group discussion, perhaps based on the thought that "There but for the grace of God go I." Ironically, given that a robust quality improvement program has great potential for reducing the incidence of malpractice, fear that their discussions and conclusions could be subject to discovery if the adverse outcome under consideration becomes the subject of a malpractice claim often causes physicians to mute their criticisms of a colleague's patient management. In some states protection of peer review is under attack, and physicians are reluctant to trust the courts. Thus, the professional and ethical obligation to engage in activities that improve and advance the quality of patient care is subverted by fears of the legal system.

Disclosure of errors

If physicians are sometimes disinclined to engage in frank discussions among themselves of adverse outcomes and the errors that contributed to them, the question of disclosing such errors to patients and families engenders even greater anxiety. Those who do so act out of a sense of ethical obligation, hoping for the best, but recognizing the worst possibilities:

> Experience in medical negligence has shown that if a patient's care has gone wrong, then a full and frank explanation will do much to defuse the anger, upset, and resentment that the patient feels, and may reduce substantially the risk that the patient will seek redress in court. Obviously, however full the explanation, if major injury has been suffered, then patients are likely to sue to obtain damages to compensate them (eg, for loss of earnings or the cost of future care) [3].

The ethical principles underlying the impetus for disclosure have been well described:

> Failing to disclose errors to patients undermines public trust in medicine because it potentially involves deception and suggests preservation of narrow professional interests over the well-being of patients. This failure can be seen as a breach of professional ethics – a lapse in commitment to act solely in the patient's best interests.

> Furthermore, by the principle of justice or fairness, patients, when harmed, should be able to seek appropriate restitution or recompense. This ethical rationale for disclosure, based on a strong notion of autonomy, goes beyond what the law might require one to do. Nondisclosure may be

rationalized by concerns about increasing patient anxiety or confusing the patient with complicated information. This position, now largely discredited, is one of "therapeutic privilege," that is, protecting the "childlike" patient from "harmful" information [4].

Not surprisingly, physicians and patients have different views on disclosure of errors, with patients almost always wanting to be informed and most physicians disinclined to inform them [5]. Physicians might be more motivated toward disclosure if they understood that patients who discover errors on their own are, by their own report, more likely to sue [6]. In fact, a broad-based policy of disclosing errors may reduce the number of malpractice claims [7]. Thus, the physician who accepts the challenge and chooses the path of frank disclosure is both fulfilling an ethical obligation and using a valuable, proven risk management technique.

The American College of Emergency Physicians [8] has adopted a policy on disclosure of medical errors that includes the following points:

- Health care institutions should develop and implement policies and procedures for identifying and responding to medical errors, including continuous quality improvement (CQI) systems and procedures for disclosing significant errors to patients.
- Medical educators should develop and incorporate into their curricula programs on identifying and preventing medical errors and on communicating truthfully and sensitively with patients and their representatives about errors.
- ED [emergency department] directors, chairs, quality managers, and other leaders in emergency medicine should play a leading role in developing institutional and ED policies for prompt error identification, responsible reporting, and proper remediation.
- Society should adopt tort reforms and system changes that improve patient safety by encouraging disclosure of medical errors.

Guidelines for disclosing errors have been published [4] and may be helpful to the clinician:

- Disclose promptly what you know about the event. Concentrate on what happened and the possible consequences.
- Take the lead in disclosure; don't wait for the patient to ask.
- Outline a plan of care to rectify the harm and prevent recurrence.
- Offer to get prompt second opinions where appropriate.
- Offer the option of a family meeting and the option of having lawyers present.
- Document important discussions.
- Offer the option of follow-up meetings.
- Be prepared for strong emotions.
- Accept responsibility for outcomes, but avoid attributions of blame.
- Apologies and expressions of sorrow are appropriate.

Clinical guidelines

The use of clinical guidelines may present ethical issues that are not, at first blush, readily apparent. Motivations for the use of clinical guidelines include standardizing (and, it is hoped, improving) patient care; complying with the dictates of managed care organizations and other third-party players; and reducing the risk of liability exposure, inasmuch as following clinical guidelines will demonstrate adherence to a standard of care.

Conflicts arise, however, when the guidelines themselves are suspect, in the view of the physician. Sometimes a given guideline has been developed by a professional organization representing another specialty and fails to take into account the unique perspective of the practitioner of emergency medicine. Guidelines may be consensus-based, rather than evidence-based; the physician's knowledge of the medical literature may conflict with elements of such guidelines and lead to a lack of confidence in the wisdom of following them. Finally, the physician may be aware of the fact that those involved in developing guidelines are sometimes biased by intellectual or financial conflicts of interest. A medical investigative journalist writing for the British Medical Journal concluded, "Seemingly impartial organizations that issue professional guidelines may have ties to the manufacturers of recommended interventions" [9].

When guidelines are suspect, the emergency physician is faced with a conflict between the advantages of following them and the duty to the patient to adhere to the principles of best medical practice. Such conflicts can be difficult and time-consuming to resolve. They typically require careful documentation so that anyone reviewing the record can see that the physician was familiar with the guideline in question and had explained clearly the reasons for deviating from it. And, in some cases, the physician may feel obligated to have a discussion with the patient about available interventions recommended, according to certain clinical guidelines, but which the emergency physician does not believe would serve the patient well. Although this may have some defensive advantages, it is doubtful whether there is any legal or ethical obligation to do so [10].

Against medical advice

Patients who wish to leave against medical advice (AMA) often cause the emergency physician anxiety about the possibility of an adverse outcome. This unease reflects not only concern for the patient's well-being but also an awareness of the possibility of a malpractice claim in any case in which harm comes to the patient.

Emergency physicians may use various techniques to persuade the patient to accept advice regarding hospital admission. These include a careful explanation of the risks associated with the patient's intended course of action;

exploration of the patient's reasons for making what appears to be an irrational decision against self-interest; and the enlistment of family and friends in the effort to convince the patient of the wisdom of following the physician's recommendation.

The patient's decision may arise from many sources, including denial of the potential seriousness of the medical condition; lack of confidence in the physician or institution; disagreement with the plan of management; conflicts between hospitalization and personal obligations; and financial concerns [11]. Once these elements are identified, it is possible to address them, and the basis for the patient's decision may be altered.

It has been shown that patients with mental illness and substance abuse problems are at increased risk for leaving AMA [12]. Thus, the question may arise as to whether the patient possesses decision-making capacity sufficient to understand and accept the risks associated with discharge AMA. The emergency physician may feel compelled to resort to involuntary hospitalization if the requirements of state law, which often focus on mental illness and addiction, are satisfied. Some cases may invoke an ethical obligation to pursue this avenue, such as the mentally ill or addicted patient with a life-threatening drug overdose.

The emergency physician is most likely to question a patient's decision-making capacity when the stakes are high (ie, when the risks associated with discharge AMA are great). Although this is intuitive, there is support in the literature for a "shifting standard of competency," meaning that the standard of decision-making capacity to which a person is held may vary with the magnitude of risk attendant upon the decision [13]. However, concern for the patient's autonomy cannot be dismissed lightly simply because he appears to making a very foolhardy decision.

Sometimes, physicians yield to the temptation of exaggerating the risks attendant upon the patient's choice. The patient is entitled to accurate information, and this paternalistic approach violates the principle of patient autonomy. Recognizing the primacy of the ethical principle of patient autonomy reminds the physician that, in any doctor–patient encounter, the patient is consulting the physician and is free to accept or reject the physician's advice and recommendations. When the patient's autonomy is thus respected, he is more likely to return, should he have occasion to reconsider his decision.

Finally, the physician must be aware that the ethical obligation to do what is in the patient's best interest is not terminated by the patient's refusal to follow the physician's best advice. Thus, if the patient cannot be dissuaded from leaving AMA, it is important to provide appropriate discharge instructions. The emergency physician should make a referral for further evaluation and treatment on an outpatient basis and strongly encourage follow-up. It is most important to leave the door open for the patient to return to the emergency department and to instruct the patient about what symptoms or signs should prompt such a return.

Informed consent

It is not unusual for the issue of informed consent to arise in medical malpractice cases. The most common situation is one in which an adverse outcome occurs in relation to the performance of a procedure. It may be a known risk of the procedure, yet one that occurs very infrequently. The question may arise as to whether the physician had a duty to warn the patient of this particular risk; whether the patient was, in fact, told of the risk; or even whether the patient actually understood the information being conveyed.

Informed consent is based on the ethical principle of autonomy: the right of the patient to make free choices about what happens to his/her person, including what may result from diagnostic and therapeutic interventions. Such free choices must be based on a full, or at least adequate, understanding of the nature of the proposed intervention and its potential benefits, risks, and alternatives. Thus, the patient must be presented with accurate and reliable information, and efforts must be exerted to ensure that the patient understands what he is told. In addition to honoring patient autonomy, informed consent serves the functions of protecting patients from harm and encouraging medical professionals to act responsibly in their interactions with patients [14].

Historically, the two approaches to the question of when informed consent should be obtained are the professional practice standard and the reasonable person standard [15]. Under the professional practice standard, appropriate disclosure of information is based on the traditional practices of the professional community, relying on the belief that physicians, acting in the best interests of their patients, establish (by custom) the amount and kinds of information to be disclosed. The primary objection to the professional practice standard is, of course, that it is inconsistent with the principle of patient autonomy.

The reasonable person standard, as the phrase suggests, is based on what a reasonable person would need (or want) to know. This standard has gained acceptance in most jurisdictions. According to this standard, the pertinence of a given piece of information is determined by the significance a hypothetic reasonable person would attach to it in making a decision. Thus, the determination of informational needs is shifted from physician to patient, based on the underlying belief that informed consent in law is a doctrine fashioned to permit patients to be the agents of decision making [16].

Good Samaritan laws

Few situations present such potential for conflict between ethical principles and legal concerns as when the emergency physician is in the position of the Good Samaritan. One's impulse, based on the ethical principle of beneficence, is to come to the aid of a person in distress, even though there is no legal duty to do so, and despite the fact that the setting may be far removed from the hospital emergency department where one would have the resources to provide appropriate care. As a counterweight to the impulse to do good, a number of legal questions arise. Does the law in this jurisdiction require the physician to render aid to another because of his/her qualifications to do so? (In Minnesota and a few other states, emergency physicians are required legally to respond to medical emergencies, even outside the emergency department [R. Schears, personal communication, 2005].) Does the law shield the physician from liability for a potential adverse outcome (in the absence of any evidence of intentional, malicious wrongdoing)? If not, will professional liability insurance cover him for acts performed outside the realm of his usual duties?

Obviously, knowledge of the law in one's jurisdiction, and the applicable provisions of one's insurance coverage, can be invaluable in such a situation. In the absence of such knowledge, it may be tempting to use concerns about potential legal ramifications as an excuse for falling short of the ethical ideal. It might be an interesting exercise to inquire of one's colleagues how many of them would rise from their seats and how many would sit in silence on an airplane when a flight attendant has just asked if there is a doctor on board who could come to the aid of a passenger in distress.

The author has experienced personally another sort of consequence of serving in the role of the Good Samaritan. Rising from my seat at a restaurant in response to an anguished cry, I promptly found myself at the side of a woman who had suffered a slip-and-fall accident and sustained an obvious fracture-dislocation of her ankle. I introduced myself and offered to reduce the fracture-dislocation, explaining that the reduction would be painful, after which the ankle would feel better. The woman eagerly accepted the offer. The reduction was accomplished readily with the assistance of the restaurant manager, and medics who arrived shortly thereafter applied a splint and transported her to the nearest hospital. Weeks later I received a letter from an attorney retained by the woman, asking me to serve as a witness in her lawsuit against the restaurant.

Futile (nonbeneficial) care

The concept of medical futility has existed at least since the time of Hippocrates, whose writings suggested three major goals for the practitioner of medicine: cure, relief of suffering, and withholding treatment when the patient's condition cannot be expected to respond [17]. In modern times, recognizing situations in which interventions offer no real hope for helping the patient has become increasingly challenging. In 1993, Lundberg [18] suggested that physicians define medical futility and that hospitals develop guidelines for dealing with it. Schuster [19] argued that the profession must distinguish between everything that can be done and everything that should be done.

It is precisely that distinction with which the emergency physician often wrestles in talking with the families of patients who "want everything done." Conflicts between families making such demands and the physician's belief that such measures are futile are typically resolved in favor of acceding to the family's wishes, largely because of fear of litigation. And, of course, in the emergency department or on the ward, where the emergency physician may be required to respond to cardiorespiratory arrests, there is no time for consultation with the hospital ethics committee.

Ethicists agree that the physician is under no ethical obligation to provide nonbeneficial care. However, some worry that futility is used as a trump card to overrule the autonomous wishes of patients, and harm results from failing to respect the patient's autonomy [20]. Moreover, legal considerations abound in the modern context, in which cardiopulmonary resuscitation and other forms of maximally aggressive treatment are regarded as the "default setting" in decision making about medical care.

Emergency physicians will continue to err on the side of treating aggressively. Certainly, when the patient requests an intervention, such as endotracheal intubation in the setting of end-stage chronic obstructive pulmonary disease, the physician is moved to grant the request out of respect for autonomy. When the patient is unable to participate in the decision because of critical illness or some other factors that impair decision-making capacity, thoughtful yet urgent discussion with the family must take place. Although families may respond reflexively, telling the physician to "do everything," it is often possible to redirect their thinking by explaining that they are being asked to make a "substituted judgment," that is, not to make the decision themselves about what care should be provided, but instead to reflect upon what the patient would say if able to express his wishes. The patient may never have stated explicitly a wish to avoid life-sustaining treatment without hope for meaningful recovery; however, in recent months or years, he may have said things in ordinary conversation, perhaps commenting on the illnesses and hospitalizations of friends or relatives, that reflected such feelings.

Advance directives

People in the United States are increasingly aware that hospitalized patients are subjected to maximally aggressive therapy in the absence of any clear indication that such treatment is contrary to the patient's wishes. Most say they want to participate in decisions about end-of-life care, yet most do not complete advance directives, and among those who do, most do not communicate the existence of those documents to their physicians [21].

It is a source of ongoing frustration to emergency physicians that conversations between patients with advanced chronic diseases and their primary care doctors regarding preferences for aggressive treatments and end-of-life care are not taking place. A time of crisis, such as has occasioned the patient's visit to the emergency department, clearly is not the ideal time for thoughtful reflection on the part of the patient or family. Many primary care physicians, cardiologists, pulmonologists, and even oncologists, appear to operate on the principle that if the patient wants to discuss such issues, he will bring them up.

Emergency physicians should take an active role in encouraging elderly patients with chronic diseases to engage their primary care physicians in such discussions. When a patient's wishes are known, the emergency physician is not only able to care for the patient with respect for his personal autonomy, but is also often able to provide less-than-heroic measures without fear of legal ramifications. At the same time, it is incumbent upon the physician to inquire as to the existence of advance directives and to honor them, because more and more states are enacting laws providing penalties for health care workers who knowingly violate patients' advance directives [22].

Defensive medicine versus stewardship

The ethical principle of stewardship holds that physicians have a duty not only to the individual patient but also to society as a whole. The physician should pursue the best interests of the patient and, at the same time, bear in mind the responsibility to use health care resources wisely.

Ethical conflicts may arise as a result of the potentially competing interests of the individual patient and the wise use of society's health care resources, with the physician sometimes inclined to spare no expense in the pursuit of diagnostic certainty and the provision of treatment that offers even a slight hope of benefit. This potential conflict is, however, cast into even starker relief by the pervasive practice of defensive medicine.

The Office of Technology Assessment estimates that 8% of diagnostic testing is "consciously defensive," and the results of a study of tort reform suggest that defensive medicine accounts for as much as 9% of the health care budget. Each year, there are more than 17 malpractice claims for every 100 full-time practicing physicians. It has been found that 70% to 80% of malpractice claims do not result in payment to the plaintiffs, and there appears to be no correlation between the presence or absence of medical negligence and the outcome of malpractice suits. Nevertheless, each paid claim against a physician is "immortalized" by the National Practitioner Data Bank. The impact of these suits on a physician often results in a conscious or unconscious attempt at self-protection through the defensive practice of medicine. Because of the pervasive and widespread incursion of defensive medicine into the clinical environment, these practices have actually come to represent the standard of care, further exposing the physician to liability for failure to adhere to the "norms" imposed by a litigious society [23].

Recognition of the duty of stewardship may be found in the Code of Ethics for Emergency Physicians, adopted by the Board of Directors of the American College of Emergency Physicians (ACEP) [24]. Principle number 9 of this document states, "Emergency physicians shall act as responsible stewards of the health care resources entrusted to them." ACEP's Code of Ethics further states:

> Health care resources, including new technologies, should be used on the basis of individual patient needs and the appropriateness of the therapy as documented by medical literature. Diagnostic and therapeutic decisions should be made on the basis of potential risks and benefits of alternative treatments versus no treatment. The emergency physician has the obligation to diagnose and treat patients in a cost-effective manner and must be knowledgeable about cost-effective strategies.

Recent estimates of the cost of defensive medicine are in the range of $125 billion per year [25]. The conflict is plain between these expenditures-which are, by definition, unnecessary-and the physician's duty to be a responsible steward of societal resources. Fully aware that the practice of defensive medicine is inconsistent with the practice of cost-effective medicine, physicians rationalize their behavior in terms of the need to protect themselves from the threat of litigation. In the event of an adverse outcome, they note, no one will thank them for saving money.

But high cost, rapid growth, and increasing demand highlight the need for effective stewardship of our health care resources. Larkin [26] describes the demands of this principle in terms of moral courage: "Although we must have the moral resolve to consistently place patient welfare ahead of fiscal concerns, we also must have the courage to monitor ourselves and resist the temptation of blaming society, attorneys, bureaucrats, insurers and others for our own moral blemishes."

The role of the expert witness

Medical malpractice litigation is conducted by trial attorneys who typically have limited knowledge of the medical science underlying their clients' claims. Furthermore, their efforts to persuade a jury depend on the professional authority of physicians acting in the role of expert witness. Many states require plaintiff's counsel to submit a certification from a physician expert as to the merit of the claim being filed. On the defense side, experts will be marshaled to counter the opinions offered by those testifying for the plaintiff. The taking of depositions during the process of discovery has a powerful influence on determining the course of negotiations toward a possible settlement. When cases go to trial, the process of educating a lay jury about the medical issues involved, so that they are informed sufficiently to render a verdict, becomes a battle of the experts.

The responsibility of serving in the capacity of expert witness in a medical malpractice case brings with it a number of ethical demands. These have been summarized in the following guidelines [27]:

- The expert witness should possess current experience and ongoing knowledge in the area in which he or she is asked to testify.

- The expert witness should be willing to submit the transcripts of depositions and testimony to peer review.
- It is unethical for an expert witness to accept compensation that is contingent on the outcome of litigation.
- The expert witness should not provide expert medical testimony that is false, misleading, or without medical foundation. The key to this process is a thorough review of available and appropriate medical records and contemporaneous literature concerning the case being examined.
- After this process is completed, the expert's opinion should reflect the state of medical knowledge at the time of the incident.
- The expert witness should review the medical facts in a thorough, fair, and objective manner and should not exclude any relevant information to create a view favoring the plaintiff or the defendant.
- Expert witnesses should be chosen on the basis of their experience in the area in which they are providing testimony and not solely on the basis of offices or positions held in medical specialty societies, unless such positions are material to the witness' expertise.
- An emergency physician should not engage in advertising or solicit employment as an expert witness where such advertising or solicitation contains representations about the physician's qualifications, experience, or background that are false or deceptive.

Plaintiffs' attorneys claim that their work is made more challenging by physicians' inclination to protect their colleagues, to circle the wagons, to bury their mistakes. They cite a failure of the profession to police itself as a major contributing factor to the occurrence of medical malpractice and assert that the physician who is willing to testify as an expert witness for a plaintiff is courageously defying the profession's behavioral expectations in order to help secure just compensation for an injured victim of medical negligence.

Most physicians hold a strikingly different view: they regard many physicians who testify for plaintiffs as hired guns who will say anything on the witness stand to help make the case for the attorney who is paying them generously for their services. Increasingly, medical professional organizations are scrutinizing the testimony given by their members to see if it measures up to the ethical standards they have established. The American Association of Neurological Surgeons has led the way in disciplining its members for unethical expert witness testimony, notwithstanding the potential for the organization to be subject to retaliatory lawsuits (see, for example, Donald C. Austin, MD vs. American Association of Neurological Surgeons [28]). The American College of Emergency Physicians has a process in place to do the same.

Tort reform: the problem

During the last 50 years, tort costs in the United States have increased more than a hundredfold. In contrast, overall economic production (as measured by GDP) has grown by a factor of 37, and population has grown by a factor of less than two. Between 1975 (the first year for which insured medical malpractice costs were identified separately) and 2003, the increase in medical malpractice costs outpaced increases in overall United States tort costs. Medical malpractice costs rose an average of 11.8% per year, compared with an average annual increase of 9.2% per year for all other tort costs. The compounded impact of this 28-year difference in growth rates is that medical malpractice costs rose by a factor of 23 between 1975 and 2003, whereas all other tort costs grew by a factor of 12. The estimated cost of the medical malpractice tort system in 2003 was approximately $26.5 billion [29].

As of this writing, 27 states have enacted tort reforms that include caps on noneconomic damages, and 20 others remain on the American Medical Association's list of crisis states, states in which the association regards the lack of tort reform as a threat to patients' access to care. A recent study found that implementation of caps on noneconomic damages is associated with an increase in the supply of physicians, with the most pronounced differences in high-risk specialties [30].

Tort reform: getting it right

Most of the medical profession's efforts in the realm of tort reform have been directed toward reducing the number of medical malpractice claims lacking in merit and limiting payments for claims that are pressed successfully. However, it is clear that, from an ethical standpoint, reform should be directed toward getting it right, not simply reducing losses. A fundamental requirement of the application of justice to the harms caused by medical malpractice is that all victims of medical malpractice should be compensated fairly, and those who have not truly been harmed or whose harm was not the result of negligence should be excluded.

A key study performed by Brennan and colleagues [31] at the Harvard School of Public Health demonstrates that the current system does not achieve justice. They conducted a 10-year follow-up of 51 medical malpractice claims to examine relationships between negligence and legal outcomes. A panel of impartial experts analyzed the claims in advance of resolution and determined, for each claim, whether there was an actual adverse event and whether that adverse event was the result of negligence. As of the end of 1995, 46 of the claims had been settled. Twenty-four claims, in the judgment of the investigators, did not actually involve an adverse event. Nonetheless, settlement was in favor of the plaintiff in 10 of those claims ($28,760 mean payment). Another 13 involved adverse events not caused by negligence, and 6 of those claims were settled in favor of the plaintiff ($98,192 mean payment). Only 9 of the 46 claims involved adverse events caused by negligence (an injury due to medical care that failed to meet expected standards). Those were the cases in which justice would require compensation of the victim, yet only 5 of the 9 were resolved in favor of the plaintiff ($66,944 mean payment). Seven of 8 claims involving permanent disability were closed in favor of the plaintiff ($201,250 mean payment). On multivariate analysis, neither adverse events nor negligence was related to legal outcome, and the only significant predictor of a payment being made to a plaintiff was the presence of disability. Analysis of cases in which discrepancies were noted between legal outcomes and prior expert judgment concerning the presence or absence of adverse events or negligence demonstrated the substantial role of "artful litigation."

Artful or not, litigation in our current system can hardly be regarded as producing justice when the legal outcome for 20 of 46 claims was incorrect, as judged by impartial experts. Viewed in terms of the qualifications of the persons judging the merits of claims, this is hardly surprising. The notion that it is possible, during a trial lasting 1 to 3 weeks, by the process characterized as a battle of the experts, to educate a jury of 12 members of the lay public sufficiently to allow them to produce a truly informed verdict regarding the guilt of the physician-defendant is regarded by many as nothing short of absurd.

A system is needed in which physicians and health care workers are encouraged to report medical errors; such errors are disclosed to patients and families; claims, whether resulting from such disclosure or arising independently, are evaluated by impartial panels of experts; and all patients harmed by medical negligence are compensated fairly.

It is impossible to predict with any certainty how the cost of such a system, designed to achieve justice for all victims of medical negligence, would compare with that of the current system. However, the system now in place directs only 28% of malpractice premium dollars toward indemnity, the remainder going toward attorneys' fees and administrative costs [32]. Furthermore, only 22% of money paid to resolve claims goes toward compensating victims for economic losses [33]. Thus, it would appear that the amount of money currently being wasted could fairly compensate many more deserving patients. Justice, quite arguably, is within our reach.

References

[1] Rawls J. A theory of justice. Belknap Press, New Edition 2005.
[2] Beauchamp T, Childress J. Principles of biomedical ethics. 3rd edition. Oxford University Press, 1989. p. 274.
[3] Ritchie J, Davies S. Professional negligence: a duty of candid disclosure? BMJ 1995;310: 888–9.
[4] Hébert P, Levin A, Robertson G. Bioethics for clinicians: 23. Disclosure of medical error. CMAJ 2001;164(4).
[5] Hingorani M, Wong T, Vafidis G. Patients' and doctors' attitudes to amount of information given after unintended injury during treatment: cross-sectional, questionnaire survey. BMJ 1999;318:640–1.
[6] Witman A, Park D, Hardin S. How do patients want physicians to handle mistakes? A survey of internal medicine patients in an academic setting. Arch Intern Med 1996;156:2565–9.

[7] Kraman S, Hamm G. Risk management: extreme honesty may be the best policy. Ann Intern Med 1999;131:963–7.

[8] American College of Emergency Physicians. Disclosure of medical errors. Available at: http://www.acep.org/webportal/PracticeResources/PolicyStatementsByCategory/Ethics/DisclosureMedicalErrors.htm. Accessed June 25, 2005.

[9] Lenzer J. Alteplase for stroke: money and optimistic claims buttress the "brain attack" campaign. BMJ 2002;324:723–9.

[10] Solomon R. Quoted in: Standard of care. Emergency Physicians Monthly 2005;10(6):6–7.

[11] Jeremiah J, et al. Who leaves against medical advice? J Gen Intern Med 1995;10(7):403–5.

[12] Jeffer EK. Against medical advice: part I, a review of the literature. Mil Med 1993;158(2): 69–73.

[13] Drane JF. Competency to give informed consent. JAMA 1984;252(7):925–7.

[14] Capron A. Informed consent in catastrophic disease and treatment. University of Pennsylvania Law Review; 123:364–76.

[15] Modern status of views as to general measure of physician's duty to inform patient of risks of proposed treatment. American Law Reports 3d, 88 (1978):1008.

[16] Physician's duty to inform of risks. American Law Reports 3d, 88 (1986):1010–25.

[17] Jecker NS. Knowing when to stop: the limits of medicine. Hastings Cent Rep 1991;21: 5–8.

[18] Lundberg GD. American health care system management objectives. The aura of inevitability becomes incarnate. JAMA 1993;269:2554–5.

[19] Schuster DP. Everything that should be done – not everything that can be done. Am Rev Respir Dis 1992;145:508–9.

[20] Ardagh M. Futility has no utility in resuscitation medicine. J Med Ethics 2000;26:396–9.

[21] Golin CE, Wenger NS, Liu H, et al. A prospective study of patient-physician communication about resuscitation. J Am Geriatr Soc 2000;48:S52–60.

[22] Hickey DP. The disutility of advance directives: we know the problems, but are there solutions? J Health Law 2003;36(3):455–73.

[23] Anderson RE. Billions for defense: the pervasive nature of defensive medicine. Arch Intern Med 1999;159:2399.

[24] American College of Emergency Physicians. Code of ethics for emergency physicians. Available at: http://www.acep.org/1,1118,0.html. Accessed February 14, 2005.

[25] Office of the Assistant Secretary for Planning and Evaluation, US Department of Health & Human Services. Addressing the new health care crisis: reforming the medical litigation system to improve the quality of health care 11(2003).

[26] Larkin GL, Weber JE, Moskop JC. Resource utilization in the emergency department: the duty of stewardship. J Emerg Med 1998;16:499–503.

[27] American College of Emergency Physicians. Expert witness guidelines for the specialty of emergency medicine. Available at: http//www.acep.org/1,560,0.html. Accessed February 14, 2005.

[28] Donald C. Austin, MD vs. American Association of Neurological Surgeons, 253 F.3d 967, 972–73 (7th Cir. 2001).

[29] Tillinghast-Towers Perrin. US tort costs: 2004 update: trends and findings on the cost of the US tort system. Available at: http://www.towersperrin.com/tillinghast/publications/reports/Tort_2004/Tort.pdf. Accessed February 13, 2005.

[30] Encinosa WE, Hellinger FJ. Have state caps on malpractice awards increased the supply of physicians? Health Affairs 2005 May 31.

[31] Brennan TA, et al. Relation between negligent adverse events and the outcomes of medical malpractice litigation. N Engl J Med 1996;335(26):1963.

[32] Anderson RA. Defending the practice of medicine. Arch Intern Med 2004;164:1173–8.

[33] Tillinghast-Towers Perrin. US tort costs: 2003 update: trends and findings on the cost of the US tort system. Available at: http://www.towersperrin.com/TILLINGHAST/publications/reports/2004_Tort_Costs_Update/Tort_Costs. Accessed February 13, 2005.

ELSEVIER
SAUNDERS

Emerg Med Clin N Am
24 (2006) 749–768

EMERGENCY
MEDICINE
CLINICS OF
NORTH AMERICA

Unstable Ethical Plateaus
and Disaster Triage

Matthew D. Sztajnkrycer, MD, PhD[a,*],
Bo E. Madsen, MD[a],
Amado Alejandro Báez, MD, MSc[b]

[a]*Department of Emergency Medicine, Mayo Clinic, 200 First Street SW,
Rochester, MN 55905, USA*
[b]*Department of Emergency Medicine and Division of Trauma, Burns and Surgical
Critical Care, Brigham and Women's Hospital, Neville House, Room 226,
75 Francis Street, Boston, MA 02115, USA*

Disasters are defined medically as mass casualty incidents in which the number of patients presenting during a given time period exceeds the capacity of the responders to render effective care in a timely manner. During such circumstances, triage is instituted to allocate scarce medical resources. Current disaster triage attempts to do the most for the most, with the least amount of resources. This article reviews the nature of disasters from the standpoint of immediate medical need, and places into an ethics framework currently proposed utilitarian triage schema for prioritizing medical care of surviving disaster victims. Specific questions include whether resources truly are limited, whether specific numbers should dictate disaster response, and whether triage decisions should be based on age or social worth. The primary question the authors pose is whether disaster triage, as currently advocated and practiced in the western world, is actually ethical.

The key concepts of this article are as follows:

- Disasters are defined medically in terms of relative scarcity of medical resources, as opposed to absolute patient numbers.
- Subsequent disaster triage decisions are inherently utilitarian in nature, attempting to do the most for the most, with the least resources.

The content of this publication solely represents the views and opinions of the authors and does not necessarily reflect the official views, policies, or position of the National Disaster Medical Service, US Department of Homeland Security, or the US Government.

* Corresponding author. Department of Emergency Medicine, Mayo Clinic, 200 First Street SW, Rochester, MN 55905.

E-mail address: sztajnkrycer.matthew@may.edu (M.D. Sztajnkrycer).

doi:10.1016/j.emc.2006.05.016
emed.theclinics.com

- Most modern triage schemes use a tiered response, in which one group is deemed expectant and, therefore, not deserving of resuscitation because of consumption of scarce resources.
- Data from recent mass casualty events seem to contradict the concept of scarce resources, and suggest that these expectant patients can be managed aggressively.
- Because current triage schemes essentially constitute a societally mandated Do Not Resuscitate order, broad-level discussions involving all elements of the community should be undertaken to determine the appropriateness of these decisions.

The numbers are staggering. In the past 30 years, millions of lives have been lost to disasters, and billions of lives affected [1,2]. Approximately 62,000 people per annum die as a result of large-scale global disasters [3]. As defined by the Merriam-Webster dictionary [4], a disaster is "a sudden calamitous event bringing great damage, loss, or destruction." From a global perspective, the World Health Organization defines a disaster as a "sudden ecological phenomenon of sufficient magnitude to require external assistance" [5]. However, this definition does little to provide insight and guidance into the specific medical needs of a disaster.

The American College of Emergency Physicians' definition of disasters as "situations in which destructive effects of an event provoked by nature or human beings exceed the available resources required by a community or region in need of medical care" once again provides very little guidance to the medical community [6]. At what point are resources exceeded, for example? Moreover, a disaster may result in mass fatalities but few patients. At the institutional level, a working definition of a disaster might be a situation in which "the number of patients presenting within a given time period are such that the emergency department (or field responding units) cannot provide care for them without external assistance" [7]. More precisely, care cannot be rendered in a timely manner. For the remainder of this article, the authors will use this working definition in discussing medical care during disasters.

The principle underlying these definitions is the concept of *relative* scarcity of available resources. For example, a small community hospital may have fewer resources available to manage a multi-vehicle accident involving multiple victims than a tertiary care referral center. What constitutes a disaster for the former may in fact be routinely managed by the latter. In this way, a mass casualty incident can be distinguished from a multiple casualty incident by virtue of the former, either by the number of patients or by the nature of their injuries, exceeding the capability of the facility or responding services to adequately render care to the victims [8].

In contrast to these more subjective definitions, prehospital emergency medical services frequently define a mass casualty incident as an event involving three or more patients, or two or more responding ambulances [9]. Alternatively, a tiered system based on number of reported victims has been used by larger municipalities [10]. The advantage of this predefined approach is that responders can concentrate immediately on patient care, rather than on determining available resources.

Most disasters are brief, self-limited events that preserve the community infrastructure. In other words, the ability to care for patients remains intact, albeit stressed by the rate of casualty presentation (Fig. 1) [11,12]. One could further define a catastrophe or a catastrophic disaster as a circumstance where the destruction is so overwhelming that the infrastructure itself collapses, or as an "utter failure" [4]. Such a term was applied during the cold war to the results of a potential nuclear conflagration [13–15]. In more recent history, initial reports in the lay press after the 2004 South Asia tsunami indicated that all 569 medical facilities in Sri Lanka were destroyed [16]. Under such circumstances, even external assistance may be nonexistent, and care for the injured may not be an initial priority. Moreover, care for such victims may not occur in the traditional health care setting [11,14,15].

Regardless of the definition, many questions arise concerning appropriate medical care during disasters. How should we allocate resources and how do we justify these decisions? Will we treat patients with the most serious illnesses and injuries first? Will we treat on a first-come, first-served basis? Will we treat on the basis of individual "worth" to society? Will we treat the most people with the available resources, allowing that otherwise salvageable individuals will be allowed to die? The purpose of this article is to review the nature of disasters from an immediate medical need standpoint, and to place currently proposed utilitarian triage schema for prioritizing the medical care of surviving disaster victims into an ethics framework. The goal is not necessarily to provide definitive answers, but rather to raise

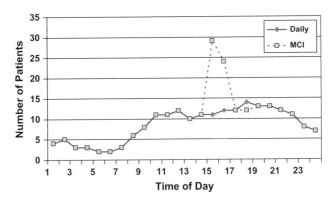

Fig. 1. Patient encounter compression during a mass casualty incident. The solid line (Daily) represents the average number of patients per hour registering to be seen in an emergency department operating under principles of daily triage. The dashed line (MCI) represents a hypothetical scenario in which an additional 30 patients present to the emergency department after a self-limited mass casualty incident. The result is a sudden spike in patient encounters over a brief period of time.

questions and encourage debate. The primary question the authors pose is whether disaster triage, as currently advocated and practiced in the western world, is actually ethical.

Triage in the disaster setting

The term triage, derived from the French verb *trier* (to sort), refers to the rapid sorting and prioritizing of patients. It is the first principle in mass casualty and disaster care [14]. The origin of modern triage is rooted in military medicine, and the work of Baron Dominique Jean Larrey, surgeon general to Napoleon's Army of the Rhine [17–19]. Larrey first implemented a system in which the wounded were prioritized for care based on need rather than rank. Moreover, initial care of the wounded occurred while on the battlefield, before transportation to a site of definitive care.

In 1846, British Naval Surgeon John Wilson developed the principles of modern mass casualty triage [18]. He postulated that in order for medical care to be truly life saving, it needed to be provided to those most in need. As a consequence, care was withheld from those for whom it was either futile or could be delayed until a later time, thereby forming the first tiered triage system. This concept in casualty care, and the term triage, was introduced subsequently to United States physicians serving in Europe in World War 1 [19,20].

In modern medical usage, the term triage more commonly refers to the concept of daily triage. From an emergency medicine perspective, this represents the prioritization of patient care during periods of the day when emergency department resources (typically beds) are scarce. It must be noted that no form of triage is needed if there is no resource limitation. Depending on the triage acuity system, patients' injuries or illnesses may range from nonurgent to life threatening [21–24]. The purpose of daily triage is to identify the latter, so as to rapidly expedite care for those most in acute need. The highest level of care is provided to these patients, even if they have a low probability of survival. A classic example would be the patient presenting in blunt traumatic arrest.

In contrast to daily triage, mass casualty or disaster triage refers to a system that occurs when available resources are insufficient to provide for the needs of all patients. Accurate casualty triage is viewed as the most important initial medical function during a mass casualty event [14,25]. It may be divided further into primary, secondary, and tertiary triage. Primary and secondary triage constitute field or prehospital triage. Primary triage occurs during the initial assessment of victims at the disaster site. Although many systems have been proposed for primary triage, the most commonly encountered in the United States is the Simple Triage and Rapid Treatment (START) system (Fig. 2) [17,18,26–32].

Regardless of the system used, patients are stratified typically into one of four categories, based on physiologic parameters (Table 1) (see Refs.

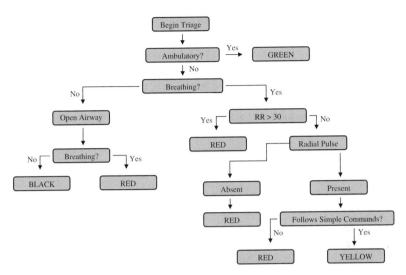

Fig. 2. START mass casualty triage algorithm. The START algorithm categorizes individuals into four categories, based on physiologic parameters and ambulatory status. RR, respiratory rate.

[12,18,26,28,30,33]). Using START terminology, ambulatory individuals are classified as GREEN. Individuals who have sustained injuries deemed not compatible with life under current resource constraints are triaged as expectant (BLACK). Immediate (RED) casualties have abnormal respiratory, perfusion, or mentation status, but are deemed as salvageable by the triage officer (see Fig. 2). Delayed individuals (YELLOW) are unable to ambulate but have normal physiologic parameters. Although they have the potential for decompensation, they require no immediate life-sustaining interventions, and treatment can be delayed typically for 4 to 6 hours [33].

Table 1
Prioritization of mass casualty victim medical need according to triage methodology

Patient category	Time to treatment	Triage methodology			
		START	Triage SIEVE	Homebush triage	John Wilson (1846)
Immediate need	Within 1 h	I (RED)	I	I (RED)	I
Urgent need	4–6 h	II (YELLOW)	II	II (GOLD)	II
Delayed/ minor need	PRN	III (GREEN)	III	III (GREEN)	II
Dying/ expectant	PRN dependent on resources	IV (BLACK)	N/A	IV (WHITE)	III
Deceased	N/A	IV (BLACK)	IV	V (BLACK)	III

Abbreviations: N/A, not considered in the context of the triage scheme; PRN, pro re nata (as needed).

Secondary triage occurs either in the field, at the site of the disaster, or at the casualty collection point, and, as such, is a field triage schema. Depending on the speed with which victims are transported to sites of definitive care, secondary triage may not be needed. Primary triage has been well described in the literature, whereas much less attention has been placed on secondary triage. Typically, such patients are either simply rescreened using a primary triage tool to assess for changes in condition, or triaged according to published trauma center referral guidelines [8]. Two dedicated secondary triage schema have been developed, Secondary Assessment of Victim Endpoint (SAVE) and Triage Sort [31,34], but have not been studied or used widely. The SAVE system was developed to identify those patients at a casualty collection point most likely to benefit from care under austere field conditions [31]. The key assumption in using SAVE is that transportation from the casualty collection point will be delayed and, therefore, definitive care is not immediately available. SAVE might therefore best be applied to catastrophic disaster circumstances. Triage Sort, as practiced in the United Kingdom, uses the revised trauma score to prioritize patient care, and assumes that care evacuation will be immediate [27,34,35].

Tertiary triage refers to patient sorting at the receiving hospital. Classically, this triage determines need for immediate resuscitation, immediate operative intervention, or intensive care unit admission, and then for admission versus discharge. The remainder of this article focuses primarily on the implications and consequences of field triage in the disaster setting.

Western medical ethical principles and principles of justice

Ethics, from the Greek *ethike* (character), may be viewed as the discipline of virtue and righteous action, an attempt to define moral principles and thereby resolve moral dilemmas [6,36,37]. As a consequence, ethics reflects the underlying moral values of society, and therefore is not absolute [38]. For example, in the context of medical ethics, if society views no moral right or value for health care, then subsequent ethical issues may be moot [39]. For the purposes of this article, the authors discuss ethics in the context of modern western society, understanding therefore that this work is not universally applicable [40]. Within western society, the concept of an underlying right to life has been upheld for several hundred years [41,42]. Although a principle of right to life may exist, the right to life in itself does not imply right to a specified length of life, nor does it imply a right or claim on resources, especially when such resources are scarce [41].

The fundamental principles of western medical ethics are respect for patient autonomy, beneficence, and nonmalfeasance [33,43–46]. A fourth principle of medical ethics is distributive justice, henceforth referred to as justice [45], which refers to the fair distribution of scarce or limited resources. The basic principle, described by Aristotle as the principle of formal justice, is that equals should be treated equally, and unequals, unequally [44].

Commonly, four ethical theories are applied to problems of justice: utilitarian, egalitarian, libertarian, and communitarian [44,47].

Utilitarian theory derives from the works of Bentham and subsequent philosophers and economists, especially Mill [48]. The underlying principle, as described by Mill in 1861, is the greatest happiness principle [48,49]. The concept is that, "Actions are right in proportion as they tend to promote happiness." The goal is actually the greatest total happiness, not necessarily the greatest happiness for the greatest number, as is often stated [44]. The most just decisions increase net usefulness to society, by both maximizing societal benefit and minimizing harm. The value of individual freedom is sacrificed for the common good. This ethical concept may be reflected in such medical terms as quality-adjusted life years and disability-adjusted life years.

Central to egalitarian theory is the concept of an equal distribution of scarce goods [48]. The theory may be refined further into strong and maximin egalitarianism. Strong egalitarianism refers to all individuals receiving an identical share. In contrast, the maximin principle, advanced by Rawls [50], accepts inequalities, provided that they benefit those worst off or that it is no longer possible to improve the lot of those worst off. The egalitarian theory articulates the concepts of fairness, equality, and opportunity in defining the ideals of a just community.

Libertarian theory may best be viewed as analogous to an economic free market concept [44,47]. The basic theory, with respect to medical ethics, postulates that the individual is the best judge of his/her own health needs. Priorities are self-determined, and reflect a capacity to pay.

Lastly, communitarian theory holds forth the concept of community standards that attempt to define virtue and good within the context of cultural traditions and society [47]. The general focus is toward creating a "good" society, and as a consequence, of selecting the right individuals to further this goal. A central conflict of this theory is who defines the concepts of "good" and "virtue." The relativist view is that each community defines its own norms within the societal context [51]. In contrast, the universalist view believes in a global concept of a good society, regardless of local cultural beliefs. A nonmedical example of the universalist view would be the importance of female education and literacy, regardless of societal context and belief.

Ethical basis of current disaster triage schema

Triage may be viewed as the means by which scarce medical resources are allocated. Unfortunately, most ethical debates concerning the triage of scarce medical resources refer to nonemergent circumstances, such as the allocation of scarce intensive care unit beds or solid organs for transplantation, or public access to hemodialysis [41,46,52–56]. Although there is an underlying concept of need in each of these cases, triage decisions affecting survival measure life span in days to months [41]. In contrast, in the disaster setting, death may be imminent, and measured in minutes to hours.

As a consequence, the traditional ethical decisions related to triage may not be applicable to the disaster setting [56].

The current concept of mass casualty triage, as developed from the work of Wilson, is clearly and unequivocally based on the concept of utilitarianism [18,56]. "Do as little as possible, for as many as possible, as quickly as possible" [57]. The intent is to maximize casualty survival, and therefore benefit society as a whole, at the expense of individual needs. The question is whether this is fair and acceptable in modern society. In essence, first responders who are typically sworn to protect and uphold the sanctity of life are now placed in the position of not performing life-saving care at the level of their ability in the interest of maximizing societal outcome [58]. The utilitarian approach, by its very nature, posits that the end does, in fact, justify the means. At the individual level, the system is not necessarily fair.

Although utilitarianism by definition subjugates, and to a certain degree infringes on, individual rights, it does so with the higher ethical principle of improving the wellness of society as a whole. Ethics is not absolute, but rather contextual. In a society that places strong emphasis on individual rights, is it just to impose what essentially amounts to a societally mandated Do Not Resuscitate order on victims of a disaster? Has modern society provided us that mandate?

Moreover, no outcome data have ever demonstrated that this triage system actually improves outcome at either the individual or societal level. Despite the decision to allow some salvageable individuals to die for the better good of society, no prospective study has ever validated the ability of mass casualty triage to achieve its stated goal of saving more lives. Retrospective sensitivity and specificity data evaluate solely the ability of the system to detect severity of injury [30]. Yet, according to international humanitarian law, triage must provide the best opportunity to survive [14].

Some data would suggest that, in fact, the current triage schema actually worsens outcomes. Undertriage refers to the inability to identify accurately all patients in need of immediate life-saving interventions, and therefore to mistriage them as lower priority patients. Traditionally, an undertriage rate less than or equal to 5% has been deemed acceptable [59]. Overtriage occurs when the severity of the injury is overestimated, and individuals less in need of care are prioritized erroneously. An overtriage rate of 50% has been advocated in an effort to minimize concomitant undertriage [60]. Overtriage passes the burden of stratifying patients downstream to higher echelons of care. It has been argued that this is fact worsens outcome by overburdening the health care system with noncritical patients whose care might otherwise be delayed safely [25,61]. In the setting of mass casualty events after terrorist bombings, there is a linear increase in patient mortality related to overtriage [61].

Given the consequences of societally imposed life and death end points, triage results remain unacceptably variable. In a tabletop exercise, 70 health care teams each independently triaged a total of 45 victims. Amongst the 70 teams, the number of immediate (RED) cases ranged from 4 to 44, the number of delayed (YELLOW) cases ranged from 1 to 20, and the number of ambulatory (GREEN) cases ranged from 0 to 29. Most importantly, the number of victims triaged as expectant (BLACK) and therefore allowed to die, despite being potentially salvageable, ranged from 0 to 17 [62]. Restated, depending on field triage decisions made by first responders, as many as 37.8% of disaster victims with potentially salvageable injuries in this table-top exercise might have been allowed to die.

Triage has been mandated historically as the responsibility of the most experienced medical person available [63–66]. Is it ethical to allow a first responder with limited medical knowledge to make such stark life-and-death decisions? As stated by the ethicist Kenneth Kipnis [11], "If someone were going to decide that my wounds are too grave to treat, I would want that person to be the most competent professional around." It has even been suggested that no form of triage beyond the identification of the obviously dead should be performed in the prehospital setting, for this very reason [66,67]. As Young [68] states, "Medical staff operating at the first screening should err on the side of liberality in streaming people through to the second stage. In practice this will mean that deliberations should be confined to what are pretty clear medical considerations."

The utilitarian argument for this tiered approach to triage is that by saving more lives in a setting where not all lives may be saved, one is doing the best for society. However, it has been argued that this concept may, in fact, be false [56]. Although one has a moral obligation to save human life if one is able, that does not translate into a more-is-better argument. In fact, all are equally worth saving, and it is not required morally to save more [43].

Moreover, if life is truly a fundamental right, as put forth in Article 3 of the Universal Declaration of Human Rights [42], and an ethical obligation exists to save life, then the primary medical ethical principle of beneficence would mandate giving the benefit to the individual patient during any situation. In contrast to the utilitarian argument, it has been held forth that those in circumstances of imminent death have a special need, and so have a greater claim to scarce resources. Kilner [41] has in fact argued that only those who can benefit from scarce resources should be considered for those resources. Similarly, western society holds forth a duty to prevent death or disability of an identified individual if means are available, regardless of cost or resource use. This concept, termed the "rule of rescue," has been used to justify heroic life-saving efforts [44,45,69].

In a disaster, are resources truly limited?

The entire concept behind both the definition of disaster and the justification for utilitarian triage in the disaster setting rests on the determination that a relative scarcity of resources exists. The reality is frequently quite different [70–76]. Experience has demonstrated that resources are rarely scarce in events viewed by the general public as disasters. In one study of 29 disasters, only 2% of hospitals reported staff shortages, and only 6% reported supply shortages [70]. During the 1989 Loma Prieta earthquake, no staff shortages were reported, and, in fact, staff surplus appeared to be a problem. In a study of hospital administrators after the earthquake, 94% reported adequate supplies during the earthquake period and 87% reported sufficient supplies for the week following the earthquake [71]. A similar abundance of both supplies and medical personnel were noted after the 1989 United Airlines Flight 232 crash in Sioux City [72–74]. During the 1995 Oklahoma City terrorist bombing, at least one or two physicians were present to provide care for each patient [75,76]. During the March 11, 2004, terrorist train bombings in Madrid, 47 physicians, 159 nurses, and 390 emergency medical technicians assessed and triaged 565 patients in the field. Of these, 50 were triaged as critical, and 86 as severe [77].

Actually, the only scarce resource in patient management is time (see Fig. 1) [11,12]. In essence, the patient encounter curve is compressed, such that a larger number of patients than typical are encountered over a brief period of time. The experience has been that most patients present in the first few hours after a discrete event [66,77–80]. As such, is it acceptable ethically to allow otherwise salvageable patients to die "for the good of the many," when those many are not likely to die anyway, and can have care delayed several hours until those critically ill patients are managed?

Because of constrained resources, triage is viewed frequently as a minimalist process [57]. Dogma would state that performing complex life-sustaining procedures violates utilitarian principles by diverting scarce medical resources from the many in favor of the few. The stated objective of utilitarian triage is to maximize lives saved by limiting complex care. Yet this appears counter-intuitive. The lives to be saved are the lives immediately at risk and in need of intervention. During previous mass casualty incidents, complex life-saving interventions were performed at both the pre-hospital and hospital levels of care, despite expenditure of scarce time resources that might have been better spent treating other, less severely injured, patients. The Israeli approach to homicide bombing events includes field endotracheal intubation and needle thoracostomy [66]. Despite the presence of a mass casualty event, hospital management has been even more aggressive, including an emergency department thoracotomy.

Should the numbers dictate the response?

Statistically, despite increasing global awareness, disasters remain low-probability events for the individual community. Before the 9/11 terrorist attacks, only six discrete peace-time events in the United States resulted in more than 1000 fatalities [70]. Although the data are dated, only 10 to 15 disasters a year in the United States result in more than 40 injured victims [81]. Under these circumstances, is it ever appropriate to modify daily triage standard of care, and define a population of ordinarily salvageable victims as otherwise? If so, is there a specific number of victims that mandates the shift to a triage scheme that culls selected victims, such that others might live? Should a bus accident resulting in 28 victims be sufficient to decide that an individual in extremis should be allowed to die, especially when the other victims are either ambulatory or hemodynamically stable?

The advantage of a specific patient number in defining a disaster is that it defines more objectively the extent of the incident. However, numbers may be misleading. Experience with explosions and bombings indicates that most injuries are not imminently life threatening, and, in fact, most victims are ambulatory [78]. Only 5% to 15% of victims are in need of immediate medical care and stabilization. Similar findings were noted after the 1995 sarin attack on the Tokyo subway system [79,80]. Although 500 patients arrived during the initial 1-hour postattack period, and 640 patients were seen in the ED on the day of the attack, only 4 victims were classified as severe. Despite the large patient influx, resources were available and those in extremis were managed aggressively. Similar findings were noted after the March 11, 2004, terrorist attacks in Madrid [77]. Despite more than 1700 victims evaluated on the first day, including 177 fatalities at the scene, no patient was made expectant in the field. Patients were resuscitated aggressively both in the field and in the hospital. Therefore, the number of victims in and of itself would seem insufficient to dictate the switch to disaster triage.

At the two extremes, it has been stated that in the case of an accident, individual medical standards exist and can be sustained. As a result, no patient under these circumstances should be categorized as expectant [34]. In contrast, during a nuclear conflagration, bioterrorism event, or natural pandemic with massive numbers of casualties, the number of victims is so great and the damage to the infrastructure so dramatic, that triage will no longer effectively function regardless [11,13,14,82,83].

Are there better approaches to justice in the disaster setting?

There are some significant ethical misgivings to the use of utilitarian principles in disaster triage. As stated by Steinberg [39], "The utilitarian system significantly interferes with equality and primarily undermines those who are in greatest need of health care services." That said, it is probably fair to state that the libertarian theory of justice, as rigidly constructed, does not apply to mass casualty triage. Although patient autonomy is a guiding principle of biomedical ethics, it is unrealistic to believe that a free-market system of resource allocation, based in large part on ability to pay, has any role in resource allocation during a disaster.

The utilitarian theory, by concentrating on societal good, may place a burden of unacceptable sacrifice on individuals or subpopulations [46]. The initial concept of modern triage, as developed on the battlefield by Larre, was one of need, regardless of rank, and therefore an egalitarian concept. Arguing a strong egalitarian approach, it follows that it would be better not to treat any victim rather than to treat victims unequally; this would not appear to be an ethically tenable viewpoint. However, Larre's approach, based on need rather than rank, heralded the maximin egalitarian principles posited by Rawls [48,50]. Equality and fairness are important components of distributive justice [68]. It may not be fair that the individual is placed in a life-and-death situation involving scarce resources, but the approach to patient treatment should be fair. Moreover, an act that is fair to one patient should not be unfair to others [6]. As such, mass casualty triage should strive toward the goals of fairness, equality, and opportunity. A model based on need, where the sickest are treated first and with the most resources, might, in fact, be fairer and improve societal outcome.

Natural chance and triage

Daily triage works in part on a lottery principle, providing a natural chance (first-come, first-served) element to need-based triage [84]. In the disaster setting, it is held forth that such an approach is neither utilitarian nor egalitarian. Objections raised to the use of this triage approach include the fact that it is discriminatory to those without access to media, transportation, or health care [12,85]. However, the triage process remains, in part, based on lotteries. There is an element of chance to the order of being chosen for triage in the field, and therefore for placement in the queue for treatment and transportation, and for evacuation to definitive care. First responders may either approach those who appear most severely injured, or eschew those in favor of those able to call for help. A first responder simply may start triage at the first victim discovered. The decision may be based on age or gender (women and children first) [84]. As such, despite the misgivings of the lottery, it remains an inescapable reality of the scenario.

Should triage decisions be based on age?

Although extremely controversial, one might argue that the utilitarian triage approach, in attempting to maximize survival above all else, should discriminate against age. One could argue that it is not age, so much as the intendent comorbidities that occur with age [85,86]. It is clear that trauma outcomes are worsened with age, and, in fact, age is a criterion in determining need for trauma center evaluation [8, 87–90]. Moreover, disaster experience has demonstrated significantly worse outcomes in aged populations [91]. Data from the 1999 Taiwan Chi-Chi earthquake demonstrated that the lowest mortality rate occurred in victims in the second and third decades of life. Thereafter, mortality rate increased almost exponentially with age, such that mortality rates in patients in the ninth decade of life were approximately 10-fold higher than those in the third decade of life. Age has also been used as a rationing criterion for both organ transplantation and hemodialysis [41,46,92].

Several different justifications have been put forth to validate the concept of rationing on the basis of age. The first hinges on the concept of the tolerable death [93]. From this concept, it has been argued that life-sustaining treatment can be withheld once an individual reaches a natural life span, defined as a point at which "life's possibilities have on the whole been achieved and after which death may be understood as a sad, but nonetheless relatively acceptable event" [94]. The "fair innings" argument would state that the old have already lived more years than the young, and therefore it is only fair to give the young an opportunity to reach a similar age [95]. Although at the extremes of age this may have some intrinsic logic, it falls apart as differences in age become less extreme. A final justification for age-related triage is based on the prudential life span model, which puts forth justice between age groups. Simply stated, the concept of fair distribution between individuals is changed to one of fair distribution over the life of the single individual. As everyone ages, everyone fairly receives budgeted resources over the course of their lifespan and no unequal treatment occurs over the course of the individual lifespan [93,95]. Subsequent derivatization of this model would suggest that it is better to distribute more medical care to younger age groups.

However, there are clearly issues with age-based triage. The underlying concept is simply that older people are not as worthy of saving as younger people [41]. This view sparks of ageism, and moreover, may conflict with legal principles. The murder of a 90-year-old individual is still murder, and is treated no differently than murder of a 25-year-old. People have rights, including the right to life, which translates into equal and fair access to life-sustaining care. According to Ramsay, "The equal right of every human being to live, and not the relative personal or social worth, should be the ruling principle. When not all can be saved, and all need not die, the ruling principle can be applied only or best by a random choice among equals" [55].

The final issue with age-related triage in the disaster setting is the practical aspect of age determination. Not all individuals age equally. In allocating solid organs or hemodialysis, one has the luxury of time to weigh all the circumstances that define the tolerable death and to determine the actual age of the patient. Such time does not exist in a disaster. If one decides to triage based on age at a disaster, then does one base it on actual age, which may be difficult to determine, or on apparent age, which may be quite misleading?

Should a social lottery exist in triage?

The term "social lottery" refers to the concept of unequal allocation of societal resources based on chance. One cannot always choose one's position in life or one's underlying health, although one's decisions may change it for the better or worse. In the setting of a disaster, should social worth weigh into triage decisions? The communitarian theory might, in fact, support such an argument, as a "good" society is built by "good" individuals. However, most would hold that social position should not weigh into triage decisions [96,97].

One specific aspect of social worth that may have a role in disasters is the ability to provide medical care. It has been argued that individuals with training in medical care provision should receive preferential triage and treatment. If medical care is scarce, then the ability to provide such care is a resource and should not be squandered. By rapidly treating these individuals, and allowing them to provide care, one may enhance the ability to treat other victims. This concept is referred to as the "multiplier effect" [11,12,41,85]. Therefore, a utilitarian argument would be that allowing these individuals to jump the queue would in fact serve a greater social good in the long run and be the ethically just choice. However, this argument has a flaw. Medical resources usually are not limited and therefore the medically skilled victim does not augment a scarce resource. Moreover, because most disasters are discrete, time-limited events, the amount of time required to treat and return to duty an injured medically skilled individual will probably exceed the time of the disaster.

As a society, we ask first responders and emergency medical technicians to enter into hazardous environments. No one is required ethically to put one's own life in danger to assist others. A basic ethical principle is that health care providers should look first to their own safety, then that of their team, and lastly that of the patient [12,98]. Therefore, a more sound ethical argument might be that as a good and just society, we have an ethical responsibility to care for those who risk their lives in the name of society [12].

The final decision to prioritize these patients may fall more to practical concerns than to ethical debate. If a first responder is injured, it may be prudent to evacuate rapidly, to place the minds of his/her peers at ease. First responders who are preoccupied with the health of their injured colleague will be less likely to focus on the task at hand. Moreover, from a morale standpoint, witnessing the care provided to a downed colleague will reassure the remaining responders that they will be well cared for if injured, and allow them to focus on the task at hand.

Triage in catastrophe

To this point, the scope of this article has involved mass casualty incidents and disasters in which the fabric of society remains intact. It is an unfortunate reality of modern life that disasters may occur at such a catastrophic scale that society may cease to function effectively. The past 5 years have borne witness to the utter destruction of Bam, Iran, and to the South Asia tsunami. It has been estimated that in a nuclear war, millions of severely injured people would be left to die [14,15,83]. It has been argued that any attempt to help the injured after nuclear conflagration would be futile, and therefore the utilitarian approach would be to focus on care of the uninjured [13]. In the setting of complex humanitarian emergencies, the decision has been made to treat only those left standing [14].

How would western society respond to a bioterror event involving 100,000 inhalational anthrax casualties? Such doomsday scenarios, in addition to their massive scale, are no longer self-limited. At the peak of the Toronto, Canada, SARS epidemic, 292 paramedics were quarantined for a total of 1637 quarantine days [99]. The rules of triage may no longer even apply [14,100,101]. Under such circumstances, hospitals no longer may be capable of serving as sites of patient care [11,14]. The issues raised by such an event are beyond the scope of the current work. However, the Agency for Healthcare Research and Quality and the Office of Public Health Emergency Preparedness have released a white paper recently to address some of these concerns [101].

Where now triage?

In this article, many questions have been raised and, unfortunately, few answers provided. What is clear is that much more discussion is needed on this difficult topic, and not simply at the medical level. Previous experience with hemodialysis rationing panels has demonstrated that lack of open communication about the allocation process leads to controversy and resentment [44,102]. Public outcry over perceived biases in hemodialysis allocation essentially forced the US government to fund an expensive therapy, a decidedly nonutilitarian approach, despite its support from society [44].

The current schema essentially constitutes a societal waiver of informed consent, under the guise that such a waiver is necessary under extraordinary circumstances for the betterment of society as a whole. Is it not possible that a similar public outcry would occur if the general public was aware that decisions potentially depriving loved ones of life were being made by a group of physicians without their input? It has been suggested that the consequences of triage would not be accepted by western society [17,103]. Rationing, defined as intentionally withholding beneficial care from patients on the basis of cost or limited resources, is not a well-tolerated concept in this society [104]. If such is the case, and because our mandate comes from the community and society as a whole, then is the current triage methodology acceptable?

The time to address or resolve these complex issues is not during or after a disaster, but rather in the preparatory phase. The discussion must be transparent and reflect the cultural, ethical, and moral makeup of the community as a whole, to avoid both the tyranny of the majority (especially in regards to such issues as age-related rationing and specific ethnic or religious beliefs) and the tyranny of experts [46]. Stakeholders in these discussions must not only represent their diverse interests effectively, but be accountable for their representation.

Such discussions would allow the community to see triage consequences from multiple ethical and moral perspectives, to better comprehend the so-called "tragic choices." It may be that society deems the utilitarian theory to be the most just means of triage for mass casualty incidents, despite its potential for unfairness at the individual level. Such open discussion may, in fact, reveal that society has no support for the triage scheme that the health care community has developed to protect the many at the expense of the few. A mandate to ration lives must come from, and be accepted by, the community the triage decisions are designed to protect.

On a concluding note, Domres [33] has argued that disaster triage is ethical only under extreme situations, where unexpected numbers of victims could not be foreseen and planned for. If such is the case, then does it not follow that failure to plan, or lack of preparation in and of itself, is unethical? As stewards of society's health care, the final responsibility is ours [105].

Author's Note:

The final version of this manuscript was submitted to Emergency Medicine Clinics of North America on 16 June 2005. On 29 August 2005, Hurricane Katrina ravaged the Gulf Coast, leaving death and destruction in its wake. In the immediate post impact phase, local and external medical teams struggled with a lack of available resources while attempting to provide care to the thousands of displaced victims. In this context, and given the more recent national discussions of allocating scarce resources in the setting of an H5N1 avian influenza pandemic, I find myself frequently reflecting upon this paper. The simple question: Given what we have recently experienced, and what we are currently planning for, is this paper still valid?

I would argue that the issues raised by this paper remain relevant. The fact is that Hurricane Katrina was no mere disaster, but truly catastrophic in its magnitude, involving complete collapse of the regional infrastructure. Similarly, current plans for pandemic avian influenza anticipate an inability of the national health care infrastructure to support the predicted number of victims. In contrast, this paper focused predominantly upon the ethics of triage in the setting of a discrete disaster rather than a catastrophe.

That said, these recent experiences highlight the on-going need for our society to openly confront the difficult ethical decisions raised in this paper. It is imperative that the public understand the limitations of the medical system during such events, and have a fair input in deciding how society, acting through its health care providers, shall determine who receives what care and when. Failure to plan and prepare for the inevitable may be the most unethical triage decision of all.

Matthew D. Sztajnkrycer, MD, PhD
1 June 2006.

References

[1] Pesik N, Keim M. Logistical considerations for emergency response resources. Pac Health Dialog 2002;9:97–103.

[2] Guha-Sapir D, Lechat MF. Reducing the impact of natural disasters: why aren't we better prepared? Health Pol Plan 1986;1:118–26.

[3] International Federation of Red Cross and Red Crescent Societies. World disaster report 2003. New York: Oxford University Press; 2004.

[4] Merriam-Webster Dictionary. 11th edition. s.v. "Disaster."

[5] Noji EK. The public health consequences of disasters. New York: Oxford University Press; 1997.

[6] Elcioglu O, Unluoglu I. Triage in terms of medicine and ethics. Saudi Med J 2004;25: 1815–9.

[7] Hogan DE, Burstein JL. Basic physics of disasters. In: Hogan DE, Burstein JL, editors. Disaster medicine. Philadelphia: Lippincott Williams and Wilkins; 2002. p. 3–9.

[8] American College of Surgeons. Advanced trauma life support. 7th edition. 2003.

[9] Lilja GP, Madsen MA, Overton J. Multiple casualty incidents. In: Prehospital systems and medical oversight. 3rd edition. Dubuque (IA): Kendall-Hunt; 2002. p. 821–7.

[10] Broward County uniform protocols 3/15/2001. Mass casualty incidents and START triage. Available at: http//www.co.broward.fl.us/browardems/tmi02700.htm. Accessed May 27, 2005.

[11] Kipnis K. Overwhelming casualties: medical ethics in a time of terror. Account Res 2003;10: 57–68.

[12] Iserson KV, Pesik N. Ethical resource distribution after biological, chemical, or radiological terrorism. Camb Q Healthc Ethics 2003;12:455–65.

[13] Pledger HG. Triage of casualties after nuclear attack. Lancet 1986;2(8508):678–9.

[14] Burkle FM. Mass casualty management of a large-scale bioterrorist event: an epidemiological approach that shapes triage decisions. Emerg Med Clin North Am 2002;20:409–36.

[15] British Medical Association. The medical effects of nuclear war: report of the British Medical Association's Board of Science and Education. Chichester (United Kingdom): John Wiley and Sons; 1983.

[16] Sztajnkrycer MD. Hospital preparedness: a public health mandate remains under-appreciated. Int J Rescue Dis Med 2005;4:2.

[17] Wiseman DB, Ellenbogen R, Shaffrey CI. Triage for the neurosurgeon. Neurosurg Focus 2002;12:1–4.

[18] Nocera A, Garner A. An Australian mass casualty incident triage system for the future based upon triage mistakes of the past: the homebush triage standard. Aust N Z J Surg 1999;69:603–8.

[19] Kennedy K, Aghababian RV, Gans L, et al. Triage: techniques and applications in decision making. Ann Emerg Med 1996;28:136–44.

[20] Rutherford W. Triage for simple compensated disasters. J Br Assoc Immed Care 1989;12: 62–7.

[21] Beveridge R, Ducharme J, Janes L, et al. Reliability of the Canadian emergency department triage and acuity scale: interrater agreement. Ann Emerg Med 1999;34:155–9.

[22] Eitel DR, Travers DA, Roseneau A, et al. The emergency severity index version 2 is reliable and valid. Acad Emerg Med 2003;10:1070–80.

[23] Jelinek GA, Little M. Inter-rater reliability of the national triage scale over 11,500 simulated occasions of triage. Emerg Med (Freemantle) 1999;8:226–30.

[24] Travers DA, Waller AE, Bowling JM, et al. Five-level triage system more effective than three-level in tertiary emergency department. J Emerg Nurs 2002;28:395–400.

[25] Frykberg ER, Tepas JJ. Terrorist bombings: lessons learned from Belfast to Beirut. Ann Surg 1988;208:569–76.

[26] Super G. START: a triage training module. Newport Beach (CA): Hoag Memorial Presbyterian; 1984.

[27] Wallis L. START is not the best triage strategy. Br J Sports Med 2002;36:473.

[28] Bozeman WP. Mass casualty incident triage. Ann Emerg Med 2003;41:582–3.

[29] Garner A, Nocera A. "Sieve", "Sort" or START. Emerg Med (Freemantle) 2001;13:477–9.

[30] Garner A, Lee A, Harrison K, et al. Comparative analysis of multiple casualty incident triage algorithms. Ann Emerg Med 2001;38:541–8.

[31] Benson DO, Koenig KL, Schultz CH. Disaster triage: START then SAVE: a new method of dynamic triage for victims of a catastrophic earthquake. Prehosp Disaster Med 1996;11: 117–24.

[32] Nocera A, Garner A. Australian disaster triage: a colour maze in the Tower of Babel. Aust N Z J Surg 1999;69:598–602.

[33] Domres B, Kock M, Manger A, et al. Ethics and triage. Prehosp Disast Med 2001;16:53–8.

[34] Sammut J, Cato D, Homer T. Major incident medical management and support (MIMMS): practical, multiple casualty, disaster-site training course for all Australian health care personnel. Emerg Med (Freemantle) 2001;13:174–80.

[35] Sammut J, Cato D, Homer T. Reply to "Sieve", "Sort", or START. Emerg Med (Freemantle) 2001;13:477–8.

[36] SAEM Ethics Committee. Virtue in emergency medicine. Acad Emerg Med 1996;3:961–6.

[37] Larkin GL, Arnold J. Ethical considerations in emergency planning, preparedness, and response to acts of terrorism. Prehosp Disast Med 2003;18:170–8.

[38] van der Wilt GJ. Cost-effectiveness analysis of health care services, and concepts of distributive justice. Health Care Anal 1994;2:296–305.

[39] Steinberg A. Allocation of scarce resources. Assia Jew Med Ethics 1995;2:14–21.

[40] Kunstadter P. Medical ethics in cross-cultural and multi-cultural perspectives. Soc Sci Med 1980;14B:289–96.

[41] Kilner JF. A moral allocation of scarce lifesaving medical resources. J Relig Ethics 1981;9: 245–85.

[42] United Nations General Assembly Resolution 217 A (III). December 1948.

[43] Beauchamp TL, Childress JF. Principles of biomedical ethics. 5th edition. New York: Oxford University Press; 2001.

[44] Lanken PN, Terry PB, Osborne ML. Ethics of allocating intensive care unit resources. New Horiz 1997;5:38–50.

[45] Cookson R, Dolan P. Principles of justice in health care rationing. J Med Ethics 2000;26: 323–9.

[46] Giacomini MK, Cook DJ, Streiner DL, et al. Using practice guidelines to allocate medical technologies. Int J Technol Assess Health Care 2000;16:987–1002.

[47] Capp S, Savage S, Clarke V. Exploring distributive justice in health care. Aust Health Rev 2001;24:40–4.

[48] Olsen JA. Theories of justice and their implications for priority setting in health care. J Health Econ 1997;16:625–39.

[49] Mill JS. Utilitarianism. 2nd edition. Indianapolis (IN): Hackett Publishing Company; 2001.

[50] Rawls J. A theory of justice (revised). New York: Oxford University Press; 1999.

[51] Roberts MJ, Reich MR. Ethical analysis in public health. Lancet 2002;359:1055–9.

[52] Society of Critical Care Medicine Ethics Committee. Consensus statement on the triage of critically ill patients. JAMA 1994;271:1200–3.

[53] Truog RD. Triage in the ICU. Hastings Cent Rep 1992;22:13–7.

[54] Weil MH, Weil CJ, Rackow EC. Guide to ethical decision-making for the critically ill: the three r's and q. c. Crit Care Med 1988;16:636–41.

[55] Stogre M. Allocating scarce resources: a question of distributive justice part II. CHAC Rev 1998;26:19–22.

[56] Bell NK. Triage in medical practices: an unacceptable model? Soc Sci Med 1981;15:151–6.

[57] Baskett PJF. Ethics in disaster medicine. Prehosp Disast Med 1994;9:4–5.

[58] Dececco J. Is TRIAGE ethical? Emergency 1986;18:60–3.

[59] Wesson DE, Scorpio R. Field triage: help or hindrance? Can J Surg 1992;35:19–21.

[60] American College of Surgeons Committee on Trauma. Field categorization of trauma victims. Bull Am Coll Surg 1986;71:17–21.

[61] Frykberg ER. Medical management of disasters and mass casualties from terrorist bombings: how can we cope? J Trauma 2002;53:201–12.
[62] The Sacco triage method. Available at: http://www.sharpthinkers.com/abc/ts_approach_triss.htm. Accessed May 27, 2005.
[63] Swan KG, Swan KG Jr. Triage: the past revisited. Mil Med 1996;161:448–52.
[64] Griffiths H. A general surgeon in Vietnam: lessons learned the hard way. Mil Med 1990;155: 228–31.
[65] Stein M, Hirschberg A. Medical consequences of terrorism. the conventional weapon threat. Surg Clin North Am 1999;79:1537–52.
[66] Almogy G, Belzberg H, Mintz Y, et al. Suicide bombing attacks: update and modifications to the protocol. Ann Surg 2004;239:295–303.
[67] Einav S, Feigenberg Z, Weissman C, et al. Evacuation priorities in mass casualty terror-related events: implications for contingency planning. Ann Surg 2004;239:304–10.
[68] Young R. Some criteria for making decisions concerning the distribution of scarce medical resources. Theory Decis 1975;6:439–55.
[69] Hope T. Rationing and life-saving treatments: should identifiable patients have higher priority? J Med Ethics 2001;27:179–85.
[70] Auf der Heide E. Principles of hospital disaster planning. In: Hogan DE, Burstein JL, editors. Disaster medicine. Philadelphia: Lippincott Williams and Wilkins; 2002. p. 57–89.
[71] Martchenke J, Pointer JE. Hospital disaster operations during the 1989 Loma Prieta earthquake. Prehosp Disas Med 1994;9:146–53.
[72] Sopher L, Petersen R, Talbott M. The crash of flight 232L: an emergency care perspective. J Emerg Nurs 1990;16:61A–6A.
[73] Kerns DE, Anderson PB. EMS response to a major aircraft incident: Sioux City, Iowa. Prehosp Disas Med 1990;5:159–66.
[74] Nordberg M. United flight 232: the story behind the rescue. Emerg Med Serv 1989;18:15, 22–31.
[75] Maningas PA, Bobison M, Mallonnee S. The EMS response to the Oklahoma City bombing. Prehosp Disas Med 1997;12:80–5.
[76] Quayle C. Lessons learned from the Oklahoma City bombing. Am Hosp Assoc News 1995; 31:7.
[77] Ortiz Alonso FJ. 2004 terrorist bombings in Madrid: an analysis of clinical management. Presented at the 2005 NDMS Conference. Orlando (FL), May 3, 2005.
[78] Severance HW. Mass-casualty victim "surge" management. preparing for combings and blast-related injuries with possibility of hazardous materials exposure. N C Med J 2002; 63:242–6.
[79] Okumura T, Suzuki K, Fukuda A, et al. The Tokyo subway sarin attack: disaster management, pt 1: community emergency response. Acad Emerg Med 1998;5:613–7.
[80] Okumura T, Suzuki K, Fukuda A, et al. The Tokyo subway sarin attack: disaster management, pt 2: hospital response. Acad Emerg Med 1998;5:618–24.
[81] Wright JE. The prevalence and effectiveness of centralized medical responses to mass casualty disasters. Mass Emerg 1977;2:189–94.
[82] Asaeda G. The day that the START triage system came to a STOP: observations from the World Trade Center disaster. Acad Emerg Med 2002;9:255–6.
[83] Leaning J. Physicians, triage, and nuclear war. Lancet 1988;2(8605):269–70.
[84] Hall W. Social class and survival on the S.S. Titanic. Soc Sci Med 1986;22:687–90.
[85] Pesik N, Keim ME, Iserson KV. Terrorism and the ethics of emergency medical care. Ann Emerg Med 2001;37:642–6.
[86] Tan CP, Ng A, Civil I. Co-morbidities in trauma patients: common and significant. N Z Med J 2004;10:U1044.
[87] MacLeod J, Lynn M, McKenney MG, et al. Predictors of mortality in trauma patients. Am Surg 2004;70:805–10.

[88] Demetriades D, Murray J, Martin M, et al. Pedestrians injured by automobiles: relationship of age to injury type and severity. J Am Coll Surg 2004;199:382–7.

[89] Nirula R, Gentilello LM. Futility of resuscitation criteria for the "young" old and the "old" old trauma patient: a national trauma data bank analysis. J Trauma 2004;57:37–41.

[90] Aldrian S, Nau T, Koenig F, et al. Geriatric polytrauma. Wien Klin Wonchenschr 2005; 117:145–9.

[91] Liang NJ, Shih YT, Shih FY, et al. Disaster epidemiology and medical response in the Chi-Chi earthquake in Taiwan. Ann Emerg Med 2001;38:549–55.

[92] Tauber AI. Medicine, public health, and the ethics of rationing. Perspect Biol Med 2002;45: 16–30.

[93] Jecker NS. Should we ration health care. J Med Humanit 1989;10:77–90.

[94] Callahan D. Setting limits: medical goals in an aging society with "a response to my critics." Washington D.C.: Georgetown University Press; 1995.

[95] Clarke CM. Rationing scarce life-sustaining resources on the basis of age. J Adv Nurs 2001; 35:799–804.

[96] American Medical Association Council on Ethical and Judicial Affairs. Ethical considerations in the allocation of organs and scarce medical resources among patients. Arch Intern Med 1995;5:29–39.

[97] Diekma DS. The preferential treatment of VIPs in the emergency department. Am J Emerg Med 1996;14:226–9.

[98] Iserson KV. Threatening situations. In: Isoerson KV, Sanders AB, Mathieu D, editors. Ethics in emergency medicine. 2nd edition. Tucson (AZ): Galen Press; 1995. p. 383–6.

[99] Verbeek PR, McClelland IW, Silverman AC, et al. Loss of paramedic availability in an urban emergency medical services system during a severe acute respiratory syndrome outbreak. Acad Emerg Med 2004;11:973–8.

[100] Hocking F. Psychiatric aspects of extreme environmental stress. Dis Nerv Syst 1970;31: 544–5.

[101] Agency for Healthcare Research and Quality. Altered standards of care in mass casualty events. AHRQ Publication No. 05–0043. Rockville (MD). April 2005.

[102] Iglehart J. Health policy report: the American health care system: the end-stage renal disease program. N Engl J Med 1993;328:366–71.

[103] Department of the Army. NATO handbook on the medical aspects of NBC defensive operations. Washington, DC: AMED P-6; 1987. Draft No. 1986–87:17–19.

[104] Aaron H, Schwartz WB. Rationing health care: the choice before us. Science 1990;247: 418–22.

[105] ACEP Ethics Committee. Code of ethics for emergency physicians. Ann Emerg Med 2004; 43:686–94.

ELSEVIER
SAUNDERS

Emerg Med Clin N Am
24 (2006) 769–784

EMERGENCY
MEDICINE
CLINICS OF
NORTH AMERICA

The Interface: Ethical Decision Making, Medical Toxicology, and Emergency Medicine

Erica Kreismann, MD[a], Maureen Gang, MD[a],
Lewis R. Goldfrank, MD[a,b,*]

[a]Department of Emergency Medicine, Bellevue Hospital/NYU Hospitals,
New York University School of Medicine, 462 First Avenue,
Room OB-345A, New York, NY 10016, USA
[b]New York City Poison Center, New York, NY 10016, USA

The emergency department is the ultimate melting pot. Physicians who choose to immerse themselves in this environment do so largely out of love—for medicine, but also for the chaos of society's reality. Emergency physicians strive to maintain their composure and compassion as they serve on the frontlines of a daily battle, struggling to provide exemplary care to underserved populations while confronted with limited resources, pressures of time, and overcrowding. Emergency physicians act as a public health safety net because so much of the health care system is inaccessible to so many. Physicians often must remind themselves that they are caring for an individual, not simply an abstract problem in an isolated moment. Physicians must remember to make decisions based not solely in science, but also in humanism. "The secret in caring for the patient is in caring for the patient" [1]. Inherent in this approach to patient care is maintaining respect for the individual patient, even when the individual reaches conclusions and makes decisions that differ from those the physician would want the patient to make. Autonomy is easy to respect when the patient is in agreement with the physician's plan. The basic principle of beneficence states that physicians must do what is best for each person, incorporating the negative obligation of nonmaleficience that physicians first must do no harm, and the positive obligation of beneficence to do that which is good [2]. Emergency physicians find themselves facing patients whom they have met moments before, knowing little about who they are or how they live and even less about what

* Corresponding author.
E-mail address: goldfl03@med.nyu.edu (L.R. Goldfrank).

matters to them. Emergency physicians must make decisions, implement care, and begin therapies for their benefit and on their behalf. Emergency physicians must care not only for the patients before them, but also for the society to which these patients ultimately return. What is the emergency physician's role at this interface of personal medicine and the needs of a society?

In cases of high acuity, it is clear: begin treatment, stabilize, sometimes save, and move on. But much of that which emergency physicians see is not what makes for good TV, and what is the physician's role then? Emergency physicians are primary care providers of last resort within a poorly constructed framework. In this respect, emergency physicians must look inward and ask, what is the role of the emergency department? Maybe not so much what it actually is, but rather, what it should be? For many emergency physicians, perhaps especially those practicing or training in large urban centers, they are not solely in the business of the stabilization and treatment of the acutely ill. Emergency physicians are the first line between the social community and the medical one. Emergency physicians are often the only point of health care access for the underserved. What is the emergency physician's responsibility to them?

The primary obligation is unquestionably to the care of the patient. But what happens when there is no clear right or wrong? When physicians are confronted with a patient whose behavior is not in his or her own self-interest? When the decisions of patients are detrimental to themselves or to the rest of society? What are physicians to do when confronted with a possibly "intoxicated" patient who is agitated and disruptive? When this patient has obvious signs of trauma? What are physicians to do when this patient is a parent, or an airline pilot, or a fellow physician? Are physicians agents of the greater good? Should they be? Or are physicians protectors of personal confidences and trusts? Is the primary obligation to the individual or to a better society?

These are issues and moral questions that arise regularly, often glossed over in the rush of decision making before moving on to the next patient, the sicker patient. A degree of ethical sophistication is required, however, in making these fundamental decisions. Physicians must be able to defend their actions, not only to society, but also to themselves. Physicians must be convinced that they are doing the right thing for the right reasons. This article addresses some of the ethical conundrums that are encountered frequently in treating patients with toxicologic emergencies. It is the authors' hope to spark conversation, debate, and even disagreement, for that is how moral growth and development occur.

Case one: alcoholism

> Emergency medical services rolls through the doors with a sorry smile and deposits one of your "regulars" in the triage bay. You recognize him immediately, not solely because he is wearing the social work outfit that you

presented to him on last night's shift. He is a patient well known to your emergency department, a chronic relapsing alcoholic, belligerent, loud, and verbally abusive when intoxicated, but who sobers into a seemingly rational and sheepish guy. He is able to maintain spotty employment and has a family that is (peripherally) involved in his life. Tonight your patient was found yelling obscenities at passersby and was brought to the emergency department by emergency medical services. He is awake and abusive to the staff, as is his routine. His speech is slurred, and his gait cannot be assessed because he is refusing to move from the gurney until he receives a dinner tray.

Patients such as this present in emergency departments throughout the United States—urban or rural—and pose a unique and frustrating set of questions and problems. These patients can be an enormous drain on already strained resources and are often disruptive and abusive, not only to staff, but also often to other patients. Yet, they have many complex medical, toxicologic, and ethical issues and often force physicians to the very brink of their humanity, patience, and kindness. This particular individual thwarts attempts at treatment and can be disruptive and even threatening to the department. His regular visits raise questions about resource allocation and futility. His decision-making capacity is questionable. The question arises regularly as to when is the appropriate time for discharge. Is this decision different on the first presentation from the fourth of that week? Is the decision different when he presents every day or every other day? Would this decision be aided in any way by documentation of a blood alcohol level?

Despite overwhelming frustrations and failures, this patient is representative of a population that serves as a prime example historically of the utility of a public health approach to toxicology and the impact that can be made by basic interventions. Wernicke's encephalopathy and Korsakoff's psychosis are now rare diseases, yet older physicians easily recall a time when they were common presentations along with severe delirium tremens. Many residents now go through their entire training without being exposed to these conditions, a direct result of the integration of public health measures into clinical practice and routine treatments. It is now the standard of care to give thiamine and folate to all patients presenting to the emergency department with any suggestion of alcohol-related problems, not only patients with stigmata of chronic alcohol abuse. Therapy with thiamine hydrochloride (vitamin B_1) is estimated to cost a few dollars per intravenous dose; this cost can be contrasted dramatically with an estimated likely cost of hundreds of thousands of dollars to society for the long-term care of a single patient with Wernicke-Korsakoff syndrome. Perhaps the sense of responsibility is shifting, and society is beginning to appreciate interconnectedness and interdependence. Substance use and abuse are among the most pervasive problems in modern culture. They are responsible for a significant portion of lost days from work, lost years of productive life, and massive social and economic burdens. The US economic cost of alcohol [3,4], tobacco [5], and other substance abuse [6] can be estimated at $500 billion per year. It reaches across all socioeconomic and educational boundaries and has been well documented in homeless psychiatric patients and college and medical students. The move away from a fatalistic assessment of individuals' interaction with their environment and toward a greater allocation of societal and personal responsibility has resulted in expansive efforts in the field of public health [7].

Although these are not the patients many physicians imagined when they first made the choice of emergency medicine, they often can be among the most challenging. They come to the doors and gurneys of emergency departments wrapped in a nearly endless list of ethical dilemmas. If little else, they require time, cumulatively, much of it, and a disproportionate number of resources. They are scanned and rescanned for every new episode of trauma. They demand to be fed, bathed, and clothed, at least at the authors' institution, on an almost regular basis [8]. What are the obligations as fellow human beings and as physicians? How has the practice of emergency medicine evolved to help physicians be better care providers and to provide more compassionate care? What are the options with patients whose abuse of self and the system takes its toll on resources, the care of other patients, and the health care providers themselves?

These patients can invoke in physicians a storm of emotions, including pity, compassion, anger, and frustration. It is important, in treating, that physicians recognize this because disregarding these emotions runs the risk of their surfacing in other ways. The emotions and anger can be multi-layered, as lofty as frustration over perceived abuse of a system of which physicians stand as staunch defenders—resource allocation, the appropriate use of an ambulance, or more appropriate allocation of increasingly scarce hospital gurneys. Or, in honest moments, physicians can acknowledge bitterness at being reduced to mere providers of food and shelter and little more. There are times when everyone feels abused. The question arises, ethically, morally, and legally: What is the right thing to do? The situation is more clear-cut when there are obvious signs of trauma or infection; under these circumstances, no one can suggest denying judicious use of the CT scanner or hospitalization, regardless of likelihood of reimbursement. This discussion of reimbursement and saving resources is most dangerous—putting physicians in the position of arbiter, determining certain patients worthy and others less so. If this were the case, the difficult patients—the ones who strain resources, who suffer chronic debilitating dependency, or who who drink or use illicit substances—would be the first to feel the biases and suffer from them even more than they currently do. The job of physicians is to care for these downtrodden patients perhaps even better than they care for themselves. These are the people who fall through the cracks, not only societally, but also medically. The scenario gets a bit more complex, although perhaps more ethically interesting as well, when the "AOB"(alcohol on breath), as they are often written on a triage board, is not sleeping peacefully in the corner, but agitated and combative and insistent on leaving. Are there any hard and fast rules?

This scenario can raise fascinating and challenging questions regarding patient autonomy and decision-making capacity. Delaying these critical analyses, decisions, and actions can place the emergency department staff and the patient in danger, so it is essential to address these issues proactively before a medical or ethical crisis ensues. These are, on the whole, not patients who can be reasoned with, although that approach is usually appropriate as a first-line attempt. If someone has suffered obvious trauma (head or other body part), if there is any question of capacity secondary to alcohol intoxication, drug use, infection, or possibly to the trauma itself, the appropriate thing to do is obtain the necessary studies even if sedation is required.

An assessment of capacity in a patient under the influence of a toxin may be impossible at times and is almost always difficult. To understand this fully, one must be clear as to the definition of capacity. The definition has two requirements: First, the patient must possess an ability to understand the medical situation and its possible consequences, and, second, the patient must show that he or she arrived at the decision rationally and with an understanding of pertinent facts and information. Capacity must be evaluated for each decision individually ("decisional capacity"). By these standards, a patient may have the capacity to make some simple health care decisions, but not other more complex ones [9]. In other words, decision-making capacity requires: "(1) possession of a set of values and goals; (2) the ability to communicate and to understand information; and (3) the ability to reason and deliberate about personal choices" [9]. It is important to distinguish this concept from that of competence. The latter is a legal standard and determined solely by a judge or court, not the treating physician. As in the case of all decisions for which capacity is required (which are virtually all decisions in medicine), one usually perceives its importance as being directly proportional to the magnitude of the problem and invoke a sliding scale of capacity. When the stakes are higher, the problem more grave, a more sophisticated understanding of the risks and benefits or alternatives is needed. Inevitably, degree of intoxication plays a role in this decision-making process.

What utility does a blood alcohol level have?

Should physicians worry in this day and age of excessive litigation about a patient whom they discharged because he woke up, ate, and ambled steadily out of the emergency department, but whose blood alcohol level was 400 mg/dL 4 hours before discharge? (As a predictive tool, even if the patient was able to metabolize alcohol at 30 mg/dL, one can still assume that he would have a level of nearly 300 mg/dL at the time of discharge.) It is the authors' belief that if the level could contribute to patient care, could guide treatment, then it is worth sending. The decision for treatment and the decision regarding cessation of therapy is a clinical one. The most relevant indicators of inebriation are not laboratory values, but rather an evaluation of the patient's clinical status: motor capacity, gait, speech, clarity of thought, and understanding of a plan. This global assessment of the clinical status must be defined to determine the appropriate time for discharge. The physician and nurse must ensure unambiguous documentation. All who will subsequently read the medical record should be clear as to the reasoning and the course of clinical decisions. Blood alcohol levels can contribute the most to the evaluation at the behavioral extremes. Valuable information is obtained when the patient is awake and eating and the blood alcohol level returns at greater than 300 mg/dL. This gives the clinician a clear indication of the severity and chronicity of the patient's problem. It does not define when discharge is safe, however. Tolerance to ethanol is toxicodynamic (change in receptor characteristics) and toxicokinetic (change in metabolic characteristics). As such, "clinical intoxication" can be defined only as a condition of impaired ability of function and should be independent of levels. If physicians kept all the patients who present with elevated blood alcohol levels until they had metabolized their alcohol to below the legal limit, the emergency department would come to a grinding halt. There would be no space for evaluation of other patients. Patients would have "iatrogenic" ethanol withdrawal, seizures, and delirium tremens, and the medical services would be overwhelmed by admissions for alcohol withdrawal. This is not a clinically appropriate or medically rational plan, and the authors do not advocate it for those reasons.

Little is known about the capacity of many of these patients. They have made prior decisions that are significantly detrimental to their health. Alcohol abuse has protean long-term effects and a neurodegenerative impact. These issues, placed in the context of a hostile social environment, raise valid concerns for the ability of the patient in case one to care for himself and make appropriate decisions. For all of society's respect for independence and autonomy, society does not permit clear self-destruction. Suicide remains illegal, as does posing a danger to self or others. Is this not a slow and painful, but clear-cut path to self-destruction? Does society have a right or a responsibility to intervene? Is there a role for involuntary psychiatric incarceration?

The arguments may be made from both sides. If a patient is able to comprehend the consequences (potential or realized) of his or her behavior and still continues to engage in it anyway, some would say that this is the patient's right. Physicians have neither the power nor the jurisdiction to intervene; to attempt to do so would overstep their bounds. Paternalism is not indicated.

The argument also can be made to the contrary. When someone engages in behavior so clearly injurious and directed at self-harm, physicians do have an obligation to intercede, just as they do with patients who are more overtly suicidal. The physicians' duty is to protect one from self-destruction, perhaps to ensure that the appropriate treatment and care—medical and psychological—are delivered. Physicians have a responsibility to remove the individual from the current environment and at least give him or her the chance to help himself or herself.

The disease of chronic alcoholism can lead to severe neurodegenerative effects that can impair one's ability to make and understand important decisions. Most clinicians would not hesitate to admit an asthmatic who returns for the third day in a row, unable to get his or her disease adequately controlled, or the patient with sickle cell disease whose pain crisis persists. Cannot the same argument be made for the disease of alcoholism? If physicians want to get at the root of the problem, they must ask themselves honestly what are the goals of therapy or discharge? Are physicians hoping to intervene or simply get this patient out of the department in the fastest or easiest way possible? Why do physicians' attitudes change so dramatically when treating chronic alcohol abusers? Would it ever be acceptable to practice medicine this way with other populations or individuals with chronic debilitating asthma or sickle cell disease?

As with other chronic illnesses, there comes a time when physicians must acknowledge that the current therapy or interventions are not achieving the desired results. Physicians must then delve deeper and pursue an underlying cause. Little is known about this patient population of "regulars" or "repeat visitors," but physicians are aware of numerous comorbidities that, if treated or addressed, would offer greatly enhanced opportunities for likely success. Mental retardation, psychiatric illness, Alzheimer's disease, and chronic central nervous system injury are often masked or confused with concurrent alcohol abuse. Little is known about the chronic effects of alcohol on the brain. It is believed that at some point in specifically selected patients after failed attempts at voluntary therapy, involuntary incarceration is indicated.

Standardized or well-defined criteria for hospital admission of alcoholics do not exist. The policy of each institution dictates a course or possible options for care, but it is the authors' recommendation that all treating physicians begin to assume responsibility for this enormous social ill. The major goals of medical management are to minimize the severity of symptoms, prevent or manage more severe withdrawal presentations, and ultimately facilitate entry into ongoing treatment programs [10]. Patients with mild symptoms often may be treated safely as outpatients, whereas patients with more severe withdrawal or coexisting conditions are often best addressed as inpatients. It is not appropriate to discharge a patient with severe tremors, unsteady gait, or hallucinations. To be appropriate for discharge, patients must have adequate mental and physical strength to cope with in the environment to which they will be returned. Physicians do not provide a service to the patient or fellow caregivers by simply trying to get the patient back out the door. The patient inevitably returns. Compelling evidence exists that there is a wide gap between patients' need for treatment and identification/referral by emergency department staff [11]. It is estimated that there are 3 to 22 million American alcoholics, but it is likely that the true number is toward the higher end of the spectrum. The gap between need and treatment is enormous.

Emergency physicians have a tendency to approach these problems as acute issues; however, change is not likely to occur until physicians reconfigure their understanding and broaden their vision. Alcohol dependency is a chronic disorder that, as with many chronic disorders, responds to medications and other interventions. Treatment requires more than detoxification and recovery and is likely to depend on continuing care, medications, and behavioral change [11]. Physicians must not be discouraged by failed attempts at assistance, for if they abandon responsibility, they will guarantee their failure as physicians.

The emergency department visit offers an opportunity for identification, brief intervention, and referral to treatment, and studies of this approach have shown varying degrees of success [12,13]. The greatest good will not come from physicians' small but valuable attempts at intervention, but from a society that addresses the problem through education and public health measures. The answer to this social problem lies in social education and health care reform.

What if the emergency department patient was not the homeless "regular" who lives on the street corner, but rather someone whose car keys fall from his pocket in the course of undressing, and he insists on leaving before achieving sobriety? The utility of a blood alcohol level is also a legal one because it determines a level at which it is no longer legal to drive. As of August 2005, all 50 states have set the legal blood alcohol limit for driving at 0.08% (80 mg/dL). From the physician's perspective, intoxication is a clinical determination, and a conservative approach is recommended if the patient in question appears intoxicated despite a "legal" level. One must not forget the limitations inherent in this test. A blood alcohol level is just that; it does not provide information on other possible coingestants. To clear a patient medically for release before clinical sobriety is achieved and to put the individual behind the wheel of a car is potentially to endanger not only the life of the patient, but also to endanger the lives of others. As with so many other ethical decisions that arise in the emergency department, clinically precise and thoughtful documentation in the medical record is essential.

What if, on that Saturday night, instead of arriving at work to find your "regular" yelling and combative, in his stead sits a young mother equally intoxicated, having been directed to the emergency department after she stumbled while walking with her daughter outside? As mentioned earlier, alcoholism and the problems of alcohol abuse cut a wide swath, crossing all socioeconomic boundaries. Although respect for patient privacy is a core value, it is subjugated to the needs and safety of the child. "The utilitarian approach to the ethics of competing rights is to balance benefits and harms. In such a balance, child safety trumps all other values" [14]. Social Services should be notified and an investigation begun.

Case two: antidotes

A 28-year-old intravenous drug user is brought to the emergency department unresponsive. His respiratory rate is 4 breaths/min, and his pupils are pinpoint. The treating resident administers 2 mg of naloxone intravenously, and within 1 minute of administration the patient is awake, alert, and insistent on leaving. The patient states that he recently used heroin and denies other ingestions. The patient insists on leaving immediately and states that he wishes to sign out against medical advice.

This case elucidates a few of the key points that must be addressed in the emergency department when caring for patients who have used toxins. It is important when treating this patient that physicians not only respect patient autonomy and independence, but also that they make use of basic principles of clinical pharmacology and medical toxicology regarding the pharmacokinetics of the antidote and the toxicokinetics of the agent used. This scenario represents a frequently encountered problem when a patient is brought to the emergency department in a clinically unstable condition after use of a toxin, which physiciains are able to reverse fully or partially, who then demands release. The right of a hospital to restrain physically or chemically an individual with an altered sensorium, to evaluate him or her, or so that an emergency intervention may be performed, is generally well respected by states and the legislature. When a patient is treated or partially treated and subsequently demands release, however, the decision regarding course of care or discharge is primarily a medical one. Few legal precedents or clear guidelines exist to aid in this decision. The staff's plan regarding further treatment must be based on a comprehensive medical assessment.

In the scenario presented, the staff must evaluate the patient in light of all of the available information. Although the patient is oriented and apparently has capacity after the administration of naloxone, the physician has information (the patient's own admission of heroin use) to suggest that he will most probably return to his prior comatose state with grave respiratory compromise. Sound practice would dictate that the hospital and medical team have a duty to prevent such an individual from leaving the emergency department if the duration of the effect of the toxin is longer than that expected of the antidote [15]. In this case, if the patient is permitted to leave, his health and even his life are placed at significant risk. It is the physician's duty to avert this situation when possible and retain the patient until medically cleared. Clear and concise documentation in the chart of therapy and clinical concern reduces liability further.

When approaching this patient, the physician ought to have some idea of his or her expectations of the situation. Given knowledge of the toxicokinetics of the toxin and pharmacokinetics of the antidote involved in this particular presentation, one can reasonably expect that beyond 1 hour, if the patient remains awake and alert, there is no toxicologic or pharmacologic reason for detaining him. If instead he becomes sedated again, predicting the clinical course becomes difficult. There is no assurance, other than the patient's history, which has proven time and again to be greatly unreliable, that the toxin truly is heroin and not some longer acting opioid, such as methadone. If this were the case, the patient likely would remain sedated for a long enough time to warrant admission and observation. Before clearance for discharge, the physician is compelled to examine the patient fully; one must carefully assess for fever in a patient with a cardiac murmur and a similar history because the clinical course and admission criteria change greatly when the possibility of bacterial endocarditis is entertained. One must watch for signs of acute lung injury and assess for suicide risk. In a patient with this presentation, it is difficult to know that the initial presentation was an unintentional overdose as opposed to an intentional overdose. Sound risk management principles dictate further observation and likely intervention to avoid the potential claims of negligence in an instance of premature release. The physician must initiate a brief substance abuse intervention to begin the discussion of drug risk assessment and therapy.

The use of longer acting reversal agents has been suggested (eg, nalmefene, half-life 2–4 hours after parenteral administration) as an alternative to the short half-life of naloxone. Because of the lack of reliable information on the ingestant and its potential duration of clinical effect, this is not recommended as an acceptable alternative. This approach is simply likely to produce a combative patient in opioid withdrawal who is just as difficult to manage as after naloxone use, but whose distress persists for a longer period.

Case three: confidentiality

> A fellow staff physician is brought to the emergency department on a Monday morning at 4 A.M. by a friend. According to the friend, your colleague had been at a party, was drinking, and had fallen and hit his head. He is grossly intoxicated, with slurred speech and acting belligerently, and he has a laceration above his left eyebrow. As he is being helped onto a stretcher, the friend disappears, and four packets of white powder are noted by you and the charge nurse to fall out of your colleague's jacket pocket. The nurse is insistent that the police department be called to investigate. Your initial inclination is to take the packets and stuff them into the sharps container.

From an ethical standpoint, this encounter presents several challenging dilemmas. What is a physician's responsibility to a patient? Are physicians violating a patient's confidentiality by reporting him or her to the police? How does this impact on the patient-physician bond of trust implicit in the care afforded patients? Would the decision differ if the physician knew that the packets were for individual use or that they were to be dispensed for monetary reimbursement at the party? Should the physician consider reporting the colleague's visit to the department Chair? Does the Health

Insurance Portability and Accountability Act (HIPAA) impact on decision making?

The physician is responsible for treating the patient's medical problems, suturing his laceration, and evaluating him for potentially serious head trauma and associated injuries. It is imperative that the physician obtain an accurate history from the patient as he becomes more alert and cooperative. Is the physician responsible for protecting the patient from the ramifications of having drugs found on his person in a hospital setting? Is the physician doing him a favor, or may this ultimately cause him harm?

The Code of Ethics of the American College of Emergency Physicians states that "emergency physicians shall respect patient privacy and disclose confidential information only with consent of the patient or when required by an overriding duty such as the duty to protect others or to obey the law" [16]. It also mandates that physicians "deal fairly and honestly with colleagues and take appropriate action to protect patients from health care providers who are impaired" [16]. Both of these guidelines pertain to the physician's relationship with this particular patient. Does the physician have an overriding duty to report this patient to law enforcement officers or to a state medical society to protect others?

With regard to the drug packets, had a single packet been found on the colleague, the physician's responsibility to maintain the patient's confidentiality could be considered appropriate because one could assume that the packet was intended for his individual use. The precept of autonomy might apply. Because multiple packets were found, however, could one assume that these were not only for his use, but also were potentially for sale to others? Does complicity at this point endanger others?

The physician's first responsibility is to the health and stabilization of the patient who has entrusted himself or herself to the physician's care. The emergency department physician's primary role is in caring for the patient. When physicians take the oath of Hippocrates, they pledge not only to practice the art of medicine, but also to protect confidentiality "What I may see or hear in the course of treatment..., which on no account one must spread abroad, I will keep to myself, holding such things shameful to be spoken about" [17].

Beyond medical stabilization and immediate health risks, the waters muddy a bit. On one hand, as is touched on by the initial inclination in the scenario to stuff the packets of white powder into the sharps container, the physician's obligation lies in protecting the patient. By taking this path of action, the physician is putting an end to the potential illicit drug use aspect of the episode, clearly indicating disapproval and preventing further (immediate) harm. In doing so, the physician is not violating the patient's trust by involving the law or other authorities (although the argument could be and has been made that some trust would be broken by disposing of a potentially valued possession). The physician also has an opportunity, obligation even, for a primary intervention. The emergency department provides a frontline opportunity for counseling patients about drug use, related behavior, and possible implications, while also availing physicians with resources to make referrals for treatment. Even a brief intervention in the emergency department has been shown to decrease alcohol consumption and problem drinking in a vulnerable patient population. It is possible that these interventions and their benefits also would extend to other at-risk populations [12,13].

The involvement of the police department as being the alternative to disposing of the white powder privately can be quite problematic. This is where breach of trust and violation of the physician-patient relationship rears its head. Some have put forth that this type of betrayal ultimately would discourage individuals from seeking necessary medical attention for fear of being arrested or reported. To the authors' knowledge, no studies have been done showing this effect.

The physician is clearly violating the patient's confidentiality by reporting him to the police, but there are times and circumstances when this is deemed not only acceptable, but even morally indicated. The real sticking point in this particular scenario is whether or not it is morally justifiable. For some, the issue changes with the patient's intent: single packet intended for personal consumption might raise issues of personal judgment and impairment, but the scope of the issue and the potential for harm widen dramatically with multiple packets and intent to distribute drugs. Some would argue that in weighing a patient's trust and confidence, the decision falls in favor of the patient in the first instance, but swings toward defense of greater good in the latter scenario.

Arguments supporting an ostensible violation of the physician-patient confidence are usually staunch in their defense of greater good. It is a utilitarian stand: the greatest good for the greatest number, allowing for isolated violation of a single human interaction. Defenders of the sanctity of the physician-patient relationship fear that the implications and repercussions of this breach lead inevitably to a deeper mistrust and ultimately discourage people from seeking care at all.

Physicians are human beings first, each with his or her own strengths and weaknesses. Treating physicians must not apply unrealistic expectations to colleagues and must realize that everyone is subject to life's myriad stresses. It is imperative that physicians maintain confidentiality and trust to the best of their ability. It must be ensured that physicians feel comfortable seeking the help they need without the fear of punitive measures being taken against them. Otherwise, one runs the risk of increasing despair and feelings of isolation and helplessness of physicians in need, possibly contributing to the increased risk of suicide among physicians [18].

That being stated, in the above-described scenario, one is confronted with a fellow physician who is entrusted with the care of others. It is the physician's responsibility to ensure that his or her colleague receives the help he needs so that he is able to continue to serve his patients safely. Physicians do not serve primarily as law enforcement, and it is vital to maintain a separation between legal and ethical responsibilities. A possible rational, ethical approach to this scenario would be to confiscate the patient's drug supply, notify the hospital security system, and have them, in association with the supervisor on duty, place the material in a secure location. The hospital pharmacy potentially could dispose of the material, or law enforcement officials could be notified to take possession of it with no disclosure from whom the material was obtained.

Would the approach to this patient be different if he were a body packer, a person using his body to smuggle large quantities of illicit drugs into the United States? Although it is difficult to state what amount of drug could precipitate the breach of physician-patient confidentiality, some might argue that this trust could be violated on behalf of a greater good. Others might opine that a body packer is no different from any other patient seeking care, and that the physician would be remiss for involving law enforcement officials [19].

All of these debates and concerns for confidentiality now occur in the face of federal health privacy regulations that took effect in April 2003 under HIPAA. Many misconceptions have arisen regarding the focus and scope of these regulations, and many physicians have expressed concern regarding the presumed limitations imposed, perhaps because the regulations are complex and carry civil and criminal penalties for violations. As was noted in a review on HIPAA, "it makes little ethical or clinical sense to give absolute priority to maintaining the patient's confidentiality if that jeopardizes patient care" [20]. The authors' position is clear with regard to responsibility as physicians:

> Ethically, overriding confidentiality to prevent harms to third parties is warranted when several criteria are met: the potential harm to identifiable third parties is serious and likely (necessity), the breach of confidentiality allows effective steps to prevent harm (effectiveness), there is no less restrictive alternative for protecting those at risk, disclosure is limited to what is essential to avert harm, harms to the patient are minimized and acceptable (proportionality), and policies are justified publicly (transparency) [20].

Although it is stipulated in case three that the physician has no legal duty to report the colleague's behavior, it is the physician's ethical responsibility to obtain counseling and assistance for him, not only to offer him a means to save his career, his interpersonal relationships, and perhaps his life, but also to protect his patients from the consequences of his illness. To physicians with substance abuse, the State of New York Medical Society offers confidential, nondisciplinary individualized counseling to assist in physician recovery [21]. The referral process may be initiated by a treating physician confidentially, and if deemed clinically necessary, the physician in need is enrolled in a multidisciplinary treatment program that remains confidential. As long as the physician cooperates with and is being helped by the program and has been able to care for his or her patients, the physician is not referred to the New York State Department of Health's Office of Professional Medical Conduct, which is the disciplinary office for physicians in the state. In an attempt to ensure physician-patient confidential medical care, the Joint Commission on Accreditation of Healthcare Organizations adopted a standard (MS 2.6) requiring that physician health and disciplinary actions be handled separately.

If the scenario is changed from a fellow off-duty physician to a pilot or a bus driver, how do the physician's obligations or duties change? If the physician is concerned that the patient's actions endanger the lives and welfare of others, does that impress on the physician a greater obligation? In that case, must the physician report to a higher authority, or does the autonomy and privacy of the patient still retain maximal influence over the physician's actions?

As far as the authors are aware, no legal precedent exists that broadly addresses this particular situation. The argument has been made that it is the state, not the physician, which has the primary responsibility for traffic safety (it is assumed that this would include air traffic as well because the two situations are greatly analogous).

> The American Society of Addiction Medicine stresses the societal stigma affecting persons with substance related disorders and the critical importance of confidentiality in their treatment. It takes the position that "any reporting to authorities should be reserved only for those unusual situations in which the substance dependent patient is considered ... to pose an immediate threat to public safety," as in the case of "acute incapacitation by substances" [22].

It is the opinion of the authors, however, that this behavior, when involving a pilot, a bus driver, or another individual directly in a situation responsible for the care of others, does constitute an immediate threat to public safety, and that the circumstances also likely fall under the delineation of "unusual." The authors' recommendation in this instance in which there is also a potentially significant risk to public safety and greater good is to report the patient to a supervising authority. Ultimately the patient needs crucial social and psychological assessments and interventions. To wait until a catastrophe ensues would be morally and ethically inexcusable.

Summary

The issues raised in these scenarios and hypothetical modifications are complex yet real—they arise regularly in emergency departments across the United States [23]. Emergency physicians often have little training and few precedents for addressing these concerns. Emergency physicians must make these decisions, however, with the same incisive precision necessary to practice any other aspect of emergency medicine; these decisions have a great impact on the future of patients and likely the lives of individuals touched by them.

Each ethical dilemma is unique just as each patient brings nuances and new perspectives to old problems. There are no hard and fast rules, and often physicians are faced with difficult choices and ambiguities. The authors hope that they have created a framework within which to address some of the ethical questions that arise when toxicologic emergencies occur in the day-to-day practice of emergency medicine. Above all else, emergency physicians must retain their humanity and use this expanding medical humanism as a guide to decision making and to bettering themselves as physicians.

References

[1] Peabody F. The care of the patient. JAMA 1927;88:877.
[2] Furrow BR, Greaney TL, Johnson SH, et al. An introduction to the study of ethics and ethical theories. In: Bioethics: healthcare law and ethics. 5th edition. Minneapolis: Thomson West; 2004. p. 1–30.
[3] Mokdad AH, Marks JS, Stroup DF, et al. Actual causes of death in the United States. JAMA 2004;291:1328–45.
[4] Harwood HJ. Updating estimates of the economic costs of alcohol abuse in the United States: estimates, update methods, and data. Bethesda (MD): National Institute on Alcohol Abuse and Alcoholism; 2000.
[5] MacKenzie TD, Bartecchi CE, Schrier RW. The human costs of tobacco use. N Engl J Med 1994;330:975–80.
[6] Hoffman RS, Goldfrank LR. The impact of drug abuse and addiction on society. Emerg Med Clin N Am 1990;8:467–79.
[7] Goldfrank LR. Emergency medicine and medical toxicology: past, present and future: a very personal overview. Keynote address. Isr J Emerg Med 2005;5:10–5.
[8] Thornquist L, Biros M, Olander R, et al. Health care utilization of chronic inebriates. Acad Emerg Med 2002;9:300–8.
[9] Furrow BR, Greaney TL, Johnson SH, et al. Life and death decisions. In: Bioethics: health-care law and ethics. 5th edition. Minneapolis: Thomson West; 2004. p. 238–407.
[10] O'Connor PG, Schottenfeld RS. Patients with alcohol problems. N Engl J Med 1998;338: 592–601.
[11] D'Onofrio G. Treatment for alcohol and other drug problems. Ann Emerg Med 2003;41: 814–7.
[12] Bernstein E, Bernstein J, Leverson S. Project ASSERT: an ED-based intervention to increase access to primary care, preventive services, and substance abuse treatment system. Ann Emerg Med 1997;30:181–9.
[13] Fleming MF, Mundt MP, French MT, et al. Benefit-cost analysis of brief physician advice with problem drinkers in primary care settings. Med Care 2000;38:7–18.
[14] Seeman MV. Relational ethics: when mothers suffer from psychosis. Arch Womens Ment Health 2004;7:201–10.
[15] Kirrane BM, Drukteinis DA. Risk management and legal principles. In: Flomenbaum NE, Hoffman RS, Goldfrank LR, et al, editors. Goldfrank's toxicologic emergencies. 8th edition. New York: McGraw-Hill; 2006. p. 1879–85.
[16] American College of Emergency Physicians (ACEP). Code of ethics for emergency physicians. Ann Emerg Med 2004;43:686–94.
[17] Beauchamp TL, Childress JF. Principles of biomedical ethics. 3rd edition. New York: Oxford University Press; 1989. p. 329–34.

[18] Schernhammer E. Taking their own lives—the high rate of physician suicide. N Engl J Med 2005;352:2473–6.
[19] Traub SJ, Hoffman RS, Nelson LS. Body packing—the internal concealment of illicit drugs. N Engl J Med 2003;349:2519–26.
[20] Lo B, Dornbrand L, Dubler NN. HIPAA and patient care: the role for professional judgment. JAMA 2005;293:1766–71.
[21] Medical Society for the State of New York. Committee for Physicians' Health 2005; (February):7. Available at: http://www.mssny.org/index.htm. Accessed June 20, 2006.
[22] Leeman CP, Cohen MA, Parkas V. Should a psychiatrist report a bus driver's alcohol and drug abuse? An ethical dilemma. Gen Hosp Psychiatry 2001;23:333–6.
[23] Simon JR, Dwyer J, Goldfrank LR. Ethical issues in emergency medicine: the difficult patient. Emerg Med Clin N Am 1999;17:353–70.

ELSEVIER
SAUNDERS

Emerg Med Clin N Am
24 (2006) 785–795

EMERGENCY
MEDICINE
CLINICS OF
NORTH AMERICA

Lifelong Learning

Jon W. Schrock, MD*, Rita K. Cydulka, MD, MS

Department of Emergency Medicine, MetroHealth Medical Center,
2500 MetroHealth Drive, Cleveland, OH 44109-1998, USA

Medical progress before the twentieth century could be measured in small but important discoveries. This last century has brought an unprecedented advancement in medical knowledge with a never before seen growth in the breadth of science that forms the foundation of our understanding of medicine. The number of medical clinical trials rose from 500 annually in the 1970s to more than 10,000 in the late 1990s [1]. The amount of funding appropriated for research for the National Institutes of Health (NIH) was $300 in 1887 and reached $23.4 billion for 2002 alone [2]. This is in addition to the $32 billion spent on research by private pharmaceutical firms [3].

The allocation of science has since surpassed the human capacity to completely master it. Medical faculty, residents, and students at university and training institutions, with access to multiple specialists, researchers, and instructors, are in the optimal position to learn and use this new information in their clinic practice. In reality, most practicing clinicians do not practice in an environment that allows them to easily stay abreast of the rapid changes in medical practice. These clinicians may unknowingly practice in a manner that does not offer their patients the best possible medical care.

In the current practice environment, in which clinical, administrative, educational, and family and personal duties all compete for physicians' time, it is often difficult to continue active learning. While a number of studies have evaluated time needed to develop procedural competence, research (and research methodology) to evaluate the amount of time and the methods required for a physician to maintain overall clinical competence is lacking. This leaves the clinician with little guidance in how to maintain competence throughout a career.

While most specialists and specialty societies recognize the importance of ongoing education, including literature appraisal, many physicians lack

---

* Corresponding author. Department of Emergency Medicine, MetroHealth Medical Center, 2500 MetroHealth Drive, Cleveland, OH 44109-1998.

E-mail address: jschrock@metrohealth.org (J.W. Schrock).

doi:10.1016/j.emc.2006.05.012
emed.theclinics.com

both the time and skill set to critically assess new developments. This rapid proliferation of new medical information, coupled with the lack of time to review it all has led to the creation of commercial enterprises such as "*Journal Watch*," *Emergency Medical Abstracts*, and *American Health Consultants* that assist physicians in reviewing pertinent developments in their field.

What duty is bound of practitioners to continue to expand their medical knowledge with ongoing scientific advances? Most state medical boards require physicians to perform and document appropriate educational endeavors to maintain their medical license. The original physician covenant, the Oath of Hippocrates, addresses the teaching of medicine to willing pupils: "*I will regard his sons as my brothers and teach them the science, if they desire to learn it, without fee or contract. I will hand on precepts, lectures, and all other learning to my sons, to those of my master, and to those pupils duly apprenticed and sworn, and to none other"* [4]. There is no mention of furthering one's education for the good of the patient. Despite this, the altruistic manner of the oath implies a level of self-improvement that submits the physician to continued learning.

The directive of the physician "first, do no harm," implies ongoing learning as it may be difficult to "do no harm" if one is unaware of harm that outdated therapies may have caused. Society has come to expect this and holds physicians both legally and financially responsible for errors that result in injury and are felt to be below the community's standard of care. This places both ethical and financial motivations onto physicians to continue lifelong learning.

Standards of care change based on new research and recently developed therapeutic regimens. These advances in knowledge often leave our patients, and occasionally our physicians, confused. As the amount and quality of medical research increase, ideally, our clinical practice should incorporate that knowledge into our daily medical practice. Standard medical practices considered dogma for decades are questioned and at times, abandoned for therapies that have been proven to be safer with more extensive investigation. Cardiac drugs provide an example of rapidly advancing and evolving paradigms. Drugs once used for patients with cardiac arrhythmias were found to lead to more arrhythmias and higher mortality [5,6] and beta-blockers once taught to be contraindicated in congestive heart failure were found to offer significant benefits in survival [7]. Advances in technology also offered improvements in care unimaginable to physicians not exposed. For example, current technologies presently available might have seemed more like science fiction a few decades ago. Treatment options, such as ablation therapy for patients with uncontrolled atrial fibrillation or deep brain stimulators for patients with Parkinson's disease, are offered to patients only if the clinician is aware of them.

Therein lies the importance of lifelong learning. To be able to provide the best medical care possible, the clinician must be fully aware of all facets of the disease, including the most current. Offering dated medical care results in substandard care and may produce other undesirable consequences such as producing poor outcomes and increasing a practitioner's exposure to medical liability.

Development of medical education and board certification

Early twentieth century medical education offered little consistency in the quality of students, instructors, and clinical training [8,9]. Medical schools could be found in rural and urban centers in most every state. Their curriculum was not regulated, leading to wide variations in quality among schools. As American physicians sought additional training in Europe and obtained exposure to European systems of medical education, deficiencies in American medical education became much more pronounced. In the early part of the twentieth century, the American Medical Association asked the Carnegie Foundation for the Advancement of Teaching to evaluate medical education in the United States [10].

In 1908, the commission called upon Abraham Flexner to examine the American system of medical education and provide recommendations for improvement. Flexner was a Kentucky-born educator who spent 19 years as a secondary educator after which he completed graduate courses in education at Harvard College and the University of Berlin. At the request of the Carnegie Foundation, he spent 2 years visiting every medical school in the United States to determine ways to improve on America's medical education system. His report, *Medical Education in the United States and Canada*, completed in 1910, became a beacon for reform and was instrumental in developing the current system of modern medical education [11].

The Flexner Report, as it came to be called, pointed toward a number of problems concerning medical education and the practice of medicine, and issued a number of recommendations. He noted that the recent rush to create new American medical schools resulted in an overabundance of physicians with substandard training [11]. A large number of medical schools lacked adequate financial backing because of a lack of support from the university or because of a lack of university affiliation [11]. This meant that educational programs, such as laboratory work, were absent, leaving medical students to learn through bookwork and didactic lectures. In addition, many rural medical schools were located too far from hospitals to provide clinical experience for their students. Thus, it was not uncommon for a new physician to have never treated an ill patient until after graduating and in practice.

Recommendations issued by the Flexner Report included bedside clinical instruction through direct observation of patients, integration of research as a distinctive part of each medical school's mission, and a requirement of postsecondary education before admission. The medical community saw Flexner's report as a mea culpa, resulting in wide changes in medical education culminating in what would become the modern medical education system. The inclusion of medical education into universities led to a substantial reduction in the total number of institutions offering degrees in medicine with the closing of many of the smaller inadequately funded institutions.

The progression of the basic sciences, medical technological advances, and a larger number of physicians in urban settings through the twentieth century, allowed physicians to begin to specialize in distinct areas of medicine. Specialty societies were formed to promote scholarship and allow specialists to advance their agendas.

In 1916, the American Board of Ophthalmic Examinations was founded and offered its first board certification examination the following year. Eight years later, The American Board of Otolaryngology, the American Board of Obstetrics and Gynecology, and the American Board of Dermatology were founded. In 1933, the American Board of Medical Specialties (ABMS) was formed to perform, among other actions, "To act in an advisory capacity to these boards," and "To stimulate improvement in postgraduate medical education." Over the next 15 years, other specialties quickly developed their own representative boards. In September 1979, 63 years after the first specialty board was founded, the American Board of Emergency Medicine (ABEM) became the 23rd certification board recognized by the ABMS. ABEM offered its first emergency medicine certification examination in 1980 and certified its first diplomates in that year. Today, the ABMS is composed of 24 boards, with the American Board of Medical Genetics being the most recent member joining in 1991.

During the latter half of the twentieth century, most medical specialty boards required physicians to pass a certification examination to obtain diplomate status. Although the issue of recertification was raised by the ABMS as early as 1936, the first recertification examinations were not introduced until 1969. Over time, the ABMS came to understand that the progression of science and medicine would render the knowledge and skills measured during initial certification exams outdated over time. Despite endorsement by the ABMS, it was not until 2000 that all member boards stipulated a compulsory recertification examination to maintain status as a diplomate. Unlike most other specialties, the American Board of Emergency Medicine has always required diplomates to take a recertification examination every 10 years to remain "board certified."

The ABMS heralded a new era in ongoing medical education and certification in March, 2000, when it began the mandate of continuous certification and ongoing periodic testing to maintain certification. Additionally, requirements for evidence of lifelong learning, unrestricted professional standing, and assessment of clinical practice will be needed for physicians to continue as diplomates.

Ongoing education

The initial formalized requirement for continuing medical education (CME) began in 1934 with a mandate from the American Board of Urology as a way to augment specialist education of scientific advances [12]. At present, CME remains the principal method that practicing physicians continue their education outside of a university setting [13]. In the 1960s, the American Medical Association (AMA) created an honorary certificate that was available to physicians willing to complete 150 hours of voluntary continuing medical education [12]. Currently, 56 of 68 state and territorial licensing boards require completion of CME for recertification of their medical licenses, including all allopathic and osteopathic licensure boards in the United States and US territories.

As CME became the accepted standard for physician education after formal training, the number of institutions mandating participation grew. Companies, professional organizations, and hospital medical staff boards joined state boards in requiring that physicians complete these educational activities to maintain standing within their institution. Recent reports show physicians report spending approximately 50 hours per year in CME-related activities that are intended to improve their clinical performance [14–16]. In 2003, 2.3 million nonphysician health care providers and over 5.0 million physicians participated in some form of CME activity at a total cost of more than $1.77 billion [13].

Today CME is commercially oriented with a number of companies, known as Medical Education Services Suppliers (MESSs), acting as intermediaries. MESSs are contracted by pharmaceutical and medical organizations to arrange and perform physician educational experiences, usually in the form of grand rounds, symposiums, or publication-related activities [17]. Concern has been raised that MESSs are used by the pharmaceutical industry to give the appearance of an objective educational endeavor while the presentations may actually be biased and endorse industry products [17]. Another issue is that the cost of providing pharmaceutical industry–sponsored education results in greater expenses passed on to the general public [18,19].

Despite being used for decades as the major venue for physician education, there is little evidence that participation in CME improves patient care or outcomes [20,21]. Patel and colleagues [22] recently reported little association between patient outcome and participation in state-mandated CME when comparing the care of acute myocardial infarction in states that mandated CME with care in states that did not mandate CME [22]. Outcome measures included aspirin use, reperfusion therapy, smoking cessation programs, discharge prescriptions for aspirin and beta-blockers, and 30-day and 1-year mortality. The only therapy significantly increased in states with mandated CME was the use of thrombolytic therapy. A 1995 meta-analysis of 99 trials concluded that didactic lectures and conferences had little to no impact on changing physician practice or altering outcomes. Other forms of CME, such as reminders, outreach visits, opinion leaders, multifaceted activities, and patient-mediated interventions, have been demonstrated to alter outcomes and improve patient care [21,23–25]. Unfortunately, these more effective forms of education are the minority of CME offered.

Unfortunately, the majority of CME consists of didactics that allow for a passive form of learning and does not seem to fit the method in which most adults actively learn, ie, learner-centered and active educational programs. Other factors that may diminish the utility of CME include the physician's level of interest, prior education, and educational background in the area being taught. The mere perception of lack of clinical value of the information being taught can decrease the learner's motivation and become a barrier to change.

The impetus to change

In 1996, the Institute of Medicine (IOM) began focusing on problems ranging from education of health care personnel to health care delivery. The initial report, *To Err is Human: Building a Safer Health System*, uncovered a flawed system in which medical errors result in 44,000 patient deaths per year [26]. In this report, the authors defined the results of problems with our medical delivery system and outlined steps to build a culture of safety. Suggestions included voluntary and mandatory reporting of errors in a risk-free environment to allow for analysis and correction of these errors. While the majority of this report concentrated on patient safety issues, the initial framework for a continuous education requirement was also set in place.

[1]For most health professionals, current methods of licensing and credentialing assess knowledge, but do not assess performance skills after initial licensure. Although the state grants initial licensure, responsibility for documenting continued competence is dispersed. Competence may be considered when a licensing board reacts to a complaint. It may be evaluated when an individual applies to a health care organization for privileges or network contracting or employment. Professional certification is the current process for evaluating clinical knowledge after licensure and some programs are now starting to consider assessment of clinical skills in addition to clinical knowledge. Given the rapid pace of change in health care and the constant development of new technologies and information, existing licensing and accreditation processes should be strengthened to ensure that all health care professionals are assessed periodically on both skills and knowledge for practice [26].

In response to this IOM report, the ABMS voted to adopt a change in their recertification process for their member Boards. The new program, Maintenance of Certification, requires continuous certification, rather than episodic certification, and includes the following four components: professional standing, lifelong learning, evidence of cognitive expertise, and evaluation of performance in practice.

---

[1] *From* Kohn LT, Corrigan J, Donaldson MS. To err is human: building a safer health system. Washington, DC: National Academy Press; 2000; with permission.

This change in the certification process has already started for clinicians who wish to maintain board certification in emergency medicine. Beginning in 2004, all ABEM diplomates who intend to maintain certification past the expiration date on their current certificate must participate in such a program [27]. To comply with the lifelong learning portion of ABEM's Maintenance of Certification program, Emergency Medicine Continuous Certification program (EMCC), diplomates must complete eight lifelong learning and self-assessment modules over a 10-year period. These modules consist of approximately 20 reading references that cover content from the Model of Clinical Practice of Emergency Medicine followed by an online examination [28]. Each online exam will be available for a total of 3 years. Evidence of cognitive expertise is demonstrated by successful completion of a secure, closed book, computerized examination (Continuous Certification [ConCert]) once every 10 years. Presently, ABEM is developing the assessment practice performance component required by ABMS. These developments help promote the ongoing competence in the six core competencies.

The addition of an ongoing learning requirement by ABMS is expected to enhance the value of board certification. Time and research will be needed to ensure that these changes are producing the outcomes, including improvement in patient safety, error reduction, and modernization of practice, which the IOM recommended in their initial report in 2000.

The second published report in this series, *Crossing the Quality Chasm: A New Health System for the 21st Century*, recommended six national quality aims: safety, effectiveness, patient-centeredness, timeliness, efficiency, and equity as areas to measure future achievements. Education of health care professionals was noted as an area for reform needed to improve quality [29]. As a result of recommendations from *Crossing the Quality Chasm*, a health professions education summit to develop strategies for improving clinical education in all facets of medical education was held in the summer of 2002. The results of their recommendations were published the following year as *Health Professions Education: A Bridge to Quality*. This publication reviews the problems with educational systems for health professionals and offers focused recommendations for institutions. The IOM recommended proficiency in patient-centered care, interdisciplinary teams, evidence-based practice, quality improvement, and informatics [30]. Also included in the recommendations was a call to focus on a core set of competencies. These six competencies, advocated by the American Council for Graduate Medical Education (ACGME), consist of patient care, medical knowledge, practice-based learning and improvement, interpersonal and communication skills, professionalism, and practice. More recently, the Association of American Medical Colleges (AAMC) and the ABMS, representing the medical education oversight organizations that span a medical career from beginning to end, have adopted the original six core competencies [31].

Future directions

As society develops a better understanding of the importance of continuous education in the performance of medical professionals and the safety
of patients, more research is being produced to address these issues. Certain
obvious issues, such as lack of motivation, time, and adequate resources,
can interfere with an individual's success as an independent adult learner.
In addition, more subtle problems, such as a lack of awareness of knowledge
deficit, personal reluctance to change, ambivalence, and group mentality,
can also be significant barriers to positive educational change [32].

Most American medical students face obstacles toward lifelong learning
before they even enter medical school as the American educational culture
often promotes passive, rather than active, learning [33]. In fact, Wilcox reported that only 13% of college professors responding to a survey were supportive of self-directed learning [34]. Thus, the majority of medical students
in their preclinical years learn through the same lecture didactic format used
in undergraduate coursework. Hopefully, individual learning experiences
and support should improve as the AAMC integrates the six core competencies into medical education.

Advances in adult education and memory may provide insights into the
methods we use to educate physicians. Age can adversely affect controlled
components of memory such as actual recall impairing the ability to remember theory or design. This tends to follow predictable age-related decline
[35,36]. Conversely, other aspects of memory such as habitual tasks, vocabulary, and low-effort recall, such as remembering people in a picture, tend to
be least affected by aging [37,38]. This knowledge may be used in future aspects of physician education to provide age-appropriate curriculum.

In Great Britain, where Post-Graduate Education Allowance, the British
version of CME, is usually obtained through didactic lectures similar to the
United States, alternate avenues for postgraduate education, including
Personal Education Plans (PEPs), have been developed [39]. In PEPS,
a practitioner works with a tutor to assess educational needs and together
they develop an educational plan. The intellectual gaps named by the tutor
are largely determined by personal impression. Educational methods used to
correct knowledge and practice gaps include personal reading, practical
sessions, and coursework. Although this educational method is used by
a small fraction of the practicing physicians, it appears to gain high marks
for satisfaction [40,41]. Presently, no data are available to compare the efficacy of this new learning modality to conventional CME.

Recent attempts have been made to measure physician lifelong learning through psychometric analysis [42,43]. The factors believed to be major
features of lifelong learning include need recognition, research endeavor,
self-initiation, technical skills, and personal motivation [44]. As the operational tool has only been used in a single small study, further research is needed
to determine its reliability over time and utility with nonacademic physicians.

Technological advances, such as the computers, the Internet, and video streaming, already play a part in physician education and can be expected to grow [45]. Currently patient simulators are being used to train physicians in a variety of procedures. These include a virtual reality Pediatric Advanced Life Support (PALS) course using a "mannequin" that has a pulse, respirations, and electrical heartbeat that change in real time during training [46]. Virtual endoscopic surgery has been developed for general surgeons and gynecologists to practice in a risk-free environment [47,48]. This technology has also been extended to ocular surgery [49]. The number of physicians participating in Internet-based CME increased over 600% from 1998 to 2003 and the number of CME activities presented on the Internet has risen over 800% in the same time period. Live Internet CME activities continue to be the minority with only 275 programs in 2003. Given the ease and convenience of participating in online CME these figures are not surprising and will increase in the foreseeable future. The challenge will be to make quality physician education more available while containing cost, avoiding bias and commercial influence, and ensuring that what physicians are learning produce results in improved patient care and outcomes.

The expectation of physicians to continue their education past formal schooling has traversed from nonexistent to a requirement for all specialists expecting to maintain Board certification. This challenge is especially daunting in emergency medicine where the breadth of knowledge is vast and physicians must stay current on a wide variety of subjects, each advancing at his or her own rapid pace. Lifelong learning is a vital skill for any physician who wishes to provide current, competent, and safe medical care to his or her patients. With advancements in technology and understanding of adults as lifelong learners, more capable teaching methods are being developed. While it remains to be seen if these changes improve upon the traditional forms of CME, and actually improve patient outcome and safety, there is no escaping that the future is here.

References

[1] Chassin MR, Galvin RW. The urgent need to improve health care quality. Institute of Medicine National Roundtable on Health Care Quality. JAMA 1998;280(11):1000–5.
[2] National Institutes of Health. National Institutes of Health: An Overview. Available at: http://www.nih.gov/about/NIHoverview.html. Accessed May 17, 2004.
[3] Pharmaceutical Research and Manufacturers of America. Annual report 2004. Available at: http://www.phrma.org/publications/publications//2003-11-2-.870.pdf. Accessed Dec 14, 2004.
[4] Chadwick J, Mann WN. Hippocratic writings. Penguin Books, London, 1950.
[5] Preliminary report: effect of encainide and flecainide on mortality in a randomized trial of arrhythmia suppression after myocardial infarction. The Cardiac Arrhythmia Suppression Trial (CAST) Investigators. N Engl J Med 1989;321(6):406–12.
[6] Effect of the antiarrhythmic agent moricizine on survival after myocardial infarction. The Cardiac Arrhythmia Suppression Trial II Investigators. N Engl J Med 1992;327(4):227–33.

[7] Packer M, Coats AJ, Fowler MB, et al. Effect of carvedilol on survival in severe chronic heart failure. N Engl J Med 2001;344(22):1651–8.

[8] Bigelow HJ. Medical education in America: being the annual address read before the Massachusetts medical society. Cambridge: Welch, Bigelow, and Company; 1871.

[9] Welch WH, Burket WC. Papers and addresses. Baltimore: Johns Hopkins Press; 1920.

[10] Karabulut H, Toraman F, Evrenkaya S, et al. Clopidogrel does not increase bleeding and allogenic blood transfusion in coronary artery surgery. Eur J Cardiothorac Surg 2004; 25(3):419–23.

[11] Flexner A. Medical education in the United States and Canada. From the Carnegie Foundation for the Advancement of Teaching, Bulletin Number Four, 1910. Bull World Health Organ 2002;80(7):594–602.

[12] Josseran L, Chaperon J. [History of continuing medical education in the United States]. Presse Med 2001;30(10):493–7 [in French].

[13] (ACCME) ACfCME. ACCME Annual Report Data. Chicago: 2004:1–12.

[14] Difford F, Hughes RC. General practitioners' attendance at courses accredited for the postgraduate education allowance. Br J Gen Pract 1992;42(360):290–3.

[15] Goulet F, Gagnon RJ, Desrosiers G, et al. Participation in CME activities. Can Fam Physician 1998;44:541–8.

[16] Curry L. Learning preferences and continuing medical education. Can Med Assoc J 1981; 124(5):535–6.

[17] Ross JS, Lurie P, Wolfe SM. Health Research Group Report: Medical education service suppliers: a threat to physician education. Available at: http://www.citizen.org/publications/release.cfm?ID=7142. Accessed July 19, 2004.

[18] Relman AS. Separating continuing medical education from pharmaceutical marketing. JAMA 2001;285(15):2009–12.

[19] Drug-company influence on medical education in USA. Lancet 2000;356(9232):781.

[20] Davis DA, Taylor-Vaisey A. Translating guidelines into practice. A systematic review of theoretic concepts, practical experience and research evidence in the adoption of clinical practice guidelines. CMAJ 1997;157(4):408–16.

[21] Grimshaw JM, Russell IT. Effect of clinical guidelines on medical practice: a systematic review of rigorous evaluations. Lancet 1993;342(8883):1317–22.

[22] Patel MR, Meine TJ, Radeva J, et al. State-mandated continuing medical education and the use of proven therapies in patients with an acute myocardial infarction. J Am Coll Cardiol 2004;44(1):192–8.

[23] Davis DA, Thomson MA, Oxman AD, et al. Changing physician performance. A systematic review of the effect of continuing medical education strategies. JAMA 1995;274(9):700–5.

[24] Davis D, O'Brien MA, Freemantle N, et al. Impact of formal continuing medical education: do conferences, workshops, rounds, and other traditional continuing education activities change physician behavior or health care outcomes? JAMA 1999;282(9):867–74.

[25] Lau J, Antman EM, Jimenez-Silva J, et al. Cumulative meta-analysis of therapeutic trials for myocardial infarction. N Engl J Med 1992;327(4):248–54.

[26] Kohn LT, Corrigan J, Donaldson MS. To err is human: building a safer health system. Washington, DC: National Academy Press; 2000.

[27] McCabe JB. Emergency medicine continuous certification: why, why now, why me? Ann Emerg Med 2002;40(3):342–6.

[28] Hockberger RS, Binder LS, Graber MA, et al. The model of the clinical practice of emergency medicine. Ann Emerg Med 2001;37(6):745–70.

[29] Institute of Medicine (US). Committee on Quality of Health Care in America. Crossing the quality chasm: a new health system for the 21st century. Washington, DC: National Academy Press; 2001.

[30] Greiner A, Knebel E. Board on Health Care Services. Institute of Medicine (US). Committee on the Health Professions Education Summit. Health professions education: a bridge to quality. Washington, DC: National Academies Press; 2003.

[31] Chapman DM, Hayden S, Sanders AB, et al. Integrating the Accreditation Council for Graduate Medical Education Core competencies into the model of the clinical practice of emergency medicine. Ann Emerg Med 2004;43(6):756–69.

[32] Cabana MD, Rand CS, Powe NR, et al. Why don't physicians follow clinical practice guidelines? A framework for improvement. JAMA 1999;282(15):1458–65.

[33] Muller S. Physicians for the twenty-first century. Report of the Project Panel on the General Professional Education of the Physician and College Preparation for Medicine. J Med Educ 1984;59(11 Pt 2):7–11.

[34] Wilcox S. Fostering self-directed learning in the university setting. Stud High Educ 1996; 21(2):165–76.

[35] Jennings JM, Jacoby LL. Automatic versus intentional uses of memory: aging, attention, and control. Psychol Aging 1993;8(2):283–93.

[36] Hay JF, Jacoby LL. Separating habit and recollection in young and older adults: effects of elaborative processing and distinctiveness. Psychol Aging 1999;14(1):122–34.

[37] Schaie KW. Intellectual development in adulthood: the Seattle longitudinal study. Cambridge: Cambridge University Press; 1996.

[38] Park DC, Puglisi JT, Smith AD. Memory for pictures: does an age-related decline exist? Psychol Aging 1986;1(1):11–7.

[39] Bahrami J. Summative assessment for general practitioner registrars. Has been implemented experimentally in Yorkshire. BMJ 1995;311(7019):1573.

[40] Bahrami J, Rogers M, Singleton C. Personal education plan: a system of continuing medical education for general practitioners. Education for General Practice 1995;6:342–5.

[41] Evans A, Ali S, Singleton C, et al. The effectiveness of personal education plans in continuing professional development: an evaluation. Med Teach 2002;24(1):79–84.

[42] Six J. The generality of the underlying self-directed learning inventory. Adult Education Quarterly 1989;40:43–51.

[43] Construct FO. Validity of the Oddi Continuing Learning Inventory. Adult Education Quarterly 1990;40:139–45.

[44] Hojat M, Nasca TJ, Erdmann JB, et al. An operational measure of physician lifelong learning: its development, components and preliminary psychometric data. Med Teach 2003;25(4):433–7.

[45] Barzansky B, Etzel SI. Educational programs in US medical schools, 2000–2001. JAMA 2001;286(9):1049–55.

[46] Pediatric Education Prehospital Professionals Cincinnati Children's Hospital adds "high tech" simulator to PEPP course [newsletter]. 2002. Available at: http://www.peppsite.com/newsletter/n_03_November_2002.htm. Accessed June 1, 2004.

[47] Heinrichs WL, Srivastava S, Dev P, et al. LUCY: a 3-D pelvic model for surgical simulation. J Am Assoc Gynecol Laparosc 2004;11(3):326–31.

[48] Aggarwal R, Moorthy K, Darzi A. Laparoscopic skills training and assessment. Br J Surg 2004;91(12):1549–58.

[49] Wagner C, Schill M, Hennen M, et al. [Virtual reality in ophthalmological education]. Ophthalmologe 2001;98(4):409–13 [in German].

ELSEVIER
SAUNDERS

Emerg Med Clin N Am
24 (2006) 797–808

EMERGENCY
MEDICINE
CLINICS OF
NORTH AMERICA

Moral Moments at the End of Life

Terri A. Schmidt, MD, MS

*Department of Emergency Medicine, Center for Ethics in Health Care,
Oregon Health & Sciences University, CDW-EM, 3181 SW Sam Jackson Park Road,
Portland, OR 97239, USA*

Decision making near the end of life can be complex and laden with emotion for families and health care providers. Families and patients can prepare themselves for these difficult moments by thinking ahead about the patient's wishes and preparing clear documents that express those wishes. Health care providers can prepare themselves by being familiar with those documents, considering the goals of treatment, remembering the principles on which health care ethics are founded and knowing decision-making models that will help them to think through treatment plans and the best options for patient taking into consideration the goals of treatment.

Key concepts:

- Knowing the goals of treatment
- Communicating and honoring patient wishes
- Knowing the uses and limitations of advance directives and do not attempt resuscitation (DNAR) orders
- Ethical decision making models
- Role of futility

Three cases

The good

Eric arrives in an ambulance at 4:30 in the morning. He is a 27-year-old man who is sitting upright on the gurney, leaning forward, and in obvious severe respiratory distress. He has a Physicians Orders for Life-Sustaining Treatment (POLST) form sitting on his lap that states, "Do Not Attempt Resuscitation; Comfort Measures Only and this patient has end-stage cystic fibrosis" [1].

E-mail address: schmidtt@ohsu.edu

The bad

A 78-year-old woman with profound Alzheimer's dementia was admitted to the hospital with pneumonia. During a brief admission, her son and the doctors determined that she would not want further intervention. A decision was made to transport her home in an ambulance for end-of-life care. No written DNAR orders were provided to the emergency medical services (EMS) staff. Shortly after driving away from the hospital the patient was found to be without a pulse and not breathing.

The almost ugly

An 80-year-old man arrived in the emergency department with altered mental status. No documents were sent with the patient. He was hypotensive and his heart rate was 50 beats per minute. He could not answer any questions and no family was initially with the patient. Over the next few minutes his blood pressure continued to drop along with his oxygen saturation. Within a few minutes family arrived and were able to relay that the patient had multiple serious medical conditions. He had been hospitalized a few weeks earlier. At that time he was mentally alert and clearly expressed his wishes for no aggressive interventions. The patient was kept comfortable in the ED with family at his bedside.

In emergency medicine and EMS, all patients are presumed to desire resuscitation and life-sustaining interventions unless there is explicit information to the contrary. However, many patients with advanced illnesses may not want all interventions [2]. The emergency physician needs to determine which patients should have an attempt at cardiopulmonary resuscitation, as well as other life-sustaining interventions, and which should not. These decisions are based on the goals and ethical principles of medicine. The basic ethical principles on which modern medicine are founded include respect for patient autonomy, beneficence, nonmaleficence, and justice. Respect for patient autonomy leads to the understanding that patients may choose to limit the interventions that they wish and thus supports DNAR orders based on the patient's preferences. Both beneficence and nonmaleficence suggest that an intervention should not be performed if there is no chance that it will benefit the patient. This has been the basis for consideration of DNAR orders based on futility.

The goal of this manuscript is to describe the framework for making ethical decisions when treating patients near the end of life. To achieve those goals, the manuscript includes further discussion of the ethical principles of Western medicine, a description of methods for expressing patient preferences and two models for ethical decision making, as well as a brief discussion of the role of futility. Finally, a few comments are included on practicing procedures on the newly dead.

Methods of expressing patient preferences

Emergency physicians are frequently faced with the need to make a rapid decision about attempting resuscitation in a patient who arrives in extremis. Often the patient is unable to verbalize preferences about treatment and the physician must make these time-critical decisions based on written instructions, if available. These instructions can be either patient-initiated advance directives or health care provider–initiated DNAR orders and other treatment orders.

An advance directive is a written document, completed by the patient, expressing future wishes. It is designed to be used at a time when the patient can no longer express his or her wishes. The two main types of advance directive are living wills and durable powers of attorney for health care. The Patient Self-Determination Act, which became effective in 1991, requires that all hospitals that accept Medicare and Medicaid funds provide information about advance directives and develop policies for implementation of advance directives. There has been an increase in advance care planning since then with more patients in long-term care settings having advance directives but in many cases advance directives are still lacking when patients are transferred to emergency departments [3–6]. These forms can be cumbersome to complete and calls have been made for states to simplify the process [7]. One study found that many emergency department patients have never thought about an advance directive or prefer that families make the decision at the time of an event [8].

One type of advance directive, the living will, expresses the wishes of patients regarding life-sustaining procedures in the event of terminal illness. These documents have specific restrictions that state that the person would not want resuscitation if he or she is terminally ill, death is imminent, and resuscitation would only prolong the dying process. Because of these restrictive phrases, living wills are often of little value in the emergency and pre-hospital setting [9]. In many cases health care providers do not follow them [10] and in at least one state, they explicitly do not apply except in a hospital or clinic setting [11]. However, when the applicability and circumstances are clear, the emergency physician should respect the living will and it does provide valuable information about the patient's preferences. Often, although the document does not prevent a resuscitative effort in the emergency department, it does facilitate later decisions about withdrawal of life support in the intensive care unit.

Another form of patient-completed advance directive, the durable power of attorney for health care, gives to another person the authority to make decisions for a patient if he or she is unable to make decisions either temporarily or permanently. Under those circumstances, the person designated in the power of attorney becomes a legally recognized proxy decision maker for the patient. When a durable power of attorney exists, the emergency physician should allow the designated person to participate in decisions regarding the patient's medical care. The proxy decision maker should not base requests to initiate or withhold resuscitation on his or her own values, but make decisions according to the known wishes of the patient. Immunity is generally granted to the physician who carries out the proxy's decision in good faith. Some states allow surrogates without a specific health care power of attorney to make decisions about resuscitation and end-of-life care for incapacitated patients and others do not. Emergency physicians need to be aware of their own state laws and regulations regarding health care proxies and living wills.

Unlike living wills and health care powers of attorney, DNAR orders are written by a health care provider to indicate that resuscitation should not be started. These orders are unique in that they are directions not to do something, rather than orders that initiate a treatment. DNAR orders are one aspect of respecting patient preferences but they only apply when the patient is pulseless and apneic. However, many primary care providers believe that they apply in other circumstances and that intubation and cardioversion are not appropriate in a patient with DNAR orders [12]. A 1997 report found that most emergency physicians are willing to honor written directives regarding resuscitation but would not withhold resuscitation based on unofficial documents or verbal reports.

Just as emergency physicians must consider patient preferences when deciding when to attempt resuscitation, EMS systems and out-of-hospital providers face these same decisions [13]. Similarly to physicians in the emergency department, patient-initiated advance directives are difficult for emergency medical technicians (EMTs) to apply to decisions about specific life-support measures [14]. Physician DNAR orders are often more successful. Most states now have out-of-hospital DNAR programs, consistent with the American College of Emergency Physicians' position that, "Each emergency medical services (EMS) system should have a well-defined, comprehensive policy for dealing with out-of-hospital 'do not attempt resuscitation' (DNAR) directives" [15]. The number of states authorizing out-of-hospital DNR orders has increased from 11 states in 1992 [16] to 42 states in 1999 [17]. A Canadian study found that nearly 10% of cardiac arrest calls were for patients with a terminal illness. In 63% of these cases, there was either a verbal (by family) or written request for no resuscitation [18]. A recent survey found that 89% of a national sample of EMTs were willing to honor a state-approved DNR order and that 77% had local protocols for termination of resuscitation in the prehospital setting [19]. However, another study found that 21% of patients with DNAR orders in long-term care facilities had resuscitation attempts when EMS was called. Thus, states have had success with their DNR programs [20] but problems remain. For example, Connecticut has a DNR bracelet program requiring EMTs to honor these DNR orders and provides immunity from liability for honoring the order [21]. However, one study suggests that bracelet DNR programs are used infrequently [14]. In addition, advance directives and DNR orders may not be available when EMS arrives and often do not accompany patients to the emergency department [4,22,23]. Further, out-of-hospital DNAR programs typically provide only orders about resuscitation with no guidance for patients who are breathing and have a pulse. It is often harder for physicians and prehospital providers to know what interventions are or are not appropriate for the seriously ill patient who is not in cardiopulmonary arrest but cannot speak for him or herself, and does not have a surrogate present to express the patient's wishes.

Physician Orders for Life-Sustaining Treatment paradigm

In 1991, a group of Oregon health care providers and organizations formed what became known as the Physician Orders for Life-Sustaining Treatment (POLST) Task Force to develop methods of honoring patient treatment choices near the end of life [24,25]. The goal of this program is to communicate patient preferences for treatment in the form of medical orders as patients transition between multiple care settings such as from home or long-term care to the emergency department. The Oregon POLST Program addresses resuscitation as well as a range of medical interventions by converting patient treatment preferences about life-sustaining treatments into medical orders. The form is divided into several sections, the first two of which are especially helpful in the emergency setting (see Fig. 1). Recently, other states have begun adopting the POLST paradigm [26].

A number of studies indicate that POLST is effective in communicating patient preferences. Two studies in long-term care settings suggest the POLST Program is successful in preventing unwanted life-sustaining treatments and hospitalization, and orders regarding resuscitation are typically followed. Medical intervention orders were followed less consistently [27,28]. A recent study evaluated use of the POLST by EMTs [23]. Results suggest that the POLST Program influences treatment decisions made by EMTs. In fact, nearly three quarters of EMTs in this study had treated at least one patient with a POLST form even though this is a voluntary program. Most notably, in nearly half of the cases where a POLST form was present, EMTs used it to change the treatment plan, often avoiding interventions that the patient did not want. Thus, the POLST is one model program for expressing patient preferences and helping emergency physicians and EMS providers to determine the best level of intervention for a patient.

Remember the woman who is described in the case above who stops breathing shortly after being placed in an ambulance. No POLST form or other DNAR order was with the patient, so the paramedics began a resuscitation attempt even though they did not think this was according to the patient's wishes. This attempt included cardiopulmonary resuscitation, endotracheal intubation, and defibrillation, before her son, who was in the ambulance, was able to stop these measures by reaching the treating physician on his

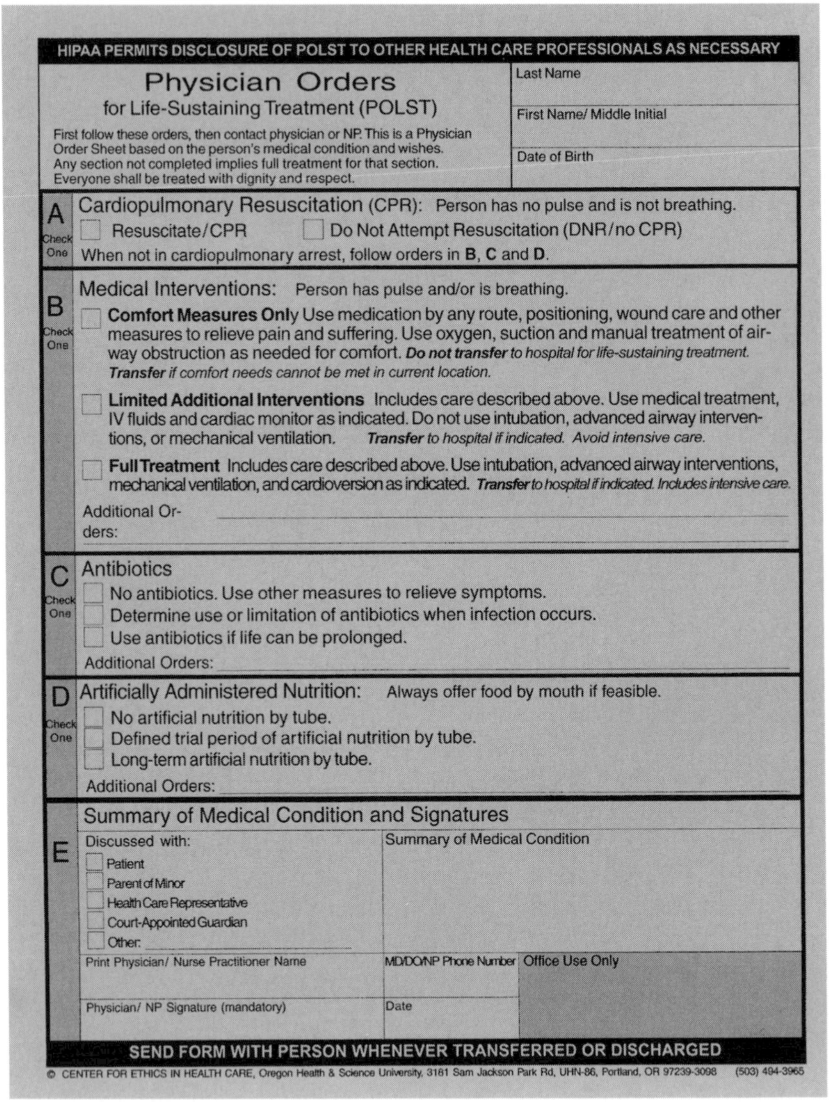

HIPAA PERMITS DISCLOSURE OF POLST TO OTHER HEALTH CARE PROFESSIONALS AS NECESSARY

Physician Orders
for Life-Sustaining Treatment (POLST)

First follow these orders, then contact physician or NP. This is a Physician Order Sheet based on the person's medical condition and wishes. Any section not completed implies full treatment for that section. Everyone shall be treated with dignity and respect.

Last Name

First Name/ Middle Initial

Date of Birth

A Check One — Cardiopulmonary Resuscitation (CPR): Person has no pulse and is not breathing.
- ☐ Resuscitate/CPR
- ☐ Do Not Attempt Resuscitation (DNR/no CPR)

When not in cardiopulmonary arrest, follow orders in **B**, **C** and **D**.

B Check One — Medical Interventions: Person has pulse and/or is breathing.
- ☐ **Comfort Measures Only** Use medication by any route, positioning, wound care and other measures to relieve pain and suffering. Use oxygen, suction and manual treatment of airway obstruction as needed for comfort. ***Do not transfer*** *to hospital for life-sustaining treatment.* ***Transfer*** *if comfort needs cannot be met in current location.*
- ☐ **Limited Additional Interventions** Includes care described above. Use medical treatment, IV fluids and cardiac monitor as indicated. Do not use intubation, advanced airway interventions, or mechanical ventilation. ***Transfer*** *to hospital if indicated. Avoid intensive care.*
- ☐ **Full Treatment** Includes care described above. Use intubation, advanced airway interventions, mechanical ventilation, and cardioversion as indicated. ***Transfer*** *to hospital if indicated. Includes intensive care.*

Additional Orders: ______

C Check One — Antibiotics
- ☐ No antibiotics. Use other measures to relieve symptoms.
- ☐ Determine use or limitation of antibiotics when infection occurs.
- ☐ Use antibiotics if life can be prolonged.

Additional Orders: ______

D Check One — Artificially Administered Nutrition: Always offer food by mouth if feasible.
- ☐ No artificial nutrition by tube.
- ☐ Defined trial period of artificial nutrition by tube.
- ☐ Long-term artificial nutrition by tube.

Additional Orders: ______

E — Summary of Medical Condition and Signatures

Discussed with:
- ☐ Patient
- ☐ Parent of Minor
- ☐ Health Care Representative
- ☐ Court-Appointed Guardian
- ☐ Other: ______

Summary of Medical Condition

Print Physician/ Nurse Practitioner Name | MD/DO/NP Phone Number | Office Use Only

Physician/ NP Signature (mandatory) | Date

SEND FORM WITH PERSON WHENEVER TRANSFERRED OR DISCHARGED

© CENTER FOR ETHICS IN HEALTH CARE, Oregon Health & Science University, 3181 Sam Jackson Park Rd, UHN-86, Portland, OR 97239-3098 (503) 494-3965

Fig. 1. Physician Orders for Life-Sustaining Treatment (POLST) form.

cell phone. All of this could have been prevented by written orders such as a DNAR order or a POLST form.

Ethical decision making

Having clear documentation can help to prevent unwanted resuscitation and respect patient wishes but conflicts and dilemmas are likely to continue to arise. When faced with an ethical dilemma, the emergency physician (or EMT) needs to know how to determine the best course of action. Knowing the goals of intervention and remembering the ethical principles on which medicine is founded are helpful but it is useful to have a framework in which to think through the problem. Often decisions must be made quickly, with limited information. Two models for ethical decision making will be presented here.

First, Ken Iserson and colleagues [29] have developed an ethical decision-making model designed for the emergency setting. The first step in this model is to ask the question, "Is this a type of ethics problem for which you have already worked out a rule or is this at least similar enough so that a rule could reasonably be extended to cover it?" If so, then follow the rule. The second step is to ask the question, "Is there an option that will buy time for deliberation without excessive risk to the patient?" If yes, buy time. Finally, if the first two steps do not yield a solution, test your proposed action against the following three rules: (1) Impartiality— Would you be willing to have this action performed if you were in the patient's place? (2) Universalizability—Would you be willing to use the same solution in all similar cases? (3) Interpersonal justifiability—Would you be willing to defend the decision to others, to share the decision in public? One way to consider the problem is to ask yourself which action you would be most willing to stand up and defend the next day.

What would happen if the emergency physician used this model to determine what to do in the case above of an 80-year-old man who arrives with altered mental status, hypotension, and bradycardia. Initially he has no advance directives or information about his preferences for treatment. He appears chronically ill but nothing is known about his quality of life or his underlying medical conditions. Using the first question, most emergency physicians agree that when no information is available about the patient's preferences we need to err on the side of intervention and attempt resuscitation. This rule could be stated as, "When in doubt regarding the patient's wishes, resuscitative efforts should be initiated." The decision to resuscitate must be an immediate "yes" or "no" decision. "Slow codes," suboptimal effort, or delayed interventions are not medically or ethically justifiable. At the same time, consider the second question. In this case there are some interventions that can be employed to buy time until more information is available. The patient could be treated with atropine or external pacing along with the use of a bag-valve mask for at least a few minutes. This would allow the family to arrive and provide more information. When the physician learns the patient's preferences he or she could either continue the resuscitation efforts or stop life-prolonging interventions. As it turns out, the family arrives after a few minutes and is able to provide information that the patient has severe congestive heart failure along with other medical problems and has completed advance directives indicting that he does not want life-sustaining treatments. Efforts at resuscitation are stopped; the social worker provides support to the family; the family members spend time with the patient in the emergency department; and he dies quietly with them in attendance. The family is grateful that they were able to be there with him when he died and that the emergency department staff treated them and their loved one with respect and dignity.

A second ethical decision-making model was developed by Jonson and colleagues [30]. The model was designed to answer a medical ethics dilemma by considering four domains: medical indications, patient preferences, quality of life, and contextual features (see Fig. 2). By considering all four of these domains the health care provider attempts to ensure that no salient features of the case are ignored.

Now, consider the story above of a man with cystic fibrosis who comes to the emergency department in respiratory distress. The medical indications are straightforward: Eric is in severe respiratory failure and in need of intubation, airway management, and ventilation. Of course, with his serious lung disease these efforts might be futile, but more on that later. In this case, his preferences are also known. He has a POLST form that indicated that he is DNAR and that he would want comfort measures only, no interventions intended to prolong his life. In fact, a brief call to his foster mom reveals that he has been very ill for the past year and his goal was to live to his 27th birthday, now 3 weeks past. This conversation also confirms that recently he has been extremely short of breath even at rest and no longer was satisfied with the quality of his life. Several of the nurses in the ED know him from previous visits and describe him as a fun-loving man with a "wicked" sense of humor. On recent visits much of the love of life seemed to be waning. Contextual features encompass any other factors that might influence a decision. Here one might consider family wishes, applicable laws, or hospital policies that have an impact on the situation. In our case, the only available family is a foster mom who was unable to come to the hospital because she was caring for others with cystic fibrosis in her

Medical Indications	Quality of Life
Patient Preferences	Contextual Features

Fig. 2. Jonsen model for ethical decision making.

home, and clearly understood that Eric might die. Based on a brief analysis, considering the four domains, I was able to determine that no attempt should be made to intubate Eric, although this meant that he was likely to die of respiratory failure in a short time. He was made as comfortable as possible, with one of the nurses or me sitting at his side. After a short while his breathing became labored and he seemed to be struggling so he was given small doses of morphine and lorazepam to keep him comfortable and he quietly and peacefully died about sunrise. His foster mom, primary physician, and I believed that his wishes had been honored and the last moments of his life were peaceful ones.

Futility

To this point, we have discussed making decisions based on patient preferences with a focus on respect for autonomy. Something needs to be said about futility in making decisions about resuscitation. Futility comes from the Latin, *futiliz,* meaning leaky or that which easily pours out [1,31]. One report found that a majority of emergency physicians had recently attempted resuscitations despite expectations that they were futile. Nonetheless, it is generally agreed that physicians should not offer or provide treatments to patients that have no chance of benefiting a patient [32]. This is based on the principles of beneficence and nonmaleficence [33,34]. To take this idea to its extreme, we would never offer surgery on the gall bladder as a treatment option for a patient who has appendicitis. The same is true of attempted resuscitation. It should not be attempted on a patient who has no chance of benefit. The problem arises when we try to define "no chance" and "benefit." Further, many physicians report that they attempt resuscitation because of legal concerns. This might be somewhat mitigated by a report from Oregon, which found that only 2.4% of families reported that too little treatment was given to a deceased family member near the end of life.

Some ethicists have suggested a probabilistic approach to defining futility. For example, if well-designed studies show a 1% or less chance of survival the treatment can be defined as futile [30]. Using this approach in the prehospital setting, in the absence of obvious signs of death (dependent lividity, rigor mortis, decapitation) there are no absolute indicators that resuscitation has no chance of success and unless there is information about patient preferences, resuscitation should be attempted [35]. However, there is a body of evidence that indicates that there have been no survivors of adult medical arrest who are not in ventricular fibrillation if a full resuscitative effort including CPR, definitive airway management, medication administration, defibrillation if necessary, and at least 20 minutes of treatment following Advanced Cardiac Life Support (ACLS) guidelines is performed [32,36,37]. In those circumstances, it is ethically justified to stop resuscitation attempts based on futility [38,39]. There is also evidence that families are generally accepting of stopping efforts without transporting the person to a hospital [40].

Many authors have pointed out the importance of determining the goals when defining futility. Marco and Larkin [31] suggest using the term "clinically nonbeneficial interventions" instead of "futility" to help clarify the intent. This allows the clinician to consider the goals of treatment. A common example is the patient for which living for a few days might be a benefit because it would allow her to say goodbye to family, or for out-of-town relatives to arrive. Thus, while some authors have argued that decisions about futility should be made by physicians and that families do not need to be consulted [41,42] to determine the goals of treatment, it makes sense to communicate with patients and families when possible. It has been noted that the use of futility to justify unilateral decisions fosters conflict.

Procedures on the newly dead

Up to this point we have considered ethical decisions in patients near the end of life. One final "moral" moment arises when teachers and trainees must make a decision on whether or not to practice procedures on the newly dead. In the past this may have been a common practice and few institutions had policies regulating the practice that occurred behind closed doors. Studies suggest that 47% to 63% of emergency programs allow the practice and that consent is rarely obtained [43–47]. These same studies indicate that few programs have written policies surrounding the practice [44,46,47]. More recently, major medical organizations have begun to address this issue, generally endorsing the need for written policies and the requirement for family consent before procedures are performed [9,48]. Recently, the Society for Academic Emergency Medicine published a position that strongly encourages all emergency medicine training programs to develop a policy and recommends that families be asked for consent before practicing procedures on the newly dead [49].

Summary

Decision making near the end of life can be complex and laden with emotion for families and health care providers. Families and patients can prepare themselves for these difficult moments by thinking ahead about the patient's wishes and preparing clear documents that express those wishes. Health care providers can prepare themselves by being familiar with those documents, considering the goals of treatment, remembering the principles on which health care ethics are founded and knowing decision-making models that will help them to think through treatment plans and the best options for patients taking into consideration the goals of treatment.

References

[1] Schmidt T. Futility-futilis-the leaky vessel. Ann Emerg Med 2000;35:615–7.

[2] Innes G, Wanger K. Dignified death or legislated resuscitation? CMAJ 1999;161:1264–5.

[3] Teno JM, Branco KJ, Mor V, et al. Changes in advance care planning in nursing homes before and after the patient Self-Determination Act: report of a 10-state survey. J Am Geriatr Soc 1997;45:939–44.

[4] Lahn M, Friedman B, Bijur P, et al. Advance directives in skilled nursing facility residents transferred to emergency departments. Acad Emerg Med 2001;8:1158–62.

[5] Jackson EA, Yarzebski JL, Goldberg RJ, et al. Do-not-resuscitate orders in patients hospitalized with acute myocardial infarction: the Worcester Heart Attack Study. Arch Intern Med 2004;164:776–83.

[6] Llovera I, Mandel FS, Ryan JG, et al. Are emergency department patients thinking about advance directives? Acad Emerg Med 1997;4:976–80.

[7] Lo B, Steinbrook R. Resuscitating advance directives. Arch Intern Med 2004;164:1501–6.

[8] Llovera I, Ward MF, Ryan JG, et al. Why don't emergency department patients have advance directives? Acad Emerg Med 1999;6:1054–60.

[9] Abramson N, de Vos R, Fallat ME, Finucane T, et al. Ethics in emergency cardiac care. Ann Emerg Med 2001;37:s195–200.

[10] Danis M, Southerland LI, Garrett JM, et al. A prospective study of advance directives for life-sustaining care. N Engl J Med 1991;324:882–8.

[11] Silveira MJ, Buell RA, Deyo RA. Prehospital DNR orders: what do physicians in Washington know? J Am Geriatr Soc 2003;51:1435–8.

[12] Lerner EB, Billittier AJ, Hallinan K. Out-of-hospital do-not-resuscitate orders by primary care physicians. J Emerg Med 2002;23:425–8.

[13] Becker LJ, Yeargin K, Rea TD, et al. Resuscitation of residents with do not resuscitate orders in long-term care facilities. Prehosp Emerg Care 2003;7:303–6.

[14] Partridge RA, Virk A, Sayah A. Field experience with prehospital advance directives. Ann Emerg Med 1998;32:589–93.

[15] American College of Emergency Physicians. "Do not attempt resuscitation" directives in the out-of-hospital setting. Ann Emerg Med 1996;27:684.

[16] Adams J. Prehospital do-not-resuscitate orders: a survey of polices in the United States. Prehospital Disaster Med 1993;8:317–22.

[17] Sabatino CP. Survey of state EMS-DNR laws and protocols. J Law Med Ethics 1999;27:297–315.

[18] Guru V, Verbeek PR, Morrison LJ. Response of paramedics to terminally ill patients with cardiac arrest: an ethical dilemma. CMAJ 1999;161:1251–4.

[19] Marco CA, Schears RM. Prehospital resuscitation practices: a survey of prehospital providers. J Emerg Med 2003;24:101–6.

[20] Iserson KV. A simplified prehospital advance directive law: Arizona's approach. Ann Emerg Med 1993;22:1703–10.

[21] Leon MD, Wilson EM. Development of a statewide protocol for the prehospital identification of DNR patients in Connecticut including new DNR regulations. Ann Emerg Med 1999;34:263–74.

[22] Morrison RS, Olson E, Mertz KR, et al. The inaccessibility of advance directives on transfer from ambulatory to acute care settings. JAMA 1995;274:478–82.

[23] Schmidt TA, Hickman S, Tolle SW, et al. The Physician Orders for Life-Sustaining Treatment (POLST) Program: Oregon emergency medical technicians' practical experiences and attitudes. J Am Geriatr Soc 2004;52:1430–4.

[24] Dunn PM, Nelson CA, Tolle SW, et al. Communicating preferences for life-sustaining treatment using a physician order form. J Gen Intern Med 1997;12(suppl):102.

[25] Dunn PM, Schmidt TA, Carley MM, et al. A method to communicate patient preferences about medically indicated life-sustaining treatment in the out-of-hospital setting. J Am Geriatr Soc 1996;44:785–91.

[26] Available at: http://www.ohsu.edu/polst/national.shtml. Accessed June 16, 2006.

[27] Tolle SW, Tilden VP, Nelson CA, et al. A prospective study of the efficacy of the physician order form for life-sustaining treatment. 1998;46:1097–102.

[28] Lee MA, Brummel-Smith K, Meyer J, et al. Physician orders for life-sustaining treatment (POLST): outcomes in a PACE program. Program of All-Inclusive Care for the Elderly. J Am Geriatr Soc 2000;48:1343–4.

[29] Iserson KV, Sanders AB, Mathieu D. Ethics in emergency medicine. 2nd ed. Tuscon, AZ: Galen Press, Ltd; 1995.

[30] Jonsen AR, Siegler M, Winslade WJ. Clinical ethics. 4th ed. New York: McGraw-Hill; 1998.

[31] Marco CA, Larkin GL. Ethics seminars: case studies in "futility"—challenges for academic emergency medicine. Acad Emerg Med 2000;7:1147–51.

[32] American Heart Association. Part 2: Ethical aspects of CPR and ECC. Resuscitation 2000; 102:17–27.

[33] Levack P. Live and let die? A structured approach to decision-making about resuscitation. Br J Anaesth 2002;89:684–5.

[34] Hilberman M, Kutner J, Parsons D, et al. Marginally effective medical care: ethical analysis of issues in cardiopulmonary resuscitation (CPR). J Med Ethics 1997;23:361–7.

[35] Pepe PE, Swor RA, Ornato JP, et al. Resuscitation in the out-of-hospital setting: medical futility criteria for on-scene pronouncement of death. Prehosp Emerg Care 2001;5:79–87.

[36] Bailey ED, Wydro GC, Cone DC. Termination of resuscitation in the prehospital setting for adult patients suffering nontraumatic cardiac arrest. National Association of EMS Physicians Standards and Clinical Practice Committee. Prehosp Emerg Care 2000;4:190–5.

[37] Bonnin MJ, Pepe PE, Kimball KT, et al. Distinct criteria for termination of resuscitation in the out-of-hospital setting. JAMA 1993;270:1457–1462.

[38] Kellerman AL, Staves DR, Hackman BB. In-hospital resuscitation following unsuccessful prehospital advanced cardiac life support: "heroic efforts" or an exercise in futility. Ann Emerg Med 1988;17:589–94.

[39] Gray WA, Capone RJ, Most AS. Unsuccessful emergency medical resuscitation: are continued efforts in the emergency department justified? N Eng J Med 1991;1991:1393–8.

[40] Schmidt TA, Harrahill MA. Family response to out-of-hospital death. Acad Emerg Med 1995;2:513–8.

[41] Schneiderman LJ, Jecker NS, Jonsen AR. Medical futility: response to critiques. Arch Intern M 1996;125:669–74.

[42] Jecker NS, Pearlman RA. Medical futility: who decides? Arch Intern Med 1992;152:1140–4.

[43] Burns JP, Reardon FE, Truog RD. Using newly deceased patients to teach resuscitation procedures. N Engl J Med 1994;331:1652–5.

[44] Morhaim DK, Heller MB. The practice of teaching endotracheal intubation on recently deceased patients. J Emerg Med 1991;9(6):515–8.

[45] Ginifer C, Kelly AM. Teaching resuscitation skills using newly deceased. Med J Aust 1996; 165:445–7.

[46] Fourre MW. Performance of procedures on the recently deceased. Acad Emerg Med 2003;9: 595–8.

[47] Knopp RK. Practicing cricothyrotomy on the newly dead. Ann Emerg Med 1995;25:694–6.

[48] The Council on Ethical and Judicial Affairs of the American Medical Association. Performing procedures on the newly dead. Acad Med 2002;77:1212–6.

[49] Schmidt TA, Abbott JT, Geiderman JM, et al. Ethics seminars: the ethical debate on practicing procedures on the newly dead. Acad Emerg Med 2004;11:962–6.

ELSEVIER
SAUNDERS

Emerg Med Clin N Am
24 (2006) 809–813

EMERGENCY
MEDICINE
CLINICS OF
NORTH AMERICA

Index

Note: Page numbers of article titles are in **boldface** type.

A

Academic freedom, publication, and
  authorship, 666–667

Adolescents, emergency department privacy
  and confidentiality and, 620–622
  emergency department visits by,
    619–620

Advance directives, 797
  medical malpractice and, 739–740

Alcohol abuse, and illicit substance abuse,
  assessment of capacity of patient and,
  771, 772–773
    decision for treatment of, 771
    emergency department response
      to, 769–774
    case illustrating, 768–769
    hospital admission in, 773–774

Alcohol testing, of minors, 623–624

American Board of Medical Specialties,
  786, 788, 789

American College of Emergency Physicians,
  principles of ethics for emergency
  physicians, 532, 599–601

American Society of Addiction Medicine,
  confidentiality and, 780

Animal research, 663–664

Authorship, publication, and academic
  freedom, 666–667

B

Beneficence, 525–526

Bioethics, application of, 529–534
  autonomy and, 522–525
  committees and consultants, 540
  definition of, and development of,
    513–514
  education in, 540–541
  law and, relationship between,
    514–516
    similarities and differences in,
      514–515

moral rules and, 516, 517
principles of, 525–527
proactive, 541–542
religion and, 516
research in, 541
"rights" and, 515–516

Biomedical industry, physician interface
  with, conflict of interest in, **671–685**

C

Care, standards of, advances in, confusion
  caused by, 784
    and treatment options,
      knowledge of, 784–785

Centers for Medicare and Medicaid,
  EMTALA and, 566, 569–572

Clinical trials, randomized, 663

Clinician values, 521–522

Communitarianism, 523

Confidentiality. See also *Privacy, and
  confidentiality.*
  American Society of Addiction
    Medicine and, 780
  case illustrating, 776–779
  definition of, 634
  versus privacy, 526–527

Conflict of commitment, 664–666

Conflict of interest, 664–666

Continuing medical education, 784,
  787–788
  future directions in, 790–791

Culture, issues of, health care and, 687–688

D

Decision making, ethical, 800–802
  medical toxicology, and
    emergency medicine,
    767–782
  model for, 800
  medical, by minor, 628–629

Moving?

Make sure your subscription moves with you!

To notify us of your new address, find your **Clinics Account Number** (located on your mailing label above your name), and contact customer service at:

E-mail: elspcs@elsevier.com

800-654-2452 (subscribers in the U.S. & Canada)
407-345-4000 (subscribers outside of the U.S. & Canada)

Fax number: 407-363-9661

Elsevier Periodicals Customer Service
6277 Sea Harbor Drive
Orlando, FL 32887-4800

*To ensure uninterrupted delivery of your subscription, please notify us at least 4 weeks in advance of move.

ELSEVIER